MORE NOTABLE NAMES

IN

ANAESTHESIA

MORE NOTABLE NAMES

IN

ANAESTHESIA

EDITED BY

ALISTAIR G. McKENZIE

BPharm, MB, ChB, FRCA, FFPMRCA

Retired Consultant Anaesthetist, Royal Infirmary of Edinburgh, UK
President, History of Anaesthesia Society 2017-21

℗

THE CHOIR PRESS

British Library Cataloguing in Publication Data
A catalogue record for this book is available from the British Library

First published in the United Kingdom in 2021 by

The Choir Press
Gloucester GL1 5SR

ISBN 978-1-78963-170-8

Contents

viii

Contributors

Peter Charters MD MRCP FRCA
Consultant Anaesthetist, University Hospital Aintree, Liverpool, UK

Michael G. Cooper AM MB BS FANZCA FFPMANZCA
Senior Anaesthetist, The Children's Hospital at Westmead & St. George Hospital, Kogarah, Sydney, Australia and Adjunct Professor of Anaesthesiology, School of Medicine and Health Sciences, University of Papua New Guinea

Roger Eltringham MB, ChB FFARCS
Medical Director, Safe Anaesthesia Worldwide, Marden, Kent, UK

John (Iain) B. Glen BVMS PhD FRCA
GlenPharma, Knutsford, Cheshire, UK

Peter C. Gordon BSc MB, BCh FFA (SA)
Associate Professor Emeritus, Department of Anaesthesia and Perioperative Medicine, University of Cape Town, Cape Town, South Africa

Rajesh P. Haridas MB, ChB FANZCA
Sydney, New South Wales, Australia

Danielle Huckle BSc MB BS FRCA PhD
Consultant, Department of Anaesthesia, Critical Care & Pain Medicine, University Hospital Wales, Cardiff, UK and Honorary Senior Lecturer, Cardiff University

David Humphrey MB BS DA
Senior Lecturer (retired), University of Natal (now Kwazulu-Natal), Durban, South Africa

Éamon P. McCoy MD FFARCSI
Consultant Anaesthetist, Royal Victoria Hospital, Belfast, UK

Alistair G. McKenzie BPharm MB, ChB FRCA FFPMRCA
Honorary Clinical Senior Lecturer, Department of Anaesthesia, Critical Care & Pain Medicine, University of Edinburgh; Consultant Anaesthetist (retired), Royal Infirmary of Edinburgh, Edinburgh, UK

Peter Marhofer MD
Professor, Department of Anaesthesiology and Intensive Care Medicine, Medical University of Vienna, Vienna, Austria

Preface

This book is a follow on to *Notable Names in Anaesthesia* edited by Professor J. Roger Maltby (2002). In his preface to that work Roger Maltby suggested that someone else would write about the notable names he had omitted and new ones. Some years later he put this proposal to me. I readily accepted the challenge, but other commitments prevented me from fulfilling the task until I retired from clinical practice in 2019.

In selecting the notable names, I have tried to avoid those which have become obsolete in the modern practice of anaesthesiology. I have also aimed to be international, so that there are names from five continents. All the living names were given the opportunity to write their own stories or provide me with data and review my rendering. Ten living names chose not to engage with my invitation to be included in the book.

The lives in this volume cover some 240 years and include not only medical doctors and dentists, but also manufacturers, chemists, a physicist and a biologist, a libel case and even one patient who inspired her anaesthetist carer to create an award in her name. A few notable names in veterinary anaesthesia have also been included. Cross-references have been inserted where deemed appropriate to help the reader.

The book is not intended to be a comprehensive history of anaesthesia, but rather a quick reference to the eponyms. At the same time, it is hoped that the material will enrich the reader's knowledge. Applying a maximum word count to each name has meant that each entry is not the ultimate resource, but suggestions for further reading have been provided. The highs and lows in these individuals' lives are relevant to everyone's journey through life. I hope the impact of this work will be not only to revere the dead, but also to inspire the living.

Alistair G. McKenzie

October 2020

Acknowledgements

Several of the notable names selected were suggested by Roger Maltby. Many eponymous lectures and awards were revealed by the media of the various colleges and societies of anaesthesiology. A few more eponyms were found out by questioning representatives of such organizations. All suggestions were considered, but I hold myself fully accountable for the final selection.

The websites of the various colleges and societies of anaesthesiology provided much of the data for the lists of eponymous lectures and awards. Special thanks for lists of lectures and awards and for photographs go to: Caroline Hamson, Heritage Manager and Felicia El Kholi, Heritage Assistant at the AAGBI; Nuala Lucas, Chair of Education for the OAA; Rosemary Sayce, Archivist at the RCoA; David Allen, Librarian at the RSC; Peter Gordon on behalf of the SASA; Monica Cronin, Curator of the Geoffrey Kaye Museum of Anaesthetic History, ANZCA; Hirosato Kikuchi on behalf of the JSA; Raymond Roy, President of the AHA; Judith Robins, Registrar at the Wood Library-Museum of Anesthesiology.

Carmel McKenzie kindly did the end stage proof reading.

Finally, I wish to thank the Choir Press for their friendly advice and guidance in the preparation of this book.

Abbreviations

AAGBI	Association of Anaesthetists of Great Britain and Ireland
AHA	Anesthesia History Association
ANZCA	Australian and New Zealand College of Anaesthetists
ASA	American Society of Anesthesiologists
ASA	Australian Society of Anaesthetists
ASRA	American Society of Regional Anesthesia
BAO	Bachelor of the Art of Obstetrics
BCh, BChir, BS	Bachelor of Surgery, graduating medical degree (UK)
BS	Bachelor of Science (USA)
CAS	Canadian Anesthesiologists' Society
CBE	Commander of (the Order of) the British Empire
DA	Diploma in Anaesthetics (UK)
DAS	Difficult Airway Society
DDS	Doctor of Dental Surgery
ESRA	European Society of Regional Anaesthesia
FFARACS	Fellow of the Faculty of Anaesthetists of the Royal Australasian College of Surgeons
FFARCS	Fellow of the Faculty of Anaesthetists of the Royal College of Surgeons of England
FFARCSI	Fellow of the Faculty of Anaesthetists of the Royal College of Surgeons in Ireland
FFA (SA)	Fellow of the Faculty of Anaesthetics (South Africa)
FRCA	Fellow of the Royal College of Anaesthetists (formerly FFARCS)
FRCPC	Fellow of the Royal College of Physicians and Surgeons of Canada
FRCS	Fellow of the Royal College of Surgeons (of England)
HAS	History of Anaesthesia Society
JSA	Japanese Society of Anesthesiologists
LDS	Licentiate in Dental Surgery
LRCP	Licentiate of the Royal College of Physicians, graduating diploma (UK)
MB	Bachelor of Medicine, graduating medical degree (UK)
MB, ChB	Bachelor of Medicine, Bachelor of Surgery
MD	Higher degree of Doctor of Medicine (UK)
MD	Graduating degree of Doctor of Medicine (USA)
MRCP	Member of the Royal College of Physicians (higher specialist qualification)
MRCS	Member of the Royal College of Surgeons of England, graduating diploma (UK)
MRCVS	Member of the Royal College of Veterinary Surgeons
NHS	National Health Service (UK)
NZSA	New Zealand Society of Anaesthetists
OAA	Obstetric Anaesthetists' Association
OBE	Officer of (the Order of) the British Empire
RSC	Royal Society of Chemistry
SASA	South African Society of Anaesthesiologists
SOAP	Society for Obstetric Anesthesia and Perinatology
UK	United Kingdom of Great Britain and Northern Ireland
US, USA	United States of America
WFSA	World Federation of Societies of Anaesthesiologists
WHO	World Health Organization
WLM	Wood Library-Museum of Anesthesiology

AINTREE INTUBATION CATHETER

Peter Charters (1946-)

Peter Charters was born in Bootle, Merseyside, England and educated at Bootle Grammar School. He graduated MB ChB from the University of Liverpool in 1971, proceeded to resident training and passed the MRCP in 1976. Opting for a career in anaesthesia, he qualified FFARCS in 1978 and defended his MD thesis in 1984.

Charters was appointed Consultant Anaesthetist at University Hospital Aintree in Liverpool, England in 1992. His clinical and research interests included intensive care, anaesthesia for head and neck surgery, and management of the difficult airway.

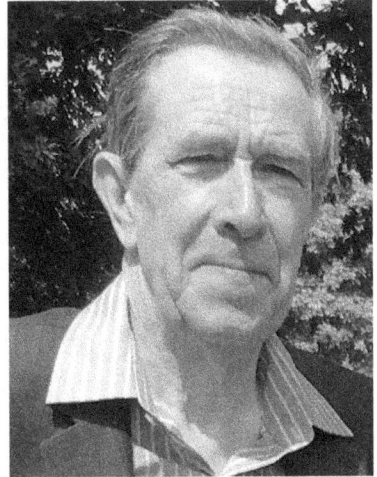

The idea for the Aintree Intubation Catheter began life in 1994 as an attempt to facilitate safe introduction to clinical use of fibrescopes in clinical practice when these were few and far between in most UK Departments, but underused because of fear of damage and the costs of repair. The laryngeal mask airway (LMA) was already in general use and while others had described "A split laryngeal mask as an aid to training in fibreoptic intubation" (1993), the aim of Charters and colleagues was to use a hollow bougie positioned over the fibrescope in order to direct it through the laryngeal mask into the trachea and subsequently to advance a tracheal tube over it (following removal of the fibrescope). They looked at what was available in their local theatre store and despite a flatus tube initially appearing to fit the bill, they settled for a jejeunostomy tube as perhaps a more aesthetic alternative. Although an initial "proof of concept" trial worked in principle, this "bougie" was far too flexible, so they turned to Cook UK for help in getting the appropriate consistency. Cook were keen to incorporate their "Rapi-Fit" connectors (Luer lock and 15mm), to allow ventilation either via a standard anaesthetic circuit or a jet ventilator system (e.g. Manujet). The first "Ventilation-Exchange Bougie", was very successful in a clinical trial (1996), but they became aware of important differences between fibrescopes, in respect of diameter and length. Cook were not keen to produce a variety of device for every fibrescope, so they eventually agreed on a modified internal diameter (1997) and this final version was called the "Aintree Intubation Catheter" (AIC) see Figure 1. This name reflected the

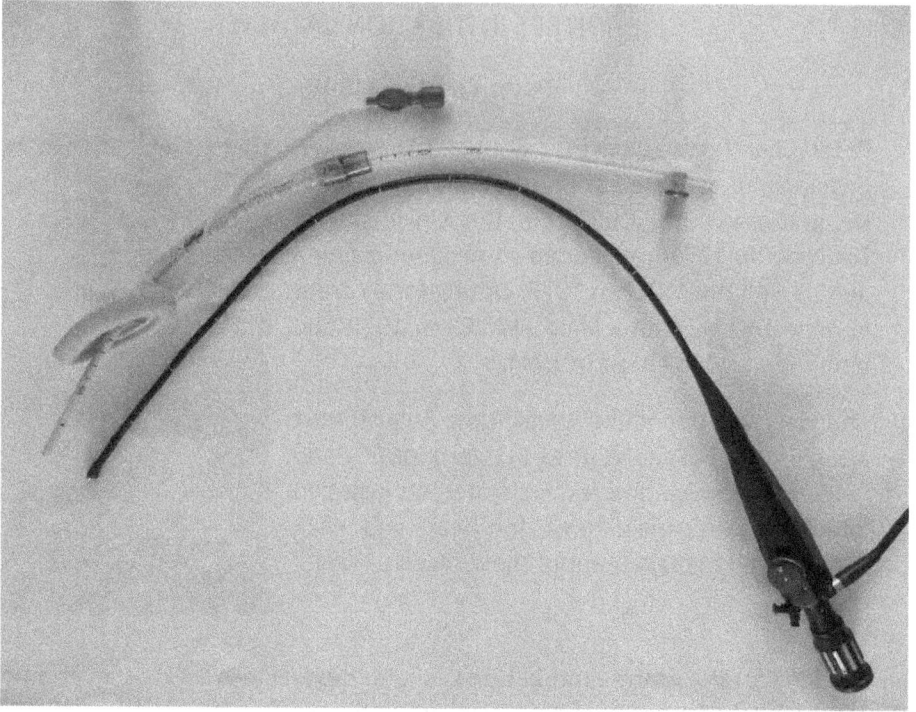

Figure 1. Aintree Intubation Catheter (AIC) inserted through a laryngeal mask airway, shown placed next to a fibrescope. For use, the AIC would be pre-loaded onto the fibrescope. Photograph by A.G. McKenzie.

relocation of the research Department from Walton to Aintree hospital. (The old Walton Hospital was in the process of closure.)

Use of the LMA/AIC technique was later (2005) advocated by others as "low skill" for those less familiar with use of the fibrescope and eventually the technique became part of the Difficult Airway Society (DAS) guidelines. In a parallel development Charters and colleagues were influenced in their approach to general training with the fibrescope by a 1992 Editorial by Dr Mason (Cardiff) who expressed concern that "none of the approaches under general anaesthesia permit the unhurried, sequential identification of the nasal, pharyngeal and laryngeal structures, which is possible in the awake subject and essential when patients with abnormal anatomy or pathology are subsequently encountered". Obviously, the Aintree Intubation Catheter could not claim to do that, but Charters and O'Sullivan had already considered the novel idea of a "dedicated airway" and eventually (1999) defined this as "An upper airway device dedicated to the maintenance of airway patency while other major airway interventions are anticipated or are in progress. The device should be compatible with spontaneous and controlled ventilation". The first incarnation of this concerned nasal fibreoptic intubation using the cuffed naso-pharyngeal airway (CNPA, Portex Ltd) in the alternative nostril as a dedicated airway. Similarly, using the AIC and fibrescope was shown to allow effective oral intubations using the cuffed oropharyngeal airway (COPA, Mallinkrodt Ltd) as a dedicated airway. Unfortunately, both the CNPA and COPA were withdrawn from clinical use within a few years of their introduction to the market. Perhaps their demise was related to the lack of investment and time for clinical refinement, particularly in comparison to the massive energy of Archie Brain in respect of laryngeal mask airway development.

There have been a number of papers from other institutions reporting favourably on the use of the AIC in unexpectedly difficult intubations but individual anaesthetists reporting their own cases by word of mouth has also been gratifying. On the other hand, Charters and colleagues have been aware of criticism to the effect that the description "low skill" is not always appropriate. Clearly there will be times when the laryngeal mask does not sit well in difficult airway patients even if ventilation remains adequate despite this. The point here is that use of the AIC/exchange technique should not be considered if ventilation is not adequate. On the other hand, less than optimal ventilation can initially be regarded as a situation that may be improved by using the fibrescope to direct laryngeal mask repositioning, for example when the epiglottis is folded down over the laryngeal inlet.

In addition to this simple option, it also occurred to Charters and colleagues that many unsatisfactory laryngeal mask placements were possible and ventilation of some sort might be possible with the majority of them, though without correction of the malposition, AIC placement might be problematic. After considering this for a while they started to deliberately misplace a 2.5 size laryngeal mask in a Trucorp mannekin. (This is the only size of LMA suitable for this situation.) The first thing that needs to happen is a systematic assessment of what the mispositioning actually meant (e.g. is the LMA stem twisted on itself, what is the position of the cuff relative to the LMA bowl and what airway landmarks are self-evident. The next thing should be an exploration of any potential spaces where it would be possible to explore the situation further. With practice it became very easy to make progress in almost all cases, i.e. it should be possible to get the AIC into the trachea over the fibrescope whatever the starting position of the LMA. Cook asked for a trade stand presentation at the first World Airway Meeting in Dublin in 2016, where these LMA misplacements were shown and their solutions demonstrated. This presentation remained available on their website when last accessed (November 2019).

Charters has been an active member of the Anaesthetic Research Society and was its Treasurer for 1998-2002. Widely recognised as a teacher, he developed the Aintree Difficult Airway Management (ADAM) courses for anticipated difficult airways and launched an associated website in 2009. He has done outstanding work for the Difficult Airway Society and was appointed DAS Professor in 2013. The Royal College of Anaesthetists awarded him the Dudley Buxton Prize (q.v. page 28) 'for meritorious work in anaesthesia' in 2014. The DAS awarded him the Macewen Medal (q.v. page 134) in 2017.

Further reading

Darling JR, Keohane M, Murray JM. A split laryngeal mask as an aid to training in fibreoptic intubation. A comparison with the Berman II intubating airway. *Anaesthesia* 1993; **48**: 1079-82.

Logan S, Charters P. Laryngeal mask and fibreoptic intubation. *Anaesthesia* 1994; **49**: 543-4.

Atherton DPL, O'Sullivan E, Lowe D, Charters P. A ventilation-exchange bougie for fibreoptic intubations with the laryngeal mask airway. *Anaesthesia* 1996; **51**: 1123-26.

Atherton DPL, O'Sullivan E, Charters P. Modification to the ventilation-exchange bougie. *Anaesthesia* 1997: **52**: 611-2.

Higgs A, Clarke E, Premraj K. Low-skill fibreoptic intubation: use of the Aintree Catheter with the classic LMA. *Anaesthesia* 2005; **60**: 915-20.

Mason RA. Learning fibreoptic intubation: fundamental problems. *Anaesthesia* 1992; **47**: 729-31.

Charters P, O'Sullivan E. The 'dedicated airway': a review of the concept and an update of current practice. *Anaesthesia* 1999; **54**: 778-86.

Ralston SJ, Charters P. Cuffed nasopharyngeal tube as a 'dedicated airway' in difficult intubation. *Anaesthesia* 1994; **49**: 133-6.

Hawkins M, O'Sullivan E, Charters P. Fibreoptic intubation using the cuffed oropharyngeal airway and Aintree intubation catheter. *Anaesthesia* 1998; **53**: 891-4.

https://www.cookmedical.com/critical-care/the-difficult-laryngeal-mask-airway-with-prof-peter-charters/ (accessed 21 November 2019).

ASA GRADE OF PHYSICAL STATUS

Meyer Saklad (1901-1979)

The ASA grading of patients for surgical procedures has been routinely used by anaesthetists practising over much of the globe for well over fifty years. The system stemmed from a publication by Meyer Saklad in 1941 based on the work of a committee of the American Society of Anesthetists Inc. (ASA) on assessment of patient risk prior to anaesthesia and surgery.

Meyer Saklad was born in Boston MA, USA in April 1901 and after schooling he undertook medical training at Tufts University (Medford MA). He graduated MD in 1924 and proceeded to internship at the Memorial Hospital, Pawtucket until 1925. Then, in general practice his experience of administering anaesthesia drew him to specialise in that field.

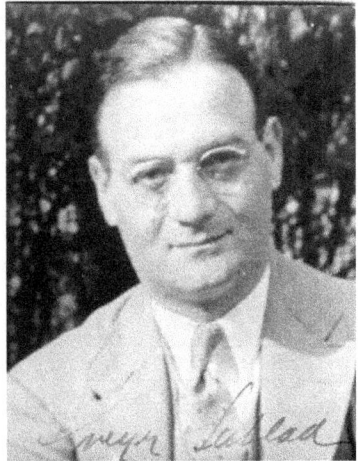

Meyer Saklad. Image courtesy of the Wood Library-Museum of Anesthesiology.

Saklad did anaesthetic preceptorships under Albert Miller at the Rhode Island Hospital, Gaston Labat in New York and M. Kappis in Hanover, Germany. Furthermore, he learned endotracheal anaesthesia from Paluel Flagg. In 1939 he was admitted to the American Board of Anesthesiology and in that year he was appointed Chief of the Anesthesiology Department at Rhode Island Hospital (RIH) in Providence RI.

In 1941 Saklad was recruited by the ASA to serve with Emery A. Rovenstine and Ivan B. Taylor on a committee to devise a system of data collection in anaesthesia for classification of operative risk. Recognising the huge number of variables in "operative risk", they decided that it would be best to grade patients in relation to their physical state alone. In his eloquent paper of May 1941 Saklad listed six Classes of "Physical State", although Classes 5 and 6 were simply the addition of emergency surgery (Table 1). For Classes 1 to 4 helpful examples were given, including levels of functional capacity. Definitions of these grades of "Physical State" were presented in a booklet published by the ASA. Saklad clearly grasped the importance of comparing like with like. He pointed out that instead of "operative risk", the idea of "Physical State" was adopted, with the aim of tabulation of statistical data to compare the patients' preoperative condition with the results of the surgery (now known as outcomes). The system was called the 'ASA Classification of Physical Status'.

Table 1. Original ASA Classification of Physical Status (1941)

Class	Definition
1	**No** organic pathology or patients in whom the pathological process is localized and does not cause any systemic disturbance or abnormality.
2	A moderate but **definite systemic disturbance**, caused either by the condition that is to be treated by surgical intervention or which is caused by other existing pathological processes, forms this group.
3	**Severe** systemic disturbance from any cause or causes. It is not possible to state an absolute measure of severity, as this is a matter of clinical judgment.
4	**Extreme** systemic disorders which have already become an eminent threat to life regardless of the type of treatment. Because of their duration or nature there has already been damage to the organism that is irreversible. This class is intended to include only patients that are in an extremely poor physical state.
5	Emergencies that would otherwise be graded in Class 1 or Class 2.
6	Emergencies that would otherwise be graded as Class 3 or Class 4.

Soon after, the ASA House of Delegates added Class 7: "a moribund patient expected to die in 24 hours with or without operation". In 1942 R.C. Adams and J.S. Lundy published on a slightly different classification of operative risk, introduced at the Mayo Clinic; this did not gain much acceptance, being rather eclipsed by the ASA system. In 1945 the name 'American Society of Anesthetists' was changed to the 'American Society of Anesthesiologists' (ASA).

The 1957 textbook *Introduction to Anesthesia - The Principles of Safe Practice* by Dripps, Eckenhoff and Vandam, contained a chapter on Physical Status or "Risk" in which the ASA classification was given. However, the authors stated that at the University of Pennsylvania, just five classes were used: 1 – 4 and 7; in emergency situations they just added the letter E. In 1961 Dripps *et al* published a study on the role of anaesthesia in surgical mortality, in which they used the classification of Physical Status from their 1957 book – but changing the wording in the definitions for Classes 1-4: for "none, definite, severe, and extreme systemic disturbance" they substituted "normal healthy, mild, severe, and incapacitating systemic disease". They concluded that the contribution of anaesthesia to death was related to the physical condition of the patient: as the physical condition deteriorated, mortality increased.

In 1962 the House of Delegates of the ASA amended the Classification of Physical Status to conform with the system of Dripps and colleagues, using simpler language (Table 2). Examples were no longer given. This ASA grading began to appear in British textbooks of anaesthesia later in the 1960s. Later the grading was utilised by anaesthetists worldwide and incorporated into anaesthetic charts.

Table 2. 1962 ASA Classification of Physical Status

Class	Definition
1	A normal healthy patient.
2	A patient with a mild systemic disease.
3	A patient with a severe systemic disease that limits activity, but is not incapacitating.
4	A patient with an incapacitating systemic disease that is a constant threat to life.
5	A moribund patient not expected to survive 24 hours with or without operation.

In the event of emergency operation, precede the number with an E.

After his work on the ASA grading system, Saklad went on to become chairman of the American Board of Anesthesiology's examining system. During the Second World War he expanded his interest in pulmonary ventilation. In 1948 he was sponsored by the World Health Organisation to participate in an anaesthesia training programme for physicians in Poland and Finland. Notably in 1950, under the auspices of the Unitarian Service Committee (USC), he went to Japan to lecture and teach the principles and techniques of anaesthesiology. In 1953 he published a book *Inhalation Therapy and Resuscitation*. His final mission with the USC was to Peru in 1961.

Meyer Saklad retired as Chief of Anesthesiology at RIH in 1962; his successor was his brother, Elihu Saklad. However, Meyer then became physician in charge of the hospital's Division of Anesthesia Research. He developed principles and techniques of evaluating ventilatory apparatus and in 1964 he accepted the chairmanship of the Z79 ventilator standards subcommittee. Then in 1967 he became Chairman of the International Ventilator Standards Committee, of International Standards Organization (ISO). His work led to a US standard for lung ventilators being published in 1976. He also laid the groundwork in the application of computers to the monitoring of ventilation.

In his lifetime Saklad was elected President of the American Board of Anesthesiology, President of the New England Society of Anesthesiologists, and President of the Rhode Island Society of Anesthesiologists. He was a keen amateur photographer and his photographs were often displayed at the Providence Art Club. He died in July 1979.

The year before Saklad's death, W.D. Owens *et al* published an assessment which indicated that different anaesthetists did not always agree about the

ASA physical status grading, i.e. it was inconsistent. This paper was based on a questionnaire sent to a random selection of anaesthetists, who were asked to read brief descriptions of ten hypothetical patients and then grade each one according to the ASA Physical Status Classification. Although 92% of the respondents stated that they used the classification routinely, 60% had not read the definitions recently. An accompanying Editorial by Arthur S. Keats scolded the authors for not properly crediting Saklad *et al* as the originators.

Following the development of criteria for diagnosing brainstem death, in 1980 a Physical Status Class 6 was added to the ASA classification to take account of the brainstem-dead organ donor. Over the next three decades further studies indicated inconsistency in recording ASA grades. Seeming to recognise the problem, in 2014 the ASA House of Delegates revised the classification again with restoration of examples, as in the original design by Saklad *et al*. At least one study has shown that the re-introduction of examples into the definitions has reduced inconsistency in assigning ASA grades by clinicians trained in anaesthesia.

Further reading

Saklad M. Grading of patients for surgical procedures. *Anesthesiology* 1941; **2**: 281-4.

Dripps RD, Lamont A, Eckenhoff JE. The role of anesthesia in surgical mortality. *Journal of the American Medical Association* 1961; **178**: 261-6.

New Classification of Physical Status. *Anesthesiology* 1963; **24**: 111.

We Salute Dr. Meyer Saklad. *Anesthesia and Analgesia* 1969; **48**: 217-18.

Obituary Dr. Meyer Saklad. *The Rhode Island Herald*, 2 August 1979; 2.

Owens WD, Felts JA, Spitznagel EL. ASA Physical Status Classifications: A Study of Consistency Ratings. *Anesthesiology* 1978; **49**: 239-43.

Keats AS. Editorial. The ASA Classification of Physical Status – A Recapitulation. *Anesthesiology* 1978; **49**: 233-6.

Mayhew D, Mendonca V, Murthy BVS. A review of ASA physical status – historical perspectives and modern developments. *Anaesthesia* 2019; **74**: 373-9.

THE RICHARD BAILEY LIBRARY

Richard John Bailey (1932 -)

Richard John Bailey was born in rural Moree, New South Wales, Australia in 1932. He was the first son after five daughters the family later moving to Sydney. He started medicine in 1949 at the University of Sydney, graduating in 1956, with his first exposure to anaesthesia being the requirement to perform ten open ether anaesthetics prior to graduation. His diary entry for 21 January 1954 says: *Gave an anaesthetic today, my second. Fellow in 2nd stage for a long time ... coughed a lot!* After three years residency at St Vincent's Hospital, Sydney, The Women's Hospital at Crown Street and the Children's Hospital at Camperdown, Richard became the second anaesthetic registrar in 1959 at the Children's Hospital (officially named the Royal Alexandra Hospital for Children).

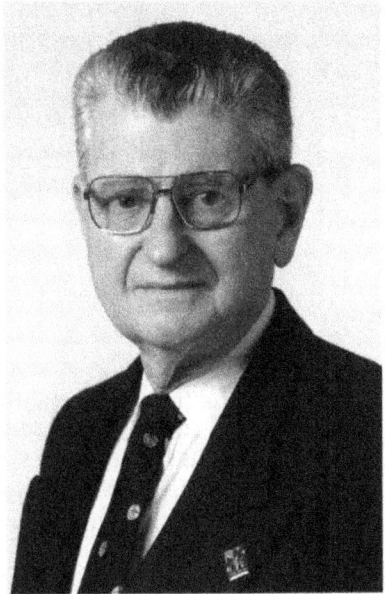

Richard Bailey in 2009. Image courtesy of Australian Society of Anaesthetists.

Bailey returned to St Vincent's Hospital to finish his anaesthetic training, attaining his Fellowship (FFARACS) in 1962. He then spent two years as the Wellcome Research Fellow at the Montefiore Medical Center in New York working with Foldes, Duncalf and Nagashima, gaining research experience in plasma cholinesterases, myasthenia gravis, opioids and their antagonists. Included in this time was a visiting fellowship at the Albert Einstein Medical School. Following this was six months further training at Addenbrooke's Hospital in Cambridge mentored by Ronald Millar, Aileen Adams and John Farman, attaining the English Fellowship (FFARCS) in January 1966.

After returning to Sydney in July 1966, Richard commenced at St Vincent's Hospital where he was to remain for 32 years. This also included work with the Elizabeth Bay private group, the United Dental Hospital and Prince of Wales/Prince Henry Hospitals. In 1968 he started a long association with St Margaret's Children's Hospital. In 1969 he rejoined the anaesthetic department of the Royal Alexandra Hospital for Children, Camperdown where he was to continue until retirement from clinical anaesthesia in 1998.

He then worked as medical advisor to the Department of Veterans' Affairs until full retirement in 2002.

Bailey's clinical work was unusual for the time in that he had a lifelong involvement with paediatric and adult cardiac anaesthesia. This included involvement with the first bypass operation at the Children's Hospital at Camperdown in 1959, the first Australian heart transplant at St Vincent's by Dr Harry Windsor in 1968, the third in 1976 and the current transplant programme commenced by Dr Victor Chang in 1984. His first patient in this programme is still alive 36 years later. He was also closely involved in the developing and challenging field of paediatric airway endoscopy with Dr Bruce Benjamin for many years. Another area of expertise was the provision of anaesthesia for electrocochleography and cochlear implant in deaf children. This was ground-breaking technology for these children led by Prof Bill Gibson, Bailey documenting over 1000 anaesthetics for these children over the first 13 years of this very successful programme.

Bailey has been a noted bibliophile and collector for many years specifically in the history of anaesthesia and medicine. He also has diverse and eclectic interests in book binding, campanology, botany and ornithology - it being no surprise that his bookplate shows the Australian Regent Bowerbird – a bird renowned for collecting items to decorate its bower! He is also a great believer in serendipity – his grandfather was an editor of a small rural newspaper, the *Maitland Mercury*, which was the first NSW newspaper to report on painless surgery in 1847. Richard Bailey was assistant to the editor of the *Anaesthesia and Intensive Care History Supplement* for many years from its inception in 2005, achieving a David M. Little Award (q.v. page 123) in 2009. He has had long standing correspondence with many other anaesthesia historians globally over the years, including his friend Patrick Sim of the Wood Library-Museum of the American Society of Anesthesiology.

Richard Bailey has had a long involvement in the acquisition, promotion and research into books, equipment, archives and ephemera relating to the history of anaesthesia in Australia. He was appointed Honorary Librarian and Archivist in 1981 and also later Honorary Curator to the Harry Daly Museum (q.v. page 37) at the Australian Society of Anaesthetists (ASA). Currently he is Honorary Archivist. Since retirement he has also been involved with the NSW Retired Anaesthetists Group. He was awarded life membership of the Australian Society of Anaesthetists in 2009 and has been a member for 55 years.

The Library

The ASA decided at its second annual general meeting in 1937 to establish a library, aiming at being a practical reference library. It was initially housed at Geoffrey Kaye's house which was also the home of the Society. In 1946, the Library (and Museum) were housed at the Department of Physiology at the University of Melbourne before locating to 49 Mathoura Rd, Melbourne, which was rented to the ASA by Kaye who served as Curator and Librarian from 1951-1955. After this the collections were moved to the Royal Australasian College of Surgeons in Spring St, Melbourne. For some years the ASA headquarters moved from state to state before finally being established in Sydney in the early 1970s.

In June 1980, a library with an historical bent was established at the ASA's first real home in Paddington, Sydney, with the purchase of John Snow's original monograph *On the Inhalation of the Vapour of Ether*. The library has slowly grown since this time with mostly donations and a very limited budget, becoming deliberately orientated towards the history of anaesthesia rather than just another medical library with journals and textbooks, which could be easily accessed in hospital and university libraries and now on-line.

The library at the Australian Society of Anaesthetists was named **the Richard Bailey Library** at the opening of the Society's extended headquarters at Edgecliff in Sydney in 1994. This was a very fitting honour as the collection of books, pamphlets and ephemera on the history of anaesthesia is one of the best in the region with its focus on national and international material. There are many items in the library and the Harry Daly Museum that have been donated by Richard over the years. Other significant book donations have been made by early prominent Australian anaesthesia historians such as Gwen Wilson and Harry Daly.

There are close to 3000 titles in the library covering many aspects of the history of anaesthesia, resuscitation, intensive care and pain medicine and other related fields. Of international standing is a collection of 300 titles relating to mesmerism – a particular area of expertise of Dr Bailey. There are also over 250 pamphlets and letters. Australian authors who publish contemporary textbooks are encouraged to donate a copy to the library. Bailey and colleagues reproduced a rare facsimile – Nathan Rice's *Trials of a Public Benefactor* (1859) for the 11th World Congress of Anaesthesiology which was held in Sydney in 1996.

Other valuable highlights of the collection include:

- A first edition (1800) of Humphry Davy's *Researches ...concerning nitrous oxide or dephlogisticated nitrous air* (q.v. page 44)

- Original reprint of HJ Bigelow's publication in the *Boston & Medical Surgical Journal*, Nov 18, 1846, *Insensibility during surgical operations produced by inhalation*. This was originally from Bigelow's estate and was donated to the ASA by the Francis A Countway Library of Medicine, Boston.

The Richard Bailey Library collection can be seen at:
https://ehive.com/collections/5441/richard-bailey-library

The library is presided over by the History of Anaesthesia Library Museum and Archives (HALMA) Committee which is now establishing a History of Anaesthesia Research Unit (HARU).

The Richard Bailey Library along with the Harry Daly Museum has exhibited displays at many major national Australian meetings promoting the history of anaesthesia. In recent years it has also been the venue for an annual History of Anaesthesia Seminar which is planned to continue at the new headquarters at 86 Chandos St, Naremburn in Sydney, just north of the Sydney Harbour Bridge. It is hoped the move to the new ASA Headquarters will be completed by early 2021.

Richard Bailey has always had a fascination for Latin and its modern usage. So, it is fitting to conclude with
Haec laudem celebrat bibliotheca tuam
(This library sings your praises).

Further reading

Wilson G. *Fifty years. The Australian Society of Anaesthetists, 1934-1984*. Australian Society of Anaesthetists, Sydney, 1987.

Bailey R. The Richard Bailey Library. *ASA Newsletter*, Australian Society of Anaesthetists. 1994 July; 94:2: p 3-4.

ASA News. Australian Society of Anaesthetists, 2009, October, p 48

Stanbury P. Storage, display and access – innovations at the Harry Daly Museum and the Richard Bailey Library of the Australian Society of Anaesthetists, Sydney. *Anaesthesia and Intensive Care* 2010: 38 (S1): 20-24.

Stanbury P. Reflections on mesmerism in literature. *Anaesthesia and Intensive Care* 2012; 40 (S1): 10-17.

Bailey R. Anaesthetist and historian. *Magazine of the Australian Society of Anaesthetists*, 2014, April, 62-63.

Curriculum Vitae. Dr Richard J Bailey. Archives, Department of Anaesthesia, The Children's Hospital at Westmead, Sydney, Australia

Stanbury P. The origin of the ASA's museum and library – and where to from here? *Magazine of the Australian Society of Anaesthetists*, June 2019, p 92-93.

Purchas JM, ed. 1956 Graduate Jubilee Book, Faculty of Medicine, University of Sydney, 2005, pp 118-121.

EVELYN BAKER AWARD

Evelyn Baker (1916-1997)

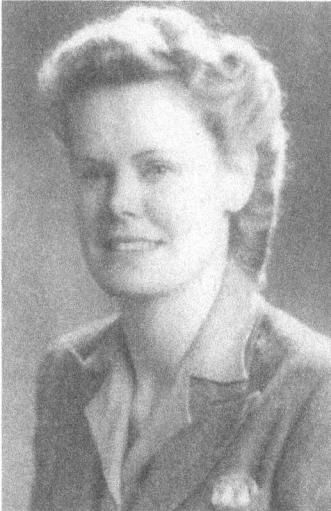

Evelyn Baker. Image courtesy of
Dr Margaret Branthwaite.

Evelyn Baker was a respiratory cripple from thoracoplasty for tuberculosis and radical mastectomy for breast cancer. The difficulties in her medical management at the Brompton Hospital in London and her resilience inspired Dr Margaret Branthwaite to endow an annual award in her memory – to anaesthetists who provide clinical excellence, but do not aspire to high academic status. This award has been presented annually by the Association of Anaesthetists of Great Britain and Ireland since 1998. The advertised calls for nomination have stated that the award recognises the 'unsung heroes' of anaesthetic departments.

Vignette which is on the scroll presented to award winners

Evelyn Willsmer was born during the First World War and spent most of her early years in London. In common with many of her generation, she developed pulmonary tuberculosis in her teens and so came under the care of the Brompton Hospital for Consumption and Diseases of the Chest. A strict regime of rest in a sanatorium, graded exercise, gold injections and a left artificial pneumothorax maintained for five years ultimately resulted in closure of a left apical cavity but that on the right persisted. In 1941 Evelyn had a right phrenic crush soon followed by a thoracoplasty – performed under local anaesthesia – by Russell Brock, later Sir Russell and finally Lord Brock. The operation was successful: Evelyn's tuberculosis never recurred and she was never prescribed antituberculous medication, but the historian of later years could not help but be moved by her description of submitting to surgery at the hands of such a dominant figure and listening, fearfully, to the sound of resection of her own ribs.

Despite chronic illness and the paternalistic caution of her physicians, Evelyn got married and spent some years in South Africa. It was there, in 1969 and while living in Johannesburg at an altitude of about 6000 feet, that she had her first episode of 'ankle swelling associated with bronchitis'. Despite short visits to England to recover from what might now be called cor pulmonale, she continued to deteriorate. In 1971, with a forced vital capacity of 1200 ml, an FEV1 of 550 ml, right ventricular hypertrophy and congestive cardiac failure, she returned permanently to the UK. Undaunted by her breathlessness she took up full-time clerical work but this respite was soon interrupted by the development of breast cancer. A left radical mastectomy left her significantly more breathless than previously. Later came ischaemic heart disease, manifest as dysrhythmias and occasional angina, and then a detached retina.

The end of the road?

In 1982 she developed symptomatic diverticulitis, a sigmoid stricture and paracolic abscess. There was no alternative to surgery but once again she survived, now with a defunctioning colostomy and in established respiratory failure. Aged 66, she was virtually bed-bound, unable to tolerate much-needed oxygen and requiring massive doses of diuretics. Was this the end of the road? She was assessed, tentatively, for non-invasive ventilatory support and expressed whole-hearted enthusiasm to try what was, at that time, relatively new and certainly uncongenial. Tall, broad shouldered and straight of back ("from breathing exercises in my teens"), Evelyn found the tank ventilator confining and claustrophobic. But she persevered, her condition improved and she sailed through surgical closure of her colostomy without complications.

She left hospital in 1982 with her heart failure under excellent control, hypoxic on exercise but, assisted by portable oxygen, able to live independently in her own house, drive her car and visit friends and relations. It was a relatively short respite and she soon needed regular elective admissions for further 'boosts' of non-invasive ventilatory support, culminating in provision of a 'pneumosuit' for use at home during sleep. This relatively simple device was inadequate to move the 'chalk thorax' of Evelyn Baker but soon a new mini-tank ventilator was marketed, suitable for home use by an unaided occupant. As always, NHS funds were limited so Evelyn bought her own, using the proceeds from the sale of her house which she had relinquished in favour of sheltered accommodation. But her room was small and the tank bulky so arrangements were made for a larger apartment on the ground floor which provided an additional benefit – Evelyn could sit out of doors even though trips further afield were becoming more difficult.

A change of system

Three years later Evelyn was persuaded to change her system of home ventilation to nasal positive pressure. She found the transition very difficult, not least because of her claustrophobia and distaste for any form of mask. But once again she persevered and succeeded, returning home to independence and enjoyment of her garden. By now contact with friends was predominantly by telephone and calls from the talkative were not always welcome because Evelyn became breathless and tired. But she retained her interest in current affairs, catered for herself and needed very little domestic assistance.

Evelyn used her ventilator overnight, with oxygen entrainment, and for short periods by day when she felt tired. Her oxygen tension while breathing air at rest was of the order of 7 kPa but speaking or moving about led to profound desaturation. The effort involved in breathing was very apparent and yet breathlessness was so much a part of her life that she lived within its limitations with far less distress than the observer would anticipate. Did she want to go on? Yes and yes again. Out-living her medical advisers became a matter of mischievous humour, as did the erroneously short prognosis of 75 years or so given as a blunt answer to a blunt question from Evelyn when she was about 70.

Two or three times during her last five years, Evelyn developed bronchitis and required hospital admission. Although poorly at first, she recuperated quickly and then enjoyed her stay, reminiscing with staff and entertaining fellow-patients with her accounts of the Brompton of a bygone era. In December 1996, aged 80 and more than 25 years after her first episode of cor pulmonale, she was admitted with pneumonia. She recovered in that her fever settled, the consolidation resolved and her sputum cleared, but this time her spirits did not lift. She was apprehensive about returning to her own home but there were few realistic alternatives. She did not have to make the decision: she faded away without difficultly or distress, tranquillity coming from within rather than from drugs.

Medical decisions

Throughout her life Evelyn was a challenge to her medical practitioners. In the early years her tuberculosis was intransigent; harsh decisions were recommended and implemented. In middle life the conflict lay between the claims of marriage and of health. Thereafter the common depredations of age took their toll, with management always compromised by profound respiratory impairment and imminent or established heart failure. She achieved something of new lease of life when non-invasive ventilation was established. It gave her 15 more years – years which she valued and used to the full, but years which were also filled with anxiety and fear as Evelyn lost friends and relatives who predeceased her and she recognised her own diminishing capabilities. An imposing and dignified figure, she earned respect, compassion and affection from all. But her medical attendants were challenged too, by the need to provide more than just science. The award in her name is in recognition of medical skills beyond mere academe.

Table 1. Evelyn Baker Award winners

Year	Recipient	Year	Recipient
1998	John R Cole	2009	Fred Roberts
1999	Meena Choksi	2010	Sudheer Medakkar
2000	Neil Schofield	2011	Keith Clayton
2001	Brian Steer	2012	John Windsor
2002	Mark Crosse	2013	Amanda Blackburn, Mike Donaldson, Andrew Kilner, Chris Vallis
2003	Paul Monks	2014	Sally Millett
2004	Margo Lewis	2015	John Leigh, Virin Sidhu, Patricia Weir
2005	Douglas Turner	2016	Rob John
2006	Martin Coates	2017	Michelle Soskin
2007	Gareth Charlton	2018	Ian Appadurai
2008	Neville Robinson	2019	Kathryn Bell, Anthony John Rampton

Further reading

Branthwaite MA. Origin and Evolution of Domiciliary Ventilation in the UK: The Responaut Study. *The History of Anaesthesia Society Proceedings* 2018; **51**: 137-42.

THOMAS BOULTON ANAESTHESIA HISTORY PRIZE

Thomas Babington Boulton (1925-2016)

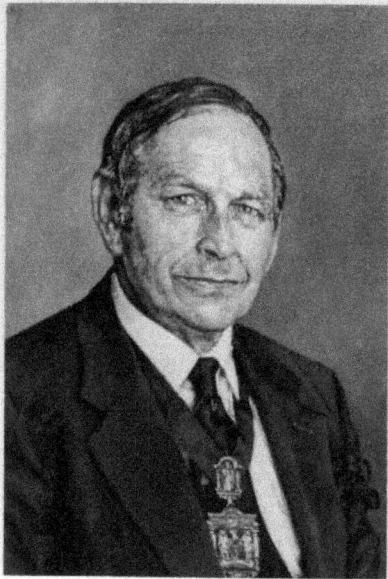

Thomas B. Boulton. Painting courtesy of The Anaesthesia Heritage Centre, AAGBI.

Thomas B. Boulton was born in Bishop Auckland, County Durham, England in 1925. He was educated at Scarborough College, followed by St Peter's School in York and then in 1943 was accepted at Emmanuel College, Cambridge University to read medicine. Qualifying at the end of 1948 he proceeded to a house officer post in 1949 at St Bartholomew's Hospital (Barts) in London, working first in surgery and then anaesthetics. From 1950 to 1952 he did National Service in the Royal Army Medical Corps (RAMC), serving in Malaya during the "campaign against the Chinese terrorists". He was obliged to take on a considerable workload in anaesthetics, becoming competent in routine and emergency cases, though largely self-taught from the 1948 *Textbook of Anaesthetics* by Minnitt and Gillies 7th edition). On demobilisation, he felt sure that his future career lay in specialising in civilian anaesthesia and he joined the Territorial Army.

Over the next six years Boulton trained in anaesthesia, passing the two parts of the Diploma in Anaesthetics (DA) and working successively at Barts, University of Michigan Hospital at Ann Arbor and finally, Southend General Hospital in Essex, England under the tutelage of J. Alfred Lee. In 1958 he took a (NHS) Consultant Anaesthetist post at the Royal Berkshire and Battle Hospitals in Reading. Although happy in this position, his ambition pushed him to move to a Consultant post at Barts in 1961, to work in the new open cardiac surgery unit. He had a successful career there for the next twelve years, introducing many improvements. During this time (1966-68), he contributed a series of eight articles in the journal *Anaesthesia* on practical anaesthesia in geographically remote and difficult situations. In 1968 also he produced the Program and the Proceedings of the Fourth World Congress of Anaesthesiologists, which was held in London that year. Then in 1969-70 he voluntarily worked at the Barsky Unit of the 'Children's Medical Relief International' in Saigon during the Vietnam War.

On invitation, in 1973 Boulton took on the mantle of Editor of *Anaesthesia*, the journal of the Association of Anaesthetists of Great Britain and Ireland (AAGBI), which meant he was on its Executive. He facilitated the time needed for this role by moving back to a Consultant post at Reading. He was Editor until 1982 and certainly encouraged articles on the history of anaesthesia. From 1976 he was contracted to work every Monday at the Churchill Hospital in Oxford and next was appointed to a Clinical Lectureship in the University of Oxford. He specialised in teaching local/regional anaesthesia and the history of anaesthesia. From 1980 he was involved in providing a course on "anaesthesia for developing countries and difficult situations". For general anaesthesia he taught the draw-over technique, which he had also suggested to the RAMC – this was subsequently developed into the "Triservice" Apparatus.

A further commitment for Boulton at this busy time was his Presidency of the Society for the Advancement of Anaesthesia in Dentistry (SAAD, predominantly dental practitioners) from 1980 to 1982. This was followed by his Presidency of the Association of Dental Anaesthetists (predominantly medical graduates) from 1983 to 1985. He tried but failed to get these two organizations to amalgamate.

In 1981 Boulton was asked to coordinate the care and cataloguing of the AAGBI's large collection of historical equipment, books, pamphlets and archives, and he was appointed Honorary Archivist the following year. He was elected President of the AAGBI 1984-86; in 1986 he set up the Charles King Collection of Anaesthetic Equipment at the Association's building – then 9 Bedford Square, London.

From 1983 he began contributing articles to the Classical File section of the bimonthly *Survey of Anesthesiology*. Some of these (e.g. on Alexander Wood and the syringe, Geoffrey Marshall and the Boyle's machine, and "balanced anaesthesia") were myth-shattering and are worth mentioning, because the journal has not been PubMed indexed: see *Further reading*.

On 7th June 1986 the inaugural meeting of the History of Anaesthesia Society (HAS) was convened by Boulton at the Royal Berkshire Hospital in Reading. In July 1987 he chaired the organising committee for the Second International Symposium on the History of Anaesthesia, held in London. Then he and Dr Richard Atkinson edited the Proceedings, which were published in 1989 as a book of nearly 700 pages – containing a wealth of information on the history of anaesthesia. Boulton was elected President of the HAS for 1988-90.

In the late 1980s Boulton was involved in the creation of the College of Anaesthetists and the design of its Coat of Arms. He retired from clinical practice in November 1990 and in that month flew to Las Vegas where he had been invited to deliver the prestigious Lewis H. Wright Memorial Lecture, at the Annual Congress of the American Society of Anesthesiologists. He was further honoured in 1991: appointment as an Officer of the Order of the British Empire (OBE), which was conferred upon him by the Queen.

In 1999 Boulton completed *The Association of Anaesthetists of Great Britain and Ireland 1932-1992 and The Development of the Specialty of Anaesthesia*, which he had been commissioned to write in 1991 – eight years of work. This book of nearly 800 pages was duly published by the AAGBI. This magnum opus formed the basis for his M.D. thesis, which degree was conferred upon him by the University of Cambridge in 1989.

Boulton was elected Wood Library-Museum Laureate in the History of Anaesthesia, jointly with Dr Norman A. Bergman in 2000. This was the second such election as the four-year Laureate had commenced in 1996. Tom was an obvious choice: besides his publications and organisational skill, he had charisma and the ability to inspire others in the history of anaesthesia.

Since 2010 the AAGBI and the HAS have jointly sponsored an annual Anaesthesia History Prize of cash and a medal for the best essay judged from essays submitted by trainee members of the AAGBI. The criteria for acceptance included "original essay of 4000-6000 words on a topic related to the history of anaesthesia, intensive care or pain management". After Tom Boulton's death it was decided that the name of this award should be changed to the Thomas Boulton Anaesthesia History Prize.

Table 1. Thomas Boulton Anaesthesia History Prize winners

Year	Recipient	Essay
2017	Sam Fosker	Come Fly with Me – taking ITU above the clouds
2018	Laura Gounon	Monitoring depth of anaesthesia, a long-standing enterprise
2019	Laura Naumann	Blood transfusion for haemorrhagic shock: have we come full circle?
2020	Serkan Cakir	Spinal Anaesthesia during the 19th and 20th Centuries – Cocaine and Controversy

Further reading

Boulton TB. The Wind Bloweth Where it Listeth. *St.John 3; viii.* A Career Carried on the Wind of Medical Progress. In: Caton D, McGoldrick KE (Eds.) *Careers in Anesthesiology X*. Park Ridge, Illinois: Wood Library-Museum, 2007; 117-300.

Boulton TB. Alexander Wood, M.D. (1817-1884) and the Use of the Syringe and Hollow Needle for Parenteral Medication. (Classical File) *Survey of Anesthesiology* 1984; **28**: 346-50.

Boulton TB. Sir Geoffrey Marshall, Shock, and Nitrous Oxide. (Classical File) *Survey of Anesthesiology* 1992; **36**: 40-45.

Boulton TB. T. Cecil Gray and the "Disintegration of the Nervous System". (Classical File) *Survey of Anesthesiology* 1994; **38**: 239-44.

GILBERT BROWN PRIZE

Gilbert Brown (1883-1960)

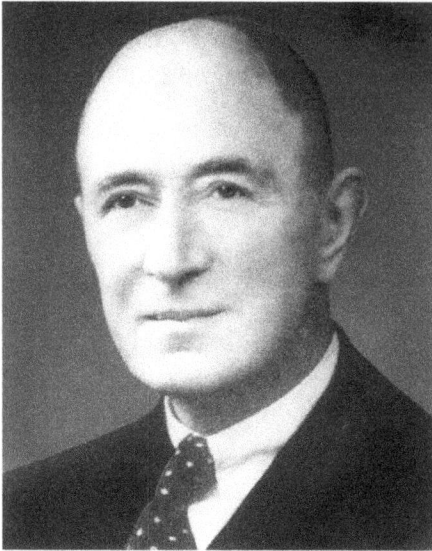

Gilbert Brown. Image courtesy of the Geoffrey Kaye Museum of Anaesthetic History, ANZCA.

Gilbert Brown was born in Wigan, England and attended the local Grammar School, followed by Waterloo High School. On his father's wishes he spent one year in the engineering course at Liverpool University, but then he insisted on changing to study medicine. He was a good athlete and captained the University Rugby football team. In 1908 he graduated MB ChB and proceeded to do junior doctor appointments in the Liverpool area.

In 1911 Brown embarked on a voyage as ship's surgeon to the Far East and the Pacific coast of the USA, almost settling in Takoma, Washington. However, the next year he visited Australia and decided to emigrate there. He went into general practice in rural South Australia, about 90 miles north of Adelaide. Having accepted his marriage proposal, Dr Marie Simpson of London duly joined him in 1914: she was a partner in the practice and acted as his anaesthetist. Because of the shortage of local doctors, Gilbert Brown was not allowed to enlist for service in the First World War until 1918: by the time he reached South Africa, the Armistice was declared and he was sent back to Western Australia, where he took charge of a quarantine station.

Brown moved to practise in Gilberton, a suburb of Adelaide in 1919 and began to concentrate on anaesthetics. In 1920 he became the anaesthetist to the surgeon Henry Newland in the plastic surgery unit of Keswick Repatriation Hospital. A year later he was appointed to the Royal Adelaide Hospital and became instructor in anaesthetics to medical and dental students. He published increasingly on various aspects of anaesthesia and in 1928 he was elected an Honorary Vice-President of the International Anaesthesia

Research Society (IARS). He led the organisation of anaesthetists in Australia by setting up for the first time a Section of Anaesthesia at the Congress of the Australian branch of the British Medical Association held in Sydney in 1929. The participants were inspired to continue the initiative by the guest of honour Francis Hoeffer McMechan, the Secretary-General of the IARS.

At the next Australasian Medical Congress held in Hobart in 1934 there was again a Section of Anaesthesia, and through the gathering Gilbert Brown instigated the formation of the Australian Society of Anaesthetists (ASA). The Society had its first meeting in Melbourne in 1935 with Brown elected President.

In 1935 Brown also went on a study tour of the UK and was made an Honorary Member of the Liverpool Anaesthetic Society. The Conjoint Board (RCP&S) awarded him the Diploma in Anaesthetics (DA) the following year. At this time, he published on post-operative pulmonary complications and attempted to initiate post-anaesthesia morbidity reporting in Australia. He pioneered the provision of an individual anaesthetic record chart for every patient with recordings of blood pressure in Australia. In 1939 he was honoured by being invited to Melbourne to deliver the triennial Embley Memorial Lecture.

During the Second World War Brown was too old for military service, but he contributed massively on the home front. He retired from the Royal Adelaide Hospital and the University in 1947, though continuing some private anaesthetic practice and he became FFARCS (England) by election in 1950. His wartime services were recognised by the award of the Insignia of a Serving Brother, the Order of St John of Jerusalem in 1953. The final accolade was Commander of the Order of the British Empire (CBE) in 1953 – the first Australian anaesthetist to be so honoured.

A year after Brown's death, the ASA liaised with the Faculty of Anaesthetists within the Royal Australasian College of Surgeons (inaugurated in 1952) to establish the Gilbert Brown Prize. This was awarded for the first time in 1963 for the best contribution to the session of the Faculty's General Scientific Meeting devoted to recent local studies and developments.

Table 1. Gilbert Brown Prize winners

Year	Recipient	Year	Recipient
1963	Bruce W. Gunner	1991	Tony Gin
1964	Trevor T. Currie	1992	Neil R. Warwick
1965	John F. Mainland	1993	Suen Ka Lok
1966	M.R. Milne	1994	Alexander L. Garden
1967	Teresa R. Brophy	1995	Katherine Leslie
1968	Trevor T. Currie	1996	Paul S. Myles
1969	NIL	1997	Warwick D. Ngan Kee
1970	Alexander W. Squire	1998	John T. Moloney
1971	NIL	1999	Philip B. Cornish
1972	John M. Gibbs	2000	Adam P. Tucker
1973	Anthony J. Newson Frank D. Pilditch	2001	Winifred J. Burnett
1974	Neville J. Davis	2002	Richard A. French
1975	Thomas A.G. Torda	2003	Kwok Ming Ho
1976	Malcolm M. Fisher	2004	Timothy McCulloch
1977	Thomas C.K. Brown	2005	Paul J. Wrigley
1978	Karl D. Alexander William B. Runciman	2006	Ashley R. Webb
1979	Robert O. Edeson	2007	Sui Cheung Yu
1980	Walter J. Russell	2008	David McIlroy
1981	Richard W. Davis	2009	David Belavy
1982	NIL	2010	Forbes McGain
1983	Peter E. Lillie	2011	Paul Sadleir
1984	Charles M. Domaingue	2012	Mary K. Hegarty
1985	Navaratnam Sivaneswaran	2013	Lawrence Weinberg
1986	Craig Nancarrow Michael Martyn	2014	Jonathan Hiller
1987	Stevenson P. Petito	2015	Dean Bunbury
1988	Edward J. McArdle	2016	Adrian Chin
1989	Mark R. Upton	2017	Jai Darvall
1990	David B.F. Cottee	2018	Rani Chahal
		2019	Verna Aykanat

Further reading

Kay G. Brown of Adelaide. *British Journal of Anaesthesia* 1950; **22**: 43-52.

Obituary Gilbert Brown, C.B.E., M.B., Ch.B., F.F.A.R.C.S. *British Medical Journal* 1960; **1**: 283.

Wilson GCM. The Tyrant Overcome: A Review of the History of Anaesthesia in Australia. *Anaesthesia and Intensive Care* 1972; **1**: 9-26.

DUDLEY BUXTON PRIZE

Dudley Wilmot Buxton (1855-1931)

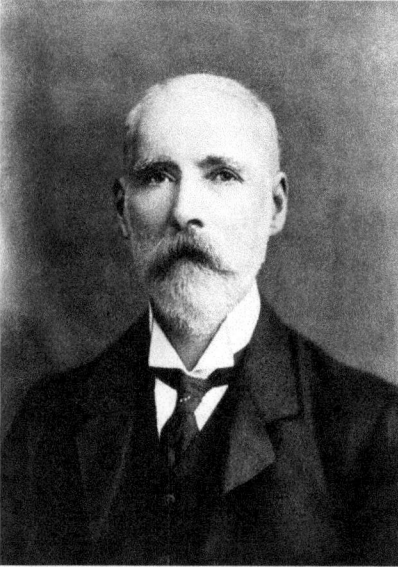

Dudley Wilmot Buxton had a marked influence on education in anaesthesia in the United Kingdom from the late 1880s to 1920. He was born in 1855 in London and educated privately. Despite a speech impediment due to a cleft palate, he studied at University College, London and from 1878 University College Hospital (UCH), qualifying in medicine with distinction in 1882. He then did house jobs at UCH and in 1884 took on laboratory work under Professor Sydney Ringer (eponym 'lactated Ringer's injection') at UCH – notably the action of drugs on involuntary and cardiac muscle in the frog; they found that the vitality of involuntary muscle persisted shorter after chloroform than after ether.

Dudley Wilmot Buxton. Credit: Wellcome Collection. Reproduced under Creative Commons Attribution (CC BY 4.0).

Thus stimulated, Buxton decided to specialise in anaesthesia and was appointed the first official anaesthetist to UCH in 1885.

Buxton immediately set about regular teaching of anaesthetics to medical students; despite this subject not being compulsory in the curriculum, his lectures were well attended – an attestation to the quality of his lectures. He carried on the late Joseph Clover's work in encouraging the use of nitrous oxide and reducing chloroform. In 1888 he published *Anaesthetics, their uses and administration*, which was both a practical and popular textbook. A whole chapter was devoted to anaesthetic mixtures, including Billroth's A.C.E., which had been introduced to prevent overdose of chloroform. Buxton advised the use of atropine for its vagolytic effect, suggesting it "might be a valuable antidote to chloroform, by preventing reflex inhibition of the heart". The book also had a chapter on medicolegal aspects of anaesthesia. Buxton went on to modify anaesthetic apparatus, improving safety. For example, with Junker's inhaler, he placed the longer afferent tube within the efferent tube, the small gap between the two acting as the outlet port. This reduced the danger of the patient inhaling liquid chloroform.

In 1890 the editor of the *Lancet* refused to believe the Report of the Second Hyderabad Chloroform Commission, and duly appointed Buxton to lead another investigation. He sent questionnaires to individual doctors in the UK and every UK hospital of over 10 beds as well as larger hospitals overseas. The data was collected through 1891, then analysed and reported in the *Lancet* 1893. In contrast to the previous report, it concluded: "It would, therefore, appear that in England and Wales chloroform is responsible for a larger number of deaths and of dangerous cases than is ether."

Meanwhile, in November 1891 the British Medical Association (BMA) Second Anaesthetic Committee (the first had been in 1880) was set up in London and Buxton was one of the executive members. Data was collected through 1892 and interim reports followed, but the final report was not until 1900. The main message was that patients given chloroform had a six to eight-fold greater risk of severe danger compared with ether. A second edition of Buxton's textbook had been published in 1892 and a third edition in 1900; use of nitrous oxide was becoming more popular.

Another event in 1892 was J.F.W. Silk's (of Guy's Hospital) suggestion in the *Lancet* that the teaching of anaesthetics be made compulsory in the undergraduate medical curriculum. Buxton made the same recommendation in the *British Medical Journal* in 1901, in which year he also was appointed secretary of a Third Chloroform Committee of the BMA, chaired by A.D. Waller. The aim was the quantitative assay of chloroform in the air and the living body. As a result, the Reader in Chemistry at Christ Church College, Oxford, A. Vernon Harcourt was co-opted onto the committee. He had devised (1899) a method of assaying the percentage of chloroform in air, by converting it into carbon dioxide and hydrochloric acid via contact with a platinum wire made red-hot by an electric current. Harcourt went on to produce his regulating chloroform inhaler in 1893. In the Report of the Committee (1910) Buxton gave a detailed description of the Vernon Harcourt inhaler, in which it was claimed that the maximum strength of chloroform vapour was automatically limited to 2% - the limit of safety.

By 1907 there was a fourth edition of Buxton's textbook. In 1909 he recommended premedication of scopolamine and morphine injections before general anaesthesia, opining that "a terrified patient after a sleepless night is in the worst condition for an anaesthetic and an operation." In 1912 the General Medical Council, perhaps heeding Buxton's call, published in the *British Medical Journal* that anaesthetics was to be included in the undergraduate curriculum.

Buxton retired from his London practice in 1919, but continued teaching. A sixth edition of his textbook appeared in 1920.

The Faculty of Anaesthetists (later to become the Royal College of Anaesthetists) established an endowed trust fund in 1967 to provide a Dudley Buxton Prize every three years. This prize is a bronze medal, which is awarded for 'meritorious work in anaesthesia or in a science contributing to the progress of anaesthesia'.

Table 1. Dudley Buxton Prize winners

Year	Recipient	Year	Recipient
1968	John Francis Nunn	2001	Peter Baskett
1971	Sir Gordon Robson	2004	Stuart Ingram
1977	Cyril Frederick Scurr	2009	Tom Clutton-Brock
1980	Sir M. Keith Sykes	2011	Mark Tooley
1983	R.J. Linden	2012	Teik Oh, Haydn Perndt
1986	James Patrick Payne	2013	Paul Gerard Murphy
1989	John Lunn	2014	Ellen O'Sullivan, Richard Griffiths, Stuart White, Peter Charters
1992	William W. Mapleson	2015	Michael Grocott
1995	Archie Brain	2016	Christopher Frerk
		2017	Ian Russell
		2019	Eugene Steffey

Further reading

Horton J. Dudley Wilmot Buxton (1855-1931). *The History of Anaesthesia Society Proceedings* 2014; **47**: 15-24.

Cartwright FF. Eminent Anaesthetists, No. 8: Dudley Wilmot Buxton. *British Journal of Anaesthesia* 1953; **25**: 68-73.

COCHRANE ANAESTHESIA REVIEW GROUP

Archibald Leman Cochrane (1909-1988)

Archie Cochrane was born in Galashiels, Scotland. When he was eight, his father was killed while soldiering in the First World War. Fortunately, he won two scholarships: first to the famous Uppingham School in England and second, in 1927, to King's College of Cambridge University. He proceeded to graduate first class in the Natural Sciences Tripos and completed the second MB in 1930.

Next Cochrane tried treatment of his severe porphyria by psycho-analysis in Berlin from Theodor Reik, whom he followed to Vienna and Leiden – studying medicine and acquiring fluency in German. He then enrolled at University College Hospital London.

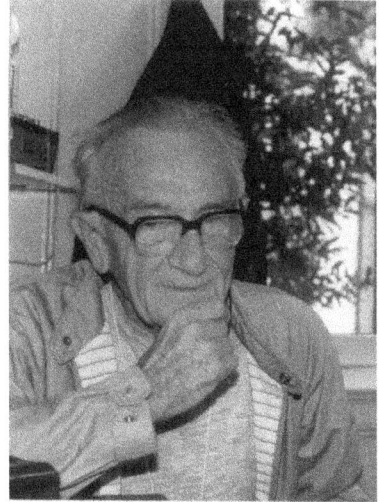

Archie Cochrane in the 1980s. Image courtesy of Cardiff University Library, Cochrane Archive, University Hospital Llandough.

In 1937 he joined the International Brigades for the Spanish Civil War, serving in the British Ambulance Unit. In his year there he learned triage at first hand. Returning to London, he qualified in medicine (1940) and joined the Royal Army Medical Corps to serve in the Second World War.

Soon he was captured in Crete and spent the next four years as a prisoner of war in Greece and East Germany, working as a Medical Officer in the camps. Under appalling conditions, he conducted his first clinical trial to show that the addition of yeast to the prisoner diet would cure oedema. Many of the prisoners had tuberculosis, so he began to become a specialist in this disease. At liberation, he was in very poor health and returned to London, where he was appointed a Member of the Most Excellent Order of the British Empire (MBE).

Cochrane studied the epidemiology of tuberculosis and was guided by Austin Bradford Hill, Director of the Medical Research Council's (MRC) Statistical

Research Unit, who first introduced randomized trials into clinical medicine. In 1948 he joined the MRC Pneumoconiosis Unit at Llandough Hospital in Wales. By 1960 he was appointed Professor of Tuberculosis and Chest Diseases at the Welsh National School of Medicine. In 1968 he was awarded the CBE for his contributions to epidemiology. Then in 1972 as Director of the MRC's Epidemiology Research Unit in Cardiff, he published *Effectiveness and efficiency: random reflections on health services* (Nuffield Provincial Hospitals Trust). This book extolled the virtues of the randomized controlled trial (RCT) and disparaged those clinicians in the National Health Service (NHS) who failed to do RCTs or ignored the results. It was very influential – in time the randomized controlled clinical trial came to be regarded as the essential tool in assessing clinical efficacy of new drugs.

After Cochrane's death, his friend Iain Chalmers in Oxford was resolved to respond to his challenge to publish periodic updates of systematic reviews of RCTs. From 1991 Chalmers proposed the 'Cochrane Centre' for international collaboration, and this was duly opened the following year. In 1993 the Cochrane Collaboration was formed to produce the Cochrane Database of Systematic Reviews – it soon became recognised as a very important source of current best evidence.

In time the main work of the Cochrane Collaboration came to be done by its Collaborative Review Groups (CRGs) which prepared and maintained the Cochrane reviews. By 2002 there were fifty CRGs, each supported by a centre – at an agreed place in the world. Thus, the Nordic Cochrane Centre is based in Copenhagen. In 1997 anaesthesiologists at Bispebjerg University Hospital in Copenhagen had the idea of forming the Cochrane Anaesthesia Review Group (CARG) supported by the Nordic Cochrane Centre. There followed preliminary meetings: at the 6th Annual Meeting of the European Society of Anaesthesiology in Barcelona, followed by the American Society of Anesthesiologists' Annual Meeting in Orlando, and at the 6th Cochrane Colloquium in Baltimore – all in 1998. Eventually CARG was established in the year 2000, with its editorial office in the Department of Anaesthesiology, Bispebjerg University Hospital, Copenhagen. The editorial team has included anaesthesiologists in Australia, Austria, Canada, China, Denmark, New Zealand, Switzerland, the UK and USA.

The scope of CARG has been review of the perioperative care of patients undergoing surgery. Topics of focus have included: preoperative assessment and optimisation, intraoperative management, postoperative complications and how to avoid them, airway management, regional anaesthesia, paediatric anaesthesia and acute pain management. It is now based in Herlev Hospital, Denmark. Its annual reports are available on the internet.

Further reading

Bosch FX (Ed.). *Archie Cochrane: Back to the Front*. Barcelona: MSD, 2003.

Pedersen T, Moller AM, Cracknell J. The Mission of the Cochrane Anesthesia Review Group: Preparing and Disseminating Systematic Reviews of the Effect of Health Care in Anesthesiology. *Anesthesia and Analgesia* 2002; **95**: 1012-18.

https://carg.cochrane.org (accessed 21 September 2019).

MICHAEL J COUSINS LECTURE

Michael J. Cousins (1939 -   )

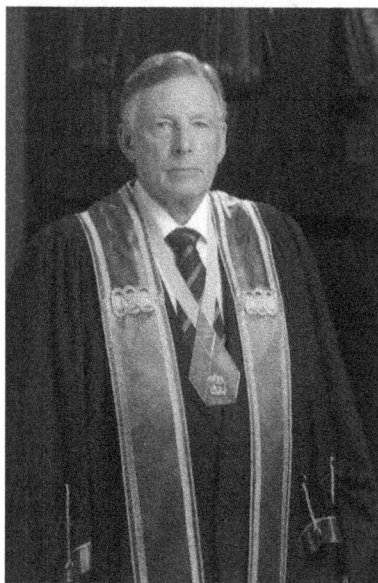

Michael Cousins. Image courtesy of the Geoffrey Kaye Museum of Anaesthetic History, ANZCA.

Michael J. Cousins was born in Sydney in 1939 and grew up in the North Shore area of that city. At the age of 14, his nose was broken in a game of rugby, and the consequent admission to hospital sparked his decision to do medicine on leaving school. He duly did the medical degree course at the University of Sydney, graduating in 1963, and proceeded to a resident post at St. George Hospital. There he was impressed by the pain suffered by two children with severe burns, and this experience convinced him that he should do intensive care; this meant he would have to first train to be an anaesthetist. So, on completion of his residency, he undertook specialist training in anaesthesia at the Royal North Shore Hospital, Sydney. Next, he embarked on research in acute pain at McGill University, Montreal, working under Professor Philip Bromage (of epidural analgesia fame). He also interacted with Ronald Melzack, who with Patrick Wall had propounded the gate control theory of pain.

In 1970 Cousins was appointed Assistant Professor of Anaesthesia at Stanford University in California, where he worked with Professor Richard Mazze to demonstrate that methoxyflurane could cause renal damage. John Bonica organised the First International Symposium on Pain in Seattle in 1973 and in the following year created the International Association for the Study of Pain (IASP). Cousins was appointed to the IASP Council and worked closely with Bonica, so embracing the multidisciplinary approach to pain management.

Cousins returned to Australia in 1975 to take up the country's first Chair of Anaesthesia and Intensive Care at Flinders University in Adelaide. In 1980 he was the Inaugural President of the Australian Pain Society. Also in that year he published the first edition of *Neural Blockade in Clinical Anesthesia and Management of Pain* with co-editor Phillip O. Bridenbaugh, Professor of Anesthesia at Cincinnati, Ohio. A second edition was published in 1988 – with more editions to come, as the book became recognised as a principal reference source for its subject. In 1984 Cousin and his colleague Laurie Mather published a review of spinal opioids in the journal *Anesthesiology*. This became one of the most cited references in the anaesthesiology and pain medicine literature. Cousins was elected President of the IASP for 1987-90.

In 1990 Cousins moved to back to Sydney to be the Foundation Professor and Head of Anaesthesia and Pain Management at the Royal North Shore Hospital. He immediately established the Pain Management Research Institute (PMRI), a not for profit, community-based centre for clinical care, teaching and research, which raised considerable funds. For the Australian and New Zealand College of Anaesthetists (ANZCA) he chaired the Joint Advisory Committee on Pain Medicine, which led to the formation of the Faculty of Pain Medicine in 1999. Unsurprisingly he served as Founding Dean of this Faculty for 1999-2002. With effect from 2003, in recognition of his contributions, the Faculty plenary session at the annual scientific meeting was named the Michael J Cousins Lecture (see Table 1).

Table 1. The Michael J Cousins lecturers and lecture titles

Year	Lecturer	Title
2003	Henrik Kehlet	Postoperative analgesia and patient outcome – the second round needs a change in tactic?
2004	Ralf Baron	Diagnosis and management of complex regional pain syndrome.
2005	Mark Sullivan	Chest pain and the mind.
2006	William Macrae	Can we prevent chronic pain after surgery?
2008	Quinn Hogan	New observations about anatomy in regional anaesthesia.
2009	Andrew Rice	Cannabinoid analgesia: future friend or dead end?
2010	Jeffrey Mogil	What's wrong with animal models of pain?
2011	Catherine Bushnell	Imaging pain: from research to clinical application.
2012	Daniel Bennett	Opiophobia, regulation and risk management: developments in the USA, a cautionary tale.
2013	Edzard Ernst	The prince and me.
2014	Audun Stubhaug	From acute to chronic pain: risk factors, genetics and possible preventative strategies.
2015	Irene Tracey	Imaging analgesia and anaesthesia.
2016	Anthony Dickenson	Novel analgesics/ future challenges.
2017	Christopher Eccleston	The psychology of physical experience: exploring the 10 neglected senses.
2018	Oscar de Leon-Casasola	The neurobiology of acute postoperative pain and the translation to postsurgical pain management guidelines.
2019	Chad Brummett	Impact of centralised pain on acute and chronic pain after surgery.

In 2004 Cousins published with Philip J. Siddall the first paper considering that chronic pain is a disease. Politically the ANZCA Faculty of Pain Medicine succeeded in getting the Australian Government to recognise Pain Medicine as a medical specialty in 2005. The University of Sydney awarded Cousins a DSc in 2006.

Cousins promoted the development of a University of Sydney Graduate Diploma and Master postgraduate degree in Pain Management, which began in 1996 and has enrolled students internationally in an Internet online education program. He headed a multidisciplinary committee which produced the book *Acute Pain Management: Scientific Evidence*, published by the National Health and Medical Research Council (NHMRC) of Australia in 1999. A third edition was published in 2010: a guideline which was endorsed world-wide by Colleges and Academies of Anaesthetists. This was followed by a fourth edition in 2015 and a fifth edition is planned for 2020.

The 13th World Congress on Pain held in Montreal in 2010 featured an inaugural International Pain Summit, which Cousins arranged. Thence came the "Declaration of Montreal" by the IASP: that access to pain management is a fundamental human right. Cousins published this in the journal *Pain* the following year. In 2012 the University of Sydney introduced Pain Medicine as a new Academic Discipline with Cousins as head; within weeks there was an Inaugural Symposium on Pain for all health care students.

Cousins took on a translational research programme with Professor John Parker and Dr Charles Brooker in 2009, which led to the first implantation of a "closed-loop" spinal cord stimulator in a human in 2015. The device has been produced commercially by the Saluda Medical company and clinical trials published.

With his fine record as an academic ambassador for Australia, Cousins justifiably received several national honours. He was awarded Member of the Order of Australia in 1995, the Robert Orton Medal (q.v. page 158) by ANZCA in 2008, and Officer of the Order of Australia in 2014. In the year of his retirement (2016) he was elected a Fellow of the Australian Academy of Health and Medical Sciences (FAAHMS). Internationally, he received the Mushin Medal (q.v. page 154) in Wales in 1986, and he delivered the Gaston Labat Lecture for the American Society of Regional Anesthesia in 1996 with the title "Pain – a persistent problem". In 1997 he delivered the Emery A. Rovenstine Lecture at the annual meeting of the American Society of Anesthesiologists with the title "Pain: the past, present, and future of anesthesiology". He was elected in 1999 to Honorary Membership of both the Pain Society of Great Britain & Ireland, and the IASP. In 2000 he delivered the Datex-Ohmeda Healthcare Lecture at the Winter Scientific Meeting of the Association of Anaesthetists of Great Britain and Ireland held in London with the title "ANZCA Faculty of Pain Medicine: the coming of age of a new field". The International Anesthesia Research Society chose Cousins for its 2005 T.H. Seldon Lectureship. Most recently he delivered the 2013 Francis Rynd Lecture (q.v. page 204) in Dublin, Ireland.

Acknowledgement

Dr Charles Brooker kindly assisted with information and read the manuscript on behalf of Professor Michael Cousins.

Further reading

Cousins MJ, Mather LE. Intrathecal and epidural administration of opioids. *Anesthesiology* 1984; **61**: 276-310.

Cousins MJ, Bridenbaugh PO (Eds.). *Neural Blockade in Clinical Anesthesia and Management of Pain* (3rd edition). Philadelphia: Lippincott-Raven, 1998.

Siddall PJ, Cousins MJ. Persistent pain as a disease entity: implications for clinical management. *Anesthesia and Analgesia* 2004; **99**: 510-20.

Interview of Michael Cousins by Michael Peschardt, 3 June 2010. http://www.abc.net.au/local/stories/2010/06/04/2918386.htm (accessed 29 September 2020).

https://blog.apsoc.org.au/2016/08/02/professor-michael-cousins-ao.retires/ (accessed 26 September 2019).

https://sydney.edu.au/medicine/museum/mwmuseum/index.php/Cousins_Michael_J (accessed 6 October 2019).

Russo M, Brooker C, Cousins MJ *et al.* Sustained long-term outcomes with closed-loop spinal cord stimulation: 12-month results of the prospective, multicenter, open-label Avalon study. *Neurosurgery* 2020; **87**: E485-E495.

HARRY DALY MUSEUM

Harry John Daly (1893-1980)

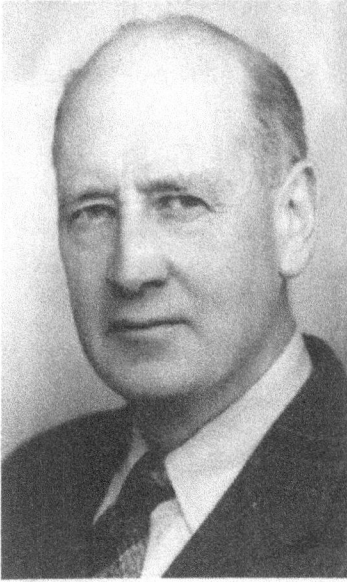

Harry Daly was born in Glebe, Sydney, in 1893, the only son of Irish migrants Henry and Victoria Daly. His secondary education was at St Ignatius College, Riverview. In 1918, Daly graduated in medicine from the University of Sydney. He was a resident medical officer at the Royal Prince Alfred Hospital for two years. In 1920, he became a general practitioner in Haberfield, Sydney. He also had an honorary appointment at Lewisham Hospital, where he became interested in specialising in anaesthesia because he was often called upon to administer anaesthesia.

In 1930, Daly was a founder member of the Section of Anaesthetics of the New South Wales Branch of the British Medical Association, and four years later he was a founder member of the Australian Society of Anaesthetists (ASA) in Hobart, Tasmania.

Harry John Daly. Photograph courtesy of the History of Medicine Library, The Royal Australasian College of Physicians.

In 1934, the Diploma in Anaesthesia, inaugurated in England, was conferred to Daly without examination. In 1935, Daly and his wife travelled overseas and met the leading anaesthetists in the United Kingdom, Europe, Canada and the United States. The trip led to enduring friendships and regular correspondence with overseas specialists, facilitating the introduction of new anaesthetic equipment and techniques, and advances in the training and organisation of anaesthetists in Australia. After returning to Australia, Daly was appointed as Honorary Anaesthetist at Sydney Hospital in 1936, and Honorary Anaesthetist to St Vincent's Hospital in 1937. He also briefly held an appointment as Honorary Anaesthetist at the Royal Prince Alfred Hospital, Sydney (1938-1939).

In August 1945, Daly became the first anaesthetist to use curare (Intocostrin, E. R. Squibb and Sons) in Australia. Daly (assisted by Stuart Marshall) administered curare for an operation for a fractured mandible at St Vincent's

Hospital in Sydney. Daly was the third President of ASA (1946-1947). He was involved in developing the curriculum and conducting examinations for the Diploma of Anaesthesia at the University of Sydney. In the 1950s, Daly was one of the founders of the Faculty of Anaesthetists within the Royal Australasian College of Surgeons. He was elected as the first Vice Dean in the new faculty in 1952, and served as the Acting Dean from 1954-1956.

Daly received honorary fellowships of the Faculty of Anaesthetists, U.K. (Hon FFARCS, 1962), the Faculty of Anaesthetists of the Royal Australasian College of Surgeons (Hon FFARACS, 1970), and the Royal Australasian College of Surgeons (Hon FRACS, 1973).

In 1966, Daly received the Companion of the Order of St Michael and St George (C.M.G.) for services to medicine and anaesthesia. In 1969, he was awarded the Orton Medal (q.v. page 158) of the Faculty of Anaesthetists of the Royal Australasian College of Surgeons for distinguished services to anaesthesia. Daly formed lasting friendships with colleagues in Australia and overseas. He was, as Gwen Wilson wrote, "perhaps the best known [of the founders of the Australian Society of Anaesthetists] and exerted the greatest influence once anaesthetics became a specialty."

The Harry Daly Museum

The Harry Daly Museum at the Australian Society of Anaesthetists was not the original museum of the Society. In 1937, Geoffrey Kaye (1903-1986), secretary of the Australian Society of Anaesthetists, was tasked with setting up an anaesthesia library and museum for the Society. Dr I. C. James of Melbourne was appointed as librarian and curator in 1939. The museum and library were housed at several locations in Melbourne before being moved in the 1990s to "Ulimaroa", a Victorian mansion acquired as the headquarters of the newly founded Australian and New Zealand College of Anaesthetists. This museum is now known as the Geoffrey Kaye Museum of Anaesthetic History.

Apart from any personal interest in the history of anaesthesia, and collecting equipment for the Society's museum, which was then located in Melbourne, there was also a practical reason for Harry Daly to maintain a collection of anaesthesia equipment in Sydney—the equipment would have been used for instruction in anaesthetic techniques. Daly had a long-standing involvement in teaching anaesthesia, and in the 1940s he was a tutor and examiner for the Diploma of Anaesthesia at the University of Sydney (the diploma was instituted in 1944).

In the late 1950s Daly donated his collection of anaesthesia equipment to the New South Wales Branch of the ASA. The problem of accommodation of Harry Daly's collection was solved in 1961 when Commonwealth Industrial Gases offered to house the collection at its premises in Alexandria, Sydney. Two honorary curators were appointed: Tony Balthasar, representing the Australian Society of Anaesthetists, and Jim Loughman, representing the Faculty of Anaesthetists. In 1965, the collection was moved to the Department of Anaesthetics at the Royal Prince Alfred Hospital, where it was curated by Harry Lorang. Around this time, a commemorative bronze plaque was struck and the collection was named in honour of Harry Daly – see Figure 1.

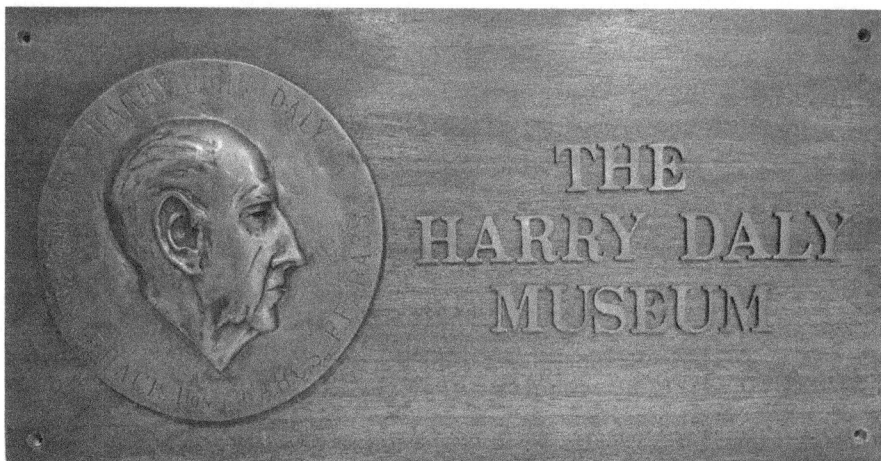

Figure 1. Bronze plaque at the entrance of the Harry Daly Museum.

In 1990 the collection was moved to the offices of the Australian Society of Anaesthetists at Edgecliff in Sydney, but there was little space to exhibit the collection. Dr Richard Bailey (q.v. page 9), honorary librarian of the Society, was appointed as honorary curator of the Harry Daly Museum in 1990. A part-time curator was employed in 1995 to assist with preparations for the 11th World Congress of Anaesthesiologists, held in Sydney in April 1996. In 2005, the Society purchased additional office space in the Edgecliff premises, which enabled an expansion of the area allocated to the museum and library. Custom-made cabinets with shelves and glass-topped drawers allowed for the display of most of 4,000 items in the museum collection – see Figure 2.

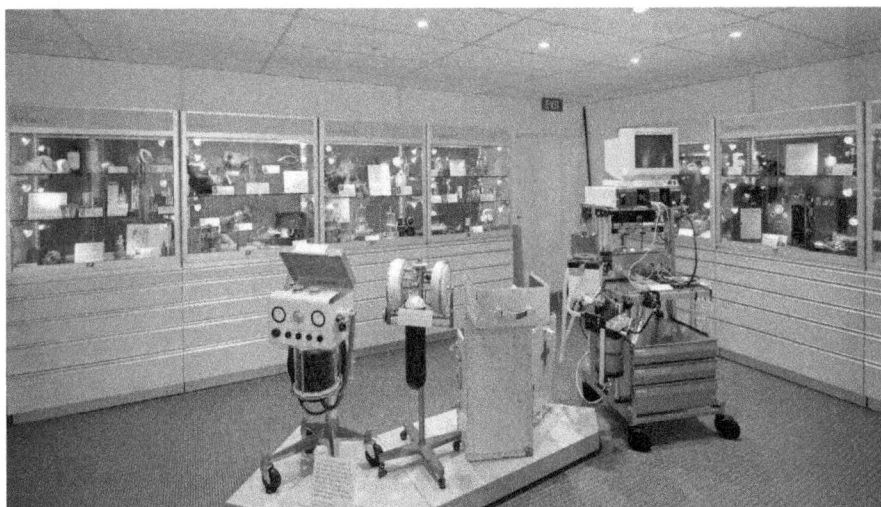

Figure 2. Interior of the Harry Daly Museum, c.2009 when it was located in Edgcliff, Sydney.

Highlights of the museum include anaesthesia equipment developed by Australians. In 1917, Hubert Ingham Clements, an engineer, collaborated with anaesthetist Dr Mark Lidwill to design an ether inhaler. Sydney anaesthetist Duncan Campbell designed a compact ventilator in the 1970s. Dr David Komesaroff (Melbourne) designed a resuscitator for use by the Mobile Intensive Care Ambulance Service in Victoria, and the Penthrox Inhaler (methoxyflurane) for analgesia in prehospital care by emergency medical personnel and in hospital emergency departments.

In 2013, the Australian Society of Anaesthetists moved its headquarters from Edgecliff, Sydney, to a multi-storey building in Walker Street, North Sydney. The Museum was relocated to 7th floor of the building, in a room adjacent to the Richard Bailey Library; the main office of the Society is located on the 8th floor. The floor space of the museum is approximately 30m^2. By early in 2021 the next move of the museum should be completed: to the new headquarters of the Society (86 Chandos Street, Naremburn, NSW, 2065).

Table 1. Honorary Curators of the Harry Daly Museum

Name of Honorary Curator	Period of curatorship
Richard J. Bailey	1990-2001
Jeanette Thirwell Jones	2001-2017
Rajesh P. Haridas	2017-2020
Michael G. Cooper	2020-

Further reading

Wilson G. Obituary: Harry J. Daly. *Anaesthesia and Intensive Care* 1981; **9**(2): 109-112.

Wilson G. *Fifty Years: The Australian Society of Anaesthetists 1934-1984*. Edgecliff, NSW: Australian Society of Anaesthetists, 1987, p. 52-53.

Wilson G (Edited by Jones JT). *One Grand Chain: The History of Anaesthesia in Australia, 1846-1962. Volume 1 (1846-1934)*. Melbourne: The Australian and New Zealand College of Anaesthetists, 1995, p. 597-598.

Daly HJ, Marshall SV. Curare in anaesthesia: a preliminary note. *Medical Journal of Australia* 1946; **2**(1): 14-16.

Stanbury P. Storage, display and access – innovations at the Harry Daly Museum and the Richard Bailey Library of the Australian Society of Anaesthetists, Sydney. *Anaesthesia and Intensive Care* 2010; **38 (Suppl 1)**: 20-24.

Webpage: https://asa.org.au/harry-daly-museum/

DAVIS TONSILLECTOMY GAG AND ITS MODIFICATIONS

Samuel Griffith Davis (1869-1943)

Samuel Griffith Davis, known to his colleagues as "Griff", was born in Hartford County, Maryland, USA in 1868. Griffith Davis was educated in private schools and at the Virginia Military Institute. He graduated MD from the University of Maryland, Baltimore in 1893 and became the first full-time anaesthetist in the state of Maryland and one of the first in the United States. He worked primarily at the Church Home and Infirmary, but also at the University of Maryland Hospital, Mercy Hospital, South Baltimore General Hospital, Union Memorial Hospital, Bon Secour Hospital, and the Hospital for Women in Maryland. He was described as "special anaesthetist" for Cushing at Johns Hopkins Hospital from 1904 until 1912 when Cushing became Harvard University's Moseley Professor of Surgery at the Peter Bent Brigham Hospital in Boston.

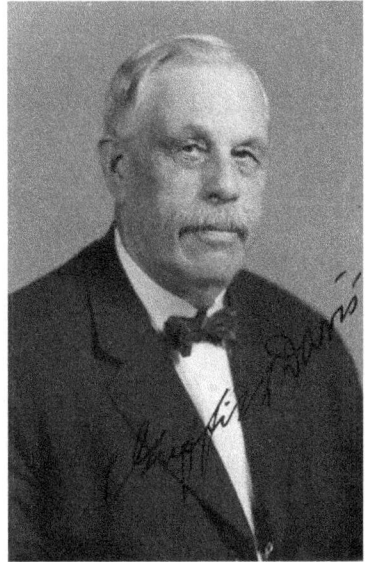

S. Griffith Davis. Image courtesy of the Wood Library-Museum of Anesthesiology.

Samuel J. Crowe (1883-1955), who graduated MD from Johns Hopkins University in 1908, was assistant surgeon to Cushing. He suggested the use of a combined mouth gag and tongue depressor, designed by Edward Sewall (1875-1957) of San Francisco for tonsillectomy. Sewall described how it pulled the base of the tongue away from the pharyngeal wall, fixed it, and allowed 'free breathing space for the patient'. In 1909-10 Crowe modified Sewall's O-shaped gag to a C-shape. Working with him, Davis added an anaesthetic delivery tube to the tongue blade: this permitted pharyngeal insufflation of ether vapour without interference in the operative field. Davis made no mention of the gag in any of his publications, but Cushing, in his book *The pituitary body and its disorders* (1910), described Davis's contribution:

"Owing to an ingenious device introduced by Dr. S.G. Davis, who has etherized nearly all of these patients [undergoing transsphenoidal hypophysectomy], it has become possible to quietly and safely anaesthetize even the individuals with an extreme lingual hypertrophy. Through a hollow metal tube, soldered to the blade which depresses and holds forward the tongue of the excellent "combined mouth-gag and adjustable tongue depressor" devised by E.C. Sewall of San Francisco, warm ether vapour is conducted directly to the opened glottis. As the pharynx is freely exposed by the apparatus, any collection of mucus can be sponged away during the course of the operation, and the anaesthetist is well away from the field. There have been no complications attributable to the etherisation in any of our thirty-two transsphenoidal operations."

Cushing moved to Boston in 1912 but Davis spent his entire career in Baltimore. Davis was appointed chief of the newly-created department of anaesthesia at the University of Maryland Hospital in 1913, and became a full professor in the department of anaesthesia at the University of Maryland in 1920. His reputation at the Church Home and Infirmary for "always inventing things" is confirmed by Gwathmey's 1914 textbook that illustrates Davis's eponymous equipment: an accurate ether dropper for insertion into an ether container; a handheld inhaler for ethyl chloride; another handheld apparatus for nitrous oxide-ether or nitrous oxide-ethyl chloride; a freestanding frame on wheels (that looks like a forerunner of later anaesthetic machines) for nitrous oxide and oxygen cylinders; a portable apparatus case that carried one oxygen and two nitrous oxide cylinders and his warm ether apparatus.

In 1921 H. Edmund G. Boyle was the official representative of the Section of Anaesthetics of the Royal Society of Medicine at the first annual meeting of the Canadian Society of Anaesthetists (held jointly with the Interstate Association of Anesthetists and the New York Society of Anesthetists in Niagara, Ontario) and at the American Society of Anesthetists' meeting in

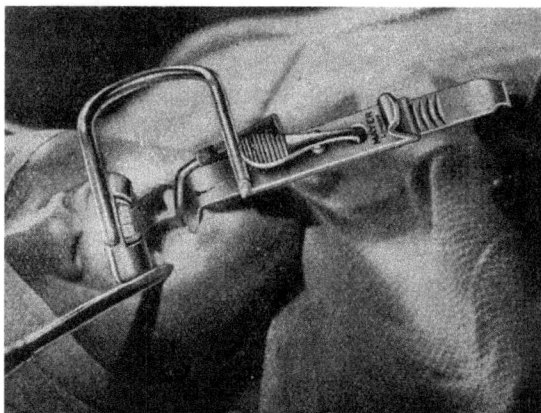

Boston, Massachusetts. While he was in Boston, he saw the gag in use for a tonsillectomy at Massachusetts General Hospital. He took one back to England and had the apparatus made for him by Mesrs. Mayer and Phelps of London with some slight modifications (Figure 1).

Figure 1. Davis combined gag and tongue depressor, introduced into England by Dr H.E.G. Boyle. From Mayer & Phelps Ltd. Catalogue, 1939.

In *The Lancet* of 25 November 1922, Boyle described how the combination of a tongue blade and gag in one instrument gave a better exposure of the tonsils than he had ever seen before, while the anaesthetic tube on the left side of the tongue blade delivered ether vapour directly to the pharynx. He referred to it as "a copy of one designed by Dr. Davis" but did not mention whether Davis was a surgeon or anaesthetist, where he practised or when he invented the gag.

It was Boyle who popularized the use of the Davis gag for tonsillectomy. Its use became almost universal in the UK within ten years of its introduction – becoming known as the Boyle-Davis gag. Boyle is more widely remembered from the eponym "Boyle machine", which is described in the first volume of *Notable Names in Anaesthesia* (2002).

In later years, after endotracheal anaesthesia became routine, the Boyle-Davis gag was further modified by Andrew Doughty (q.v. page 51), who introduced a central groove or split in the blade for an endotracheal tube. Recently it has been reported that manipulation of such a Boyle-Davis gag may displace the tracheal tube.

Further reading

Maltby JR. S Griffith Davis, inventor of the Boyle-Davis mouth gag? In: Drury PME, Armitage EN, Bacon DR et al (Eds.) *The History of Anaesthesia – Proceedings of the 6th International Symposium on the History of Anaesthesia*. Reading: Conservatree, 2007; 515-21.

Maltby JR, Robins J. Origins and modifications of the Davis mouth gag. In: Drury PME, Armitage EN, Bacon DR *et al* (Eds.) *The History of Anaesthesia – Proceedings of the 6th International Symposium on the History of Anaesthesia*. Reading: Conservatree, 2007; 523-30.

Fennessy BG, O'Connor R, Cronin M *et al*. Safety implications of the Boyle-Davis mouth gag and tracheal tube position in tonsillectomy. *British Journal of Anaesthesia* 2010; **105**: 863-6.

HUMPHRY DAVY AWARD

Humphry Davy (1778-1829)

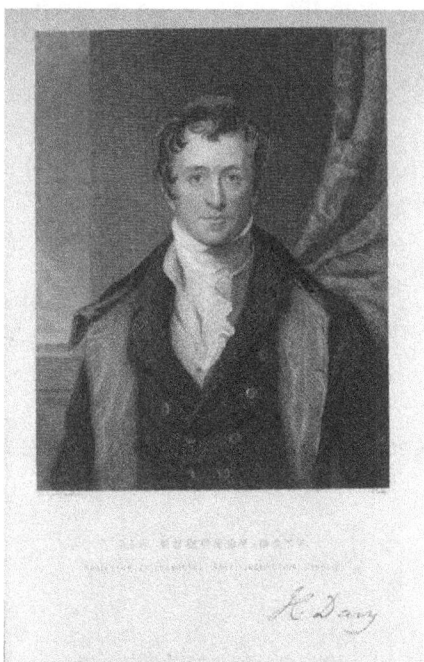

Image reproduced courtesy of the Royal Society of Chemistry Library.

From humble beginnings Humphry Davy became one of the foremost chemists of his day. In 1800 he discovered the analgesic effect of inhaling nitrous oxide and suggested that this might be used to relieve the pain of surgical operations – thus planting the seeds of modern anaesthesia.

Davy was born in 1778 in Penzance, Cornwall, England where he was educated and became especially interested in poetry. Soon after his father died, he left school aged just 16 to be apprenticed to a surgeon-apothecary in Penzance. During three years in this position from 1795-98 he read much including Lavoisier's *Traite Elementaire* and he became enthused in chemistry, conducting his own experiments on gases, heat and light.

Davy was further stimulated by Gregory Watt (son of James Watt, the pioneer of steam power), who had come to take the country air of Penzance in 1798 and boarded at the Davy household. Watt introduced Davy to Thomas Beddoes, an intellectual physician and chemist, who was planning to set up a Pneumatic Medical Institution in Bristol where there was a hot spa – for the use of 'factitious airs' to treat disease. Davy duly accepted Beddoes' invitation to be the Superintendent and went to Bristol in October 1798, although the laboratory did not open until March 1799. There apparatus for manufacturing various gases had already been prepared by James Watt in collaboration with Beddoes. Davy used Berthollet's method to manufacture nitrous oxide from ammonium nitrate, perfecting the technique. He tested the effects of this and other gases on fish, animals and humans (himself and friends).

In 1800 Davy published his results in a 580-page volume: *Researches, Chemical and Philosophical; Chiefly Concerning Nitrous Oxide or Dephlogistigated Nitrous Air and Its Respiration*. Within this work he noted the analgesic properties of nitrous oxide for headache and toothache. Notably, he wrote (page 556): "As nitrous oxide in its extensive operation appears capable of destroying physical pain, it may probably be used with advantage during surgical operations in which no great effusion of blood takes place." However, he never pursued this idea! Instead, having become acquainted with the Lakeland poets and some notable scientists who visited the Institute, he was preoccupied with them in the recreational use of nitrous oxide ('laughing gas'). However, from this time his brilliant lectures became famous.

In 1801 Davy left Bristol to become Assistant Lecturer in Chemistry, Director of the Laboratory and Assistant Editor at the Royal Institution in London. The following year at the age of twenty-three, he was elected to Professor of Chemistry. In 1807 he used electrolysis to discover the element potassium. The following year he isolated more elements: sodium, barium, strontium, calcium and magnesium.

Davy received a knighthood in 1812. But his most remembered claim to fame was still to come. Following the 1812 coal mining disaster in the north of England, he was invited to help. He then investigated how the mixture of methane and air (firedamp) explodes, and he invented the miner's safety lamp in 1815. Further honours were his election as President of the Royal Society in 1820 and re-election in 1826.

Just after being knighted in 1812, Davy married a rich widow, Jane Apreece, who had a haughty disposition. From 1813 they went on a two-year tour of continental Europe, where Davy met many of the famous scientists of the day. They were accompanied by Davy's assistant, Michael Faraday, who was treated by Lady Davy as a lowly servant. From this time Davy's status and wealth affected his character: he became jealous and tactless. In 1827 his health declined, and he went to the milder climate of Italy. There in 1829 he suffered a stroke and went to Switzerland to recuperate. He died in Geneva where he was buried.

In 1872 a statue of Davy holding the miner's safety lamp (Figure 1) was erected in Penzance. It stands in front of the Market Building (now Lloyds Bank) at the top of Market Jew Street, a main street of the town.

In 2002 the Royal College of Anaesthetists inaugurated the Humphry Davy Award, which is presented either as a medal to an individual or as a certificate to an organisation. The award is made in recognition of sustained contributions, usually in a specific activity or project, which is significant for the College. There is only one year (2007) in which this award was not presented, and in most years, there have been several recipients.

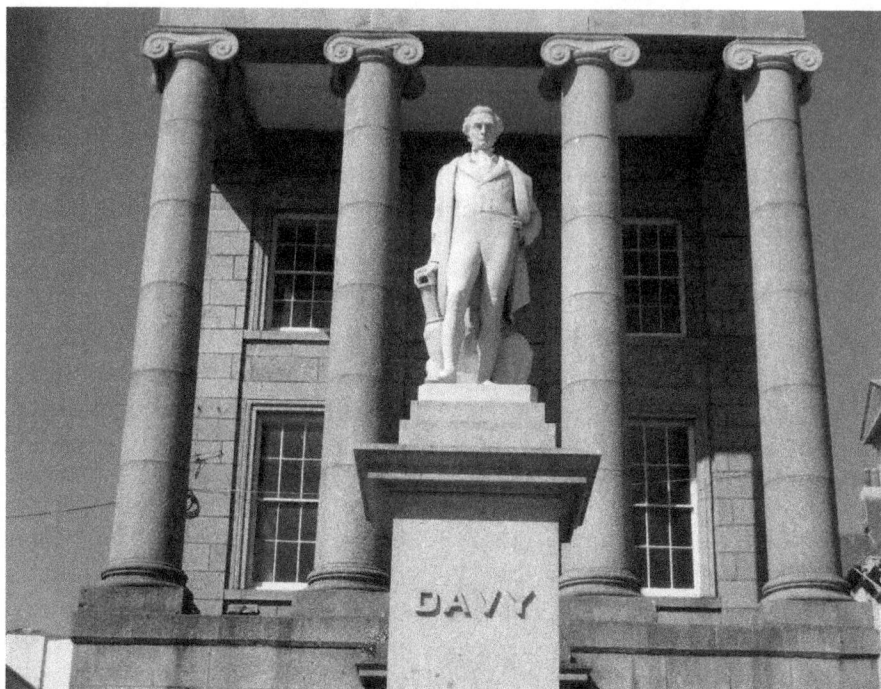

Figure 1. Statue of Humphry Davy in Penzance. Photograph by Dr John Pring.

A postage stamp of Davy, in a set of six famous names in medicine, was issued by Comoro Islands in 2008 – see Figure 2.

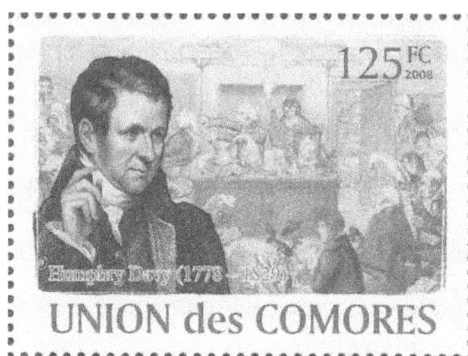

Figure 2. Humphry Davy on postage stamp of Comoro Islands. The background illustration is Gilray's cartoon of the pneumatic treatment of respiratory disease.

Table 1. Humphry Davy Award winners

Year	Recipient	Year	Recipient
2002	Helen Galley	2010	Anne Sutcliffe
2002	David Lambert	2011	Carolyn Evans
2002	Charlotte Williamson	2012	Susan Hill
2003	Abbott Laboratories	2012	Bernard Riley
2003	Datex-Ohmeda	2012	Gary Smith
2003	Clive Bray	2013	Carol Peden
2003	Leslie Shutt	2013	Jerry Cashman
2003	Jim Watt	2013	Andrew Lim
2004	Kathy Rowan	2013	Lifebox Foundation
2004	Christine Thornton	2014	Kathryn Wark
2005	Frank Walters	2014	Roger Laishley
2005	Roger Eltringham	2014	Martin Leuwer
2005	Anne Seymour	2015	Martin Kuper
2005	Janusz Liban	2015	Michael Swart
2006	Premachandran Jeyaratnam	2015	Kerri Jones
2006	Ian Smith	2015	Anil Patel
2006	Lucy White	2015	Michael Blayney
2006	Douglas Wilkinson	2015	Alexander Goodwin
2006	Ronnie Glavin	2016	Peter Brodrick
2006	Jaideep Pandit	2016	NAP5 Steering Group
2006	Christopher Rowlands	2017	GASAgain Team
2008	Helen Wise	2018	Dave Murray
2008	Madeleine Wang	2018	George Teturswamy
2008	John Colvin	2018	Eddie Wilson
2008	Gary Strichartz	2018	Jo James
2008	Timothy Cook	2018	SafeguardingPlus Working Group
2009	Julie Moore	2018	Teresa Dorman
2009	e-Learning for Health Team	2019	Fatigue Group Leadership Team
2009	K Balakrishnan	2019	Alison Cooper
2009	Tri-service Anaesthetic Society		

Further reading

Paris JA. *The Life of Sir Humphry Davy*. London: H Colburn & R Bentley, 1831

Smith WDA. A history of nitrous oxide and oxygen anaesthesia. Part i: Joseph Priestley to Humphry Davy. *British Journal of Anaesthesia* 1965; **37**: 790-8.

Knight D. *Humphry Davy: Science and Power*. Cambridge: Cambridge University Press, 1996.

DOPPLER MONITORING

Christian Andreas Doppler (1803-1853)

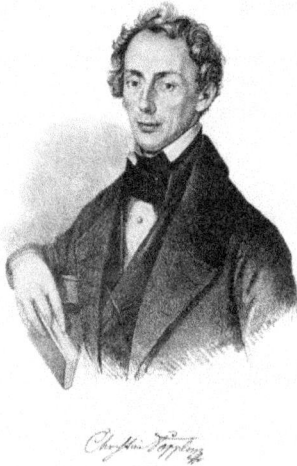

Since the 1990s flow Doppler echo-cardiography has been increasingly adopted in anaesthesia and intensive care. By means of an oesophageal probe, transoesophageal ultrasound waves reflected from flowing erythrocytes in the aorta are captured by a transducer and the frequency shift is compared with the transducer frequency. This shift is proportional to the velocity of blood flow, so that stroke volume can be calculated from the average blood velocity during a systolic cycle, the ejection time and the cross-sectional area of the aorta. Cardiac output is then obtained from the stroke volume multiplied by the heart rate.

Christian Doppler. Credit: University of Cambridge, Institute of Astronomy Library. Reproduced under Creative Commons Attribution (CC BY 4.0).

The probe of the oesophageal Doppler monitoring (ODM) device, e.g. CardioQ (Figure 1), is a 55 cm long steel spring at the distal end of which is a piezo-electric crystal emitting continuous wave Doppler ultrasound at 4 MHz. It is encased in silicone rubber and has three depth markers: 35, 40 and 45 cm from the distal end to guide insertion (the average distance from the lips in an adult being 35-40 cm). At the proximal end of the probe is a connector containing a memory device (choice of three enabling 6, 12 or 240 hours of monitoring); this is connected to the monitor which has a screen displaying both aortic waveform and digital measurements. The CardioQ incorporates a nomogram derived from the patient's age, height and weight, which are entered in the monitor at the start and stored in the memory of the probe.

In cardiac surgery intraoperative transoesophageal flow Doppler echo-cardiography is used to measure flow through the heart valves and can give a quick guide to right ventricle and left ventricle performance, including response to changes in pre- and afterload. Two Doppler techniques used are:
- continuous wave (CW) Doppler;
- pulsed waved (PW) Doppler.

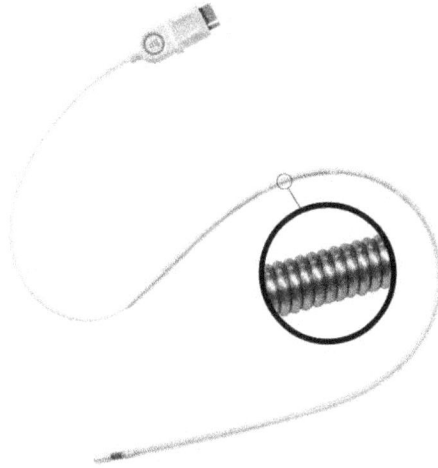

Figure 1. CardioQ probe for ODM. Image courtesy of Deltex Medical Ltd.

In abdominal surgery, oesophageal Doppler monitoring (ODM) has been used to optimise stroke volume (SV), a commonly used target being a cardiac index of greater than 4.5 litres min^{-1} for best oxygen delivery. An algorithm known as goal-directed fluid therapy (GDFT) has been claimed to improve outcome and reduce hospital stay. This involves measuring SV and if decreased by 10%, giving a fluid challenge of 200-250 mls of colloid over 5 min, then re-measuring SV aiming for a rise of >10%. A significant evidence base of randomized controlled trials (RCTs) showing outcome benefit has accumulated, but not all studies have confirmed it to be advantageous.

Christian Andreas Doppler was born in Salzburg, where he went to school. He next studied physics and mathematics at the Austrian Imperial-Royal Polytechnic Institute and in 1829 was appointed as an assistant there. He moved in 1835 to Prague where he was appointed Supplementary Professor of Higher Mathematics and Practical Geometry at the Technical Institute in 1837. This job had an extremely heavy workload with a detrimental effect on his health – perhaps the start of the disease to which he eventually succumbed. Then in 1841 he was appointed full Professor of Elementary Mathematics and Practical Geometry at the Prague Polytechnic Institute.

Doppler published a remarkable monograph in 1842: *Uebas das farbige Licht der Doppelsterne und einiger anderer Gesterne des Himmels* (English translation: On the Coloured Light of Double Stars and Certain Other Stars of the Heavens). Therein he postulated that the observed frequency of a wave depends on the relative speed of the source and the observer. By 1845 he predicted the apparent change in the frequency of sound due to relative motion between the source and the observer – this became known as the 'Doppler effect'. The French physicist, A.H.L. Fizeau, developed the mathematics of this principle with regard to light and predicted the red and blue shifts of light waves from stars.

By 1847 Doppler had published over 50 notable papers on physics, mathematics and astronomy, but he then moved again to become Professor of mathematics, physics and mechanics at the Academy of Mines and Forests in Selmebánya, Hungary (now Banska Štiavnica, Slovakia). Unfortunately, due to the Hungarian Revolution the following year, he had to flee to Vienna. In 1850 he was appointed Head of the Institute of Experimental Physics at the University of Vienna. There he had an influence on the career of a notable student, Gregor Mendel, who went on to become the father of the science of genetics. Doppler died while in Venice in 1853, seemingly from pulmonary tuberculosis.

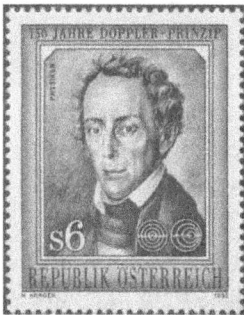

In 1896 confusion about Doppler's full name was introduced by the astronomer Julius Scheiner, who incorrectly dubbed him "Johann Christian Doppler". This mistake was copied by many and remains in many current publications! Austria issued a postage stamp of Doppler in 1992 to commemorate the 150th anniversary of the publication of his famous principle (Figure 2).

Figure 2. Christian Doppler on Austria postage stamp.

Further reading

Townend JN, Hutton P. Transoesophageal echocardiography in anaesthesia and intensive care. *British Journal of Anaesthesia* 1996; **77**: 137-9.

Singer M. Oesophageal Doppler. *Current Opinion in Critical Care* 2009; **15**: 244-48.

Challand C, Struthers R, Sneyd JR et al. Randomized controlled trial of intraoperative goal-directed fluid therapy in aerobically fit and unfit patients having major colorectal surgery. *British Journal of Anaesthesia* 2012; **108**: 53-62.

Schirmer U, Koster A. Anaesthesia for cardiac surgery. In: Hardman JG, Hopkins PM, Struys MMRF (Eds.) *Oxford Textbook of Anaesthesia*. Oxford: Oxford University Press, 2017; 939-41.

Eden A. *The Search for Christian Doppler*. Wien: Springer-Verlag, 1992.

DOUGHTY EPIDURAL TECHNIQUE

Andrew Gerard Doughty (1916-2013)

Andrew Doughty was born in Lincoln, England in 1916. After schooling at Beaumont College, Windsor, he gained entry to the University of London to read medicine. He trained at St Thomas's Hospital and qualified in 1941 during the blitz. Then he proceeded to house jobs, followed by a post of Resident Obstetrics Officer in Woking, at the evacuated St Thomas's maternity unit. Next, he joined the Royal Army Medical Corps for the Second World War effort, volunteered to do anaesthetics and was sent to train at the British General Hospital in Calcutta. In addition to patients, he anaesthetized mice for typhus research.

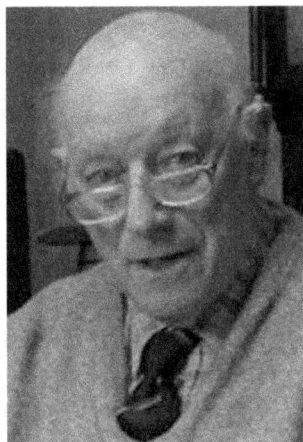

Andrew Doughty. Image courtesy of the Obstetric Anaesthetists' Association.

After the War he returned to St Thomas's Hospital as a registrar in anaesthetics and passed the Diploma in Anaesthetics (DA). In 1950 he was appointed Consultant Anaesthetist at Kingston-upon-Thames Hospital. For the operation of tonsillectomy, he introduced in 1957 a modification of the tongue-plate of the Boyle-Davis gag (q.v. page 41-43), to facilitate orotracheal intubation before placement of the gag – without the endotracheal tube (ETT) encroaching on the field of operation. A slot was cut in the distal three-quarters of the tongue-depressor and the lingual surface bevelled to accommodate the ETT, which was prevented from becoming wedged in the slot by a metal bridge at the distal end. A range of tongue-plates for use in children and adults was produced by Down Bros and by Mayer & Phelps Ltd.

Doughty set up an Intensive Care Unit at Kingston Hospital in 1966. For this he designed an intensive care record card based on the 'Nosworthy' system to enable reference and statistical analysis.

By 1968 in the UK just a few isolated enthusiasts were offering epidural analgesia in obstetrics. That year the 4th World Congress of Anaesthesiologists was held in London – obstetric epidurals were reported in the press, and on radio and television, generating much public interest. This was a catalyst for change and in the following year the Obstetric Anaesthetists' Association (OAA) was constituted, Doughty being a founder member. British obstetric opinion at this time was that epidural analgesia was associated with a high forceps delivery rate. Doughty challenged this in a report he published in the December 1969 issue of the *British Journal Anaesthesia*, being the records of over 800 deliveries he attended over the previous ten years. He claimed that while the use of selective epidural analgesia had increased, the frequency of forceps delivery had decreased. In 1971 under the auspices of the OAA, Doughty hosted a symposium on epidural analgesia in obstetrics at Kingston Hospital, which was attended by 160 anaesthetists and obstetricians from all centres of the UK.

In 1973 Doughty set up his famous epidural course at Kingston Hospital. There was just one place on the course at any one time, the trainee spending two weeks resident under close personal tuition and supervision. Some of those who attended went on to have illustrious careers in obstetric anaesthesia, for example Felicity Reynolds. The 'Doughty technique' he taught for inserting an epidural needle aimed to prevent puncture of the dura, which of course could lead to headache. As shown in Figure 1, the left (or non-dominant) hand was braced firmly against the patient's back with the fingers clasping the hub of the Tuohy needle, acting as a brake against uncontrolled advancement due to sudden loss of resistance. The fingers of the right (or dominant hand) gripped the barrel of the syringe to apply some forward movement, while maintaining greater pressure on the plunger with the metacarpal head of the right index finger (palm of the hand). Those who learned the technique from Doughty went on to teach it to others. It must be remembered that Doughty taught his technique before the days of commercially prepacked disposable epidural kits.

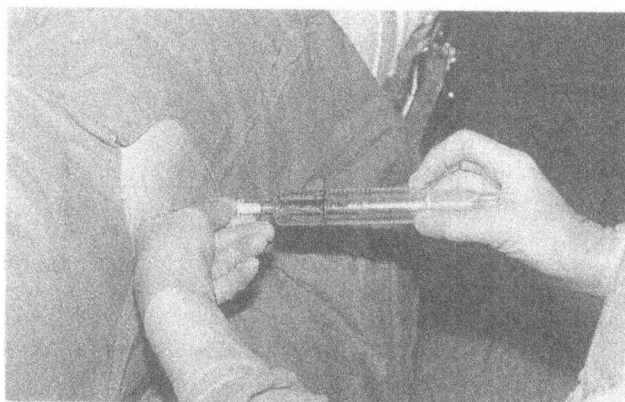

Figure 1. Doughty technique. Image reproduced with permission from Russell R. et al *Pain Relief in Labour*. London: BMJ Publishing Group, 1997.

Doughty was President of the OAA for 1979-81, although he retired from clinical practice in 1980, in which year he was elected Fellow of the Royal College of Obstetricians and Gynaecologists *ad eundem*. He was awarded the Gold Medal of the OAA in 1982. In retirement he indulged in his passion for music, taking singing lessons and performing, especially Gilbert and Sullivan. He competed as a soloist and also performed duets with Hugh F. Seeley, a retired consultant anaesthetist from St George's Hospital, London. In 1993 he was elected an Honorary Member of the Association of Anaesthetists of Great Britain and Ireland.

Further reading

Doughty A. A modification of the tongue-plate of the Boyle-Davis gag. *The Lancet* 1957; **269**: 1074.

Doughty AG. An intensive care record card. *Anaesthesia* 1969; **24**: 262-3.

Doughty A (Ed.) *Proceedings of the Symposium on Epidural Analgesia in Obstetrics.* London: BDH Pharmaceuticals Ltd., 1972.

Obituary: Andrew Doughty. *British Medical Journal* 2013; **347**: f5066.

DRÄGER ANAESTHETIC EQUIPMENT

The Dräger Family from 1902

Practising anaesthetists in many parts of the world encounter and use vaporizers, anaesthetic machines and ventilators made by the Dräger Company. This company is unique in that it has remained under the leadership of five generations of the same family since 1889.

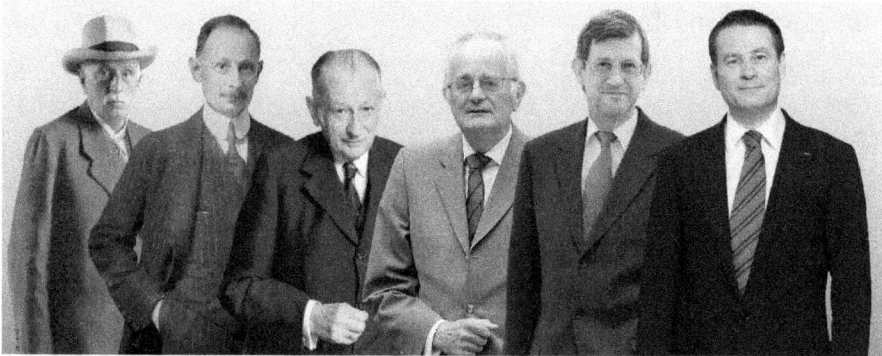

L to R: J Heinrich Dräger, A. Bernhard Dräger, Heinrich Dräger, Christian Dräger, Theo Dräger, Stefan Dräger. Image courtesy of Drägerwerk AG & Co., Lübeck.

J. Heinrich Dräger (1847-1917)

Johann Heinrich Dräger was born the son of a watchmaker in the Kirchwerder district of Hamburg, Germany and he became a talented mechanic. In 1889, with Carl Adolf Gerling, he founded the Dräger und Gerling Company in Lübeck. Within months he and his son Bernhard invented a carbon dioxide (CO_2) pressure reducing valve for use in the brewery. This 'Lubeca valve' was successful and Heinrich Dräger immediately patented it. In 1891 he became the sole owner of the company, which prospered in the production of a mechanism for automatic pressure control of CO_2 in beer pumps.

Alexander Bernhard Dräger (1870-1928)

A. Bernhard Dräger was born in Kirchwerder and after schooling at the Katharineum in Lübeck he did an apprenticeship with the Lübeck-Buechen Railway Company, qualifying as a mechanic. He joined his father's business in 1889 as a design engineer. Voluntarily he studied higher grades in science at his former school and in 1893 he attended the Technical University in Berlin, proceeding to qualify as a Dr of Engineering honoris causa. He became a partner in the Dräger firm in 1896 and he proved his worth by producing the

Finimeter, a high pressure manometer to view the fill level in oxygen cylinders, and more importantly, a reducing valve for oxygen in 1899. With his father, he developed an oxygen-driven injector, which enabled a welding torch. They then incorporated this to generate suction for drip-feed of liquid anaesthetic, working with the surgeon Dr Otto Roth, on a prototype anaesthetic apparatus.

After clinical trials at Dr Roth's hospital in Lübeck, the apparatus was demonstrated at the German Congress of Surgeons in Berlin in 1902. The Roth-Dräger mixed anaesthetic apparatus went into production the next year: see Figure 1. It was shown in 1904 as an oxygen-chloroform apparatus at the universal exposition in St Louis, USA and was awarded a diploma and silver medal. The machine went on to have successive improvements and was sold throughout the world.

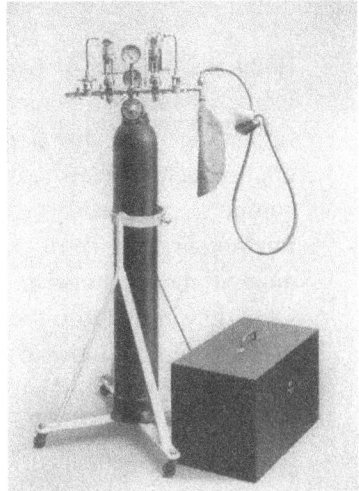

Figure 1. Roth-Dräger mixed anaesthesia apparatus 1903. Image courtesy of Drägerwerk AG & Co., Lübeck.

In 1904 Bernhard Dräger improved breathing apparatus for mine rescue and this was used in the Courrières mining disaster (France) of 1906. Heinrich Dräger in 1907 went on a business trip to Great Britain and a visit to Welsh coal mines prompted him to think of a device to pump oxygen into the lungs; this was reinforced when he witnessed the resuscitation of a man rescued from drowning in the Thames river near Tower Bridge in London. He

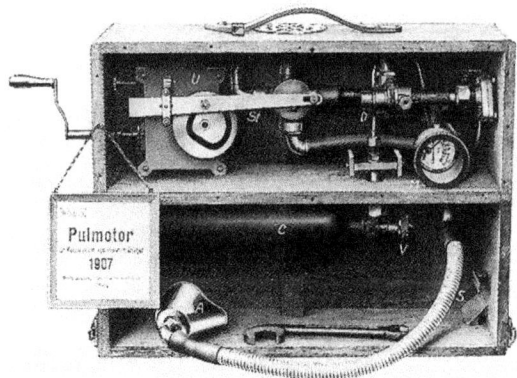

Figure 2. Dräger Pulmotor 1907. Image courtesy of Drägerwerk AG & Co., Lübeck.

designed a prototype and on his return to Lübeck, Drägerwerk built a ventilator incorporating a clockwork motor and two venturis driven by compressed oxygen – 'the Pulmotor' – see Figure 2. This was improved by 1910 and the apparatus was adopted by Fire and Police Departments for rescue operations in many countries worldwide.

In cooperation with the gynaecologist Carl J. Gauss and the chemist H. Wieland in 1924, Bernhard Dräger produced an anaesthetic circle system with a CO_2 absorber. This was used with purified acetylene (narcylene) as the inhalation anaesthetic. Bernhard Dräger was granted a patent for an anaesthetic circle system in 1927.

Heinrich Dräger (1898-1986)

Heinrich, the son of Bernhard Dräger, obtained a doctorate in agricultural economics before joining the Dräger Company in 1927. On the death of his father in 1928, he became head of the company. Improved breathing apparatus for miners was produced in 1933. During the Second World War the company produced respiratory protective devices and oxygen systems for military aircraft. Through the 1950s it was able to return to advancements in anaesthetic machines and it devised central gas supply systems in hospitals. In 1952 they introduced the Dräger Pulmomat, an automatic ventilator that could be attached to their closed-circuit anaesthetic apparatuses. From 1958 they produced the 'Vapor' vaporizer, which utilized wicks for level compensation, a large mass of copper as a heat sink and a thermometer to indicate the temperature – see Figure 3.

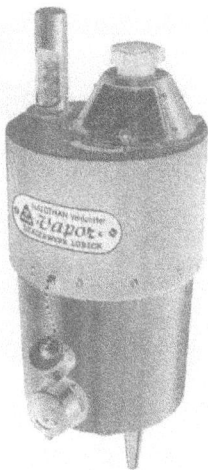

Figure 3. Dräger halothane vaporizer 1958. Image courtesy of Drägerwerk AG & Co., Lübeck.

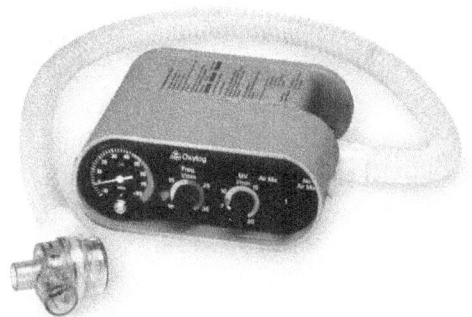

Figure 4. Oxylog emergency ventilator. Image courtesy of Drägerwerk AG & Co., Lübeck.

In the 1960s the company further improved breathing apparatus for mine rescue and firefighters. Their anaesthetic machines at this time were given the names of Roman Emperors. A notable product in the 1970s was the Oxylog emergency ventilator (Figure 4). In 1979 the company went public: Drägerwerk AG. Its first electronic ventilator EV-A was produced in 1982.

Christian Dräger (1934-)

Christian, the son of Heinrich Dräger was born in Berlin; his father sent him to a precision mechanics school in Bavaria, where he spent three years. Then he attended a local high school and proceeded to obtain a doctorate in business administration. He joined the Dräger Company in 1961 and took over the running in 1984.

Under his watch Drägerwerk AG produced the Evita intensive care ventilator in 1985, the Cicero anaesthesia workstation in 1988 and the Julian anaesthesia workstation in 1996. Christian Dräger moved to the Supervisory Board of the company in 1997. He enjoyed his retirement years by indulging his passion for art, collecting drawings of the nineteenth century and pictures of the Goethe and Romantic periods. He has shared these through public exhibitions and donations.

Theo Dräger (1938-)

Christian Dräger's younger brother, Theo took over the management of the company in 1997. Under his leadership the Zeus anaesthesia workstation was produced in 2002.

Stefan Dräger (1963-)

Stefan, the son of Christian Dräger, was born in Lübeck and after schooling he studied at the Baden-Wuerttemberg Cooperative State University, Stuttgart and graduated as an engineer. He joined the Dräger Company in 1992 and went on to develop the sale of gas monitoring systems in the US; in Lübeck he led the production of global gas monitoring systems and later the Critical Care products. He became manager (Chairman of the Executive Board) in 2005 and oversaw the marketing of the Dräger Primus anaesthesia workstation (Figure 5).

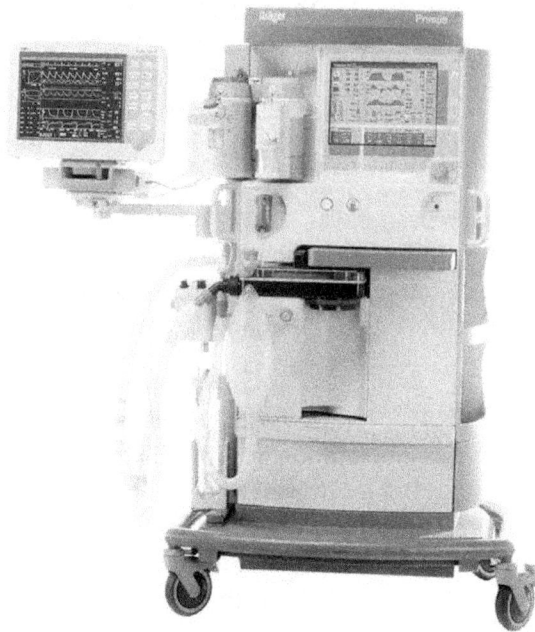

Figure 5. Dräger Primus anaesthesia workstation c.2005.
Image courtesy of Drägerwerk AG & Co., Lübeck.

Further reading

Drägerwerk AG & Co. KGaA. Dräger Technology for Life since 1889. Lübeck, 2014.

Thompson PW. The house of Dräger. In: Atkinson RS, Boulton TB (Eds.) *The History of Anaesthesia*. International Congress and Symposium Series No. 134. London: RSM Services Ltd., 1989; 298-300.

Peters A, Strätling M, Welling I, Dräger C, Schmucker P. Dr Bernhard Draeger (1870-1928): an underestimated pioneer. In: Drury PME, Armitage EN, Bacon DR et al (Eds.) *The History of Anaesthesia – Proceedings of the 6th International Symposium on the History of Anaesthesia*. Reading: Conservatree, 2007;265-70.

Baum JA. Who Introduced the Rebreathing Systems into Clinical Practice? In: Schulte am Esch J, Goerig M (Eds.) *The History of Anaesthesia – Proceedings of the 4th International Symposium on the History of Anaesthesia*. Lübeck: Dräger, 1998; 441-50.

DRUMMOND-JACKSON LIBEL CASE

Stanley Lithgow Drummond-Jackson (1909-1975)

The Drummond-Jackson libel case was a High Court Action brought by Stanley Drummond-Jackson, a London dentist, against the British Medical Association (BMA) as publishers and the authors of a report in the *British Medical Journal* (*BMJ*) on the technique of intermittent intravenous methohexitone which he promoted for sedation during conservative dentistry. Besides featuring in medical and dental journals, it was extensively publicised in the popular press from June to October 1972, dividing opinion for and against "operator-anaesthetist" dentists.

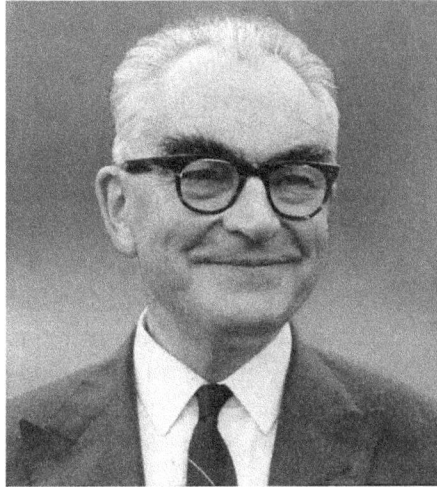

Stanley Drummond-Jackson. Image courtesy of SAAD.

Stanley L. Drummond-Jackson was born in Gosforth, Northumberland in 1909. He was educated at Barnard School and then the Dental School of the University of Edinburgh, graduating LDS in 1931. His initial practice was in Huddersfield, Yorkshire, where he became known as 'DJ'. By 1939 he established a practice in Harley Street, London, but this closed when he joined the British Army Dental Corps at the outbreak of war. Later he was seconded as an anaesthetist to a field ambulance unit of the 51st (Highland) Division.

After the Second World War, Drummond-Jackson built up a thriving dental practice at Wimpole Street in London. In 1952 he published a book on intravenous anaesthesia in dentistry. A fellow dentist Henry Mandiwall, who was also an accomplished Cinefilm maker, joined him in 1954 to produce a training film *Venepuncture in general practice.* The pair went on to produce a whole series of training films including (1957) *Intravenous anaesthesia in dentistry.* In 1957 Drummond-

Jackson founded the Society for the Advancement of Anaesthesia in Dentistry (SAAD). Initially the intravenous anaesthetic agents he used were hexobarbitone and propanidid. A review of deaths under anaesthesia in the dental surgery by Victor Goldman, Anaesthetist-in-charge at the Eastman Dental Hospital was published in 1958 – this warned against intravenous barbiturates, which was contrary to what SAAD was promoting.

In 1961 some dental surgeons in SAAD had their applications for Associate Fellowship of the Association of Anaesthetists of Great Britain & Ireland (AAGBI) rejected, which further strained relations between the two societies. By this time methohexitone had become available and Drummond-Jackson adopted it to develop a minimal incremental "ultra-light" technique. A SAAD guideline for this was available by 1966, which included that: the operator-anaesthetist should usually be assisted by two (at least one) well trained dental nurses; after a sleep dose of methohexitone, the patient be balanced by minimal increments (usually 25 mg); oxygen not required; on completion, patients could walk from the theatre with assistance after about ten minutes. Note that this technique was advocated *instead* of local anaesthesia, whereas the Jorgensen technique of intravenous sedation (developed in the USA) was intended as *an addition* to local blockade when required. Drummond-Jackson was a highly skilled dentist and he and his close colleagues insisted on a high standard of assistance; however, some dentists would attend weekend SAAD courses and return to their practices to implement the "ultra-light" technique without adequate training and staffing.

A Joint Subcommittee of the Central Health Services Council reported in 1967 on outpatient dental anaesthesia. A key recommendation of the Report was that "ideally" general dental anaesthetics should be administered by specialist (medical) anaesthetists. This was rejected by the British Dental Association.

Next in 1969 a group under John Robinson, Professor of Anaesthetics in Birmingham, published a study of 30 patients receiving minimal incremental methohexitone for dental work. They concluded that, contrary to the safety claims made by Drummond-Jackson, the technique caused clinically undetectable respiratory obstruction, depression of laryngeal reflexes, vasodilatation and arterial hypoxaemia. This paper was accompanied by an editorial in the *BMJ*, which stated that most doctors and nurses regarded the "operator-anaesthetist" technique as potentially dangerous. In response Drummond-Jackson sued the BMA and the authors of the paper for libel.

The case did not get to hearing in the High Court until June 1972. In the meantime, a Sheffield group under J.A. Thornton, Professor of Anaesthetics had published in January 1971 a study of 595 minimal incremental methohexitone administrations compared with local analgesia for conservative dentistry. The authors' findings did not support the claims of SAAD that the ultra-light methohexitone technique banished the dread of dentistry, was safer than local anaesthetic injections and produced better working conditions.

On the second day of the trial, the judge Mr Justice Ackner allowed the defendants to use the findings of Professor Thornton's team. The case dragged on until 31 October when both plaintiff and defendants agreed to discontinue and avoid many more months of evidence – all parties bearing their own costs. The gist of the agreed statements made in open Court were:

- the defendants recognised and acknowledged that Mr. S.L. Drummond-Jackson was a man of the highest integrity and skill and of outstanding ability as a dentist;
- the plaintiff withdrew any allegation against the defendants of dishonesty or impropriety; further he recognised and acknowledged that the BMJ had a right and duty to the medical profession to publish such articles.

Unfortunately, the libel case deepened the discord between the dentists of SAAD and practising anaesthetists, although clearly cooperation was the way forward. Thomas Boulton (q.v. page 18-21), the Editor of the AAGBI's journal *Anaesthesia*, became President of SAAD for 1980-82 and helped to draw the dentists and anaesthetists into harmony.

Drummond-Jackson was honoured with the Heidbrink Award (q.v. page 92) of the American Dental Association in 1968. He became President of SAAD in 1975, but sadly died in December the same year of a myocardial infarction.

Further reading

History of SAAD. http://www.saad.org.uk/history (accessed 1 November 2019).

Boulton TB. *The Association of Anaesthetists of Great Britain and Ireland 1932-1992 and the Development of the Specialty of Anaesthesia*. London: AAGBI, 1999; 238-51.

Drummond-Jackson SL. A dental-anaesthetic death. *The Lancet* 1966; I: 925.

Editorial. Intermittent Intravenous Methohexitone. *British Medical Journal* 1969; **2**: 525-6.

Wise CC, Robinson JS, Heath MJ, Tomlin PJ. Physiological Responses to Intermittent Methohexitone for Conservative Dentistry. *British Medical Journal* 1969; **2**: 540-3.

Mann PE, Hatt SD, Dixon RA, Griffin KD, Perks ER, Thornton JA. A minimal increment methohexitone technique in conservative dentistry. *Anaesthesia* 1971; 26: 3-21.

Legal Correspondent. Dentist's Libel Action Against B.M.A. *British Medical Journal* 1972; **2**: 774-5.

Legal Correspondent. End of Dentist's Libel Action. *British Medical Journal* 1972; **4**: 372-4.

Obituary. Stanley Lithgow Drummond-Jackson, TD, LDS. *British Dental Journal* 1976; **140**: 73-4.

ANGELA ENRIGHT LECTURE

Angela Clare Enright (1947 -)

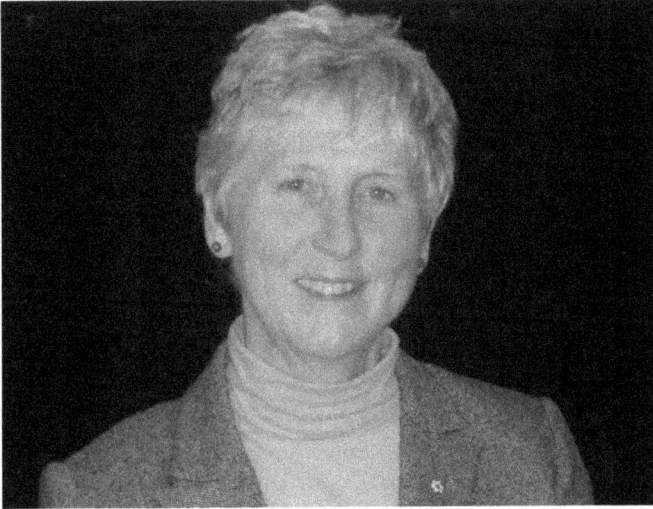

Angela Enright was born in Dublin, Ireland in 1947 and educated at Sancta Maria College, Rathfarnham, Dublin. She read medicine at University College, Dublin and graduated with MB, BCh and BAO (Honours) in 1970. After house jobs in Dublin, she moved to Canada in 1972 and worked in Ontario, doing general practice and emergency medicine and passing the Licentiate of the Medical Council of Canada in 1973. The following year she took up a resident in anaesthesia post at the Foothills Hospital, Calgary, Alberta.

After passing the FRCPC (Anesthesia) in 1977, Enright held a specialist post in Alberta through 1978 before becoming Assistant Professor of Anesthesia at the University of Saskatchewan. She was appointed Clinical Associate Professor there in 1985 and full Professor in 1995. She served as President of the Canadian Anesthesiologists' Society (CAS) for 1994-95, being the first woman to be elected to that Presidency.

In 1999 Enright moved to an anaesthesiologist post with Vancouver Island Health Authority in Victoria, British Columbia. Rising to become the Medical Director of Anaesthesia there, she was appointed Clinical Professor of Anaesthesia at the University of British Columbia in 2003. Three years later, she was appointed Professor in the Division of Medical Sciences at the University of Victoria.

In 2000 Angela Enright was President of the 12th World Congress of Anaesthesiology in Montreal. She then took over the chairmanship of the World Federation of Societies of Anaesthesiologists (WFSA) Education Committee.

Angela Enright chaired the board of the International Educational Foundation (IEF) of the CAS from 2004 to 2008. Rwanda was selected for aid: in the aftermath of the 1994 genocide there was only one anaesthesiologist left in the entire country. Through liaison of the IEF with the American Society of Anesthesiologists (ASA) and the National University of Rwanda, she started in 2007 a residency training program in anaesthesia for physicians in Rwanda. The IEF sent more than 100 volunteers to teach. By 2018 Rwanda had 18 fully-trained anaesthesiologists and 31 residents in training.

She was elected President of the WFSA in 2008 during the 14th World Congress of Anaesthesiologists in Cape Town, South Africa. By this time, continuing her interest in low resource areas, she was making a massive contribution to the global pulse oximetry project of the World Health Organisation (WHO) – part of their 'Safer Surgery Saves Lives' initiative. The project began with the WHO, WFSA and Harvard School of Public Health (HSPH) as partners: educational and training materials were developed. Before long, the WFSA accepted to take on the lead role, and further support came from the Association of Anaesthetists of Great Britain and Ireland (AAGBI). Pulse oximeters were carefully designed and produced to be affordable for areas with minimal resources and piloted in three countries, followed by launch in 2011 under the name Lifebox. Enright spent time introducing Lifebox and the Surgical Safety Checklist in several African countries.

Several honours have been bestowed on Angela Enright. In 2009 she was awarded the Gold Medal of the Irish College of Anaesthetists and in 2010 she received the Officer of the Order of Canada. Four further accolades came in 2012: the Queen's Diamond Jubilee Medal, the ASA's Nicholas Greene MD Award for Outstanding Humanitarian Contribution (q.v. page 86), the Honorary Membership of the AAGBI; and the CAS changed the name of its Annual Royal College Lecture to the 'Angela Enright Lecture' (Table 1). In 2014 she delivered the T.H. Seldon Memorial Lecture at the annual congress of the International Anesthesia Research Society (IARS) entitled "Improving Health through Discovery and Education".

Although she retired from clinical practice in 2015, Enright continued to be active in work to improve anaesthetic practice in low and middle-income countries. In that year she was appointed to the Editorial Board of *Anesthesia* and *Analgesia* for her expertise in global health, and in 2016 she became the Executive Section Editor, Global Health. She is an accomplished musician, playing piano, cello and harp.

Table 1. Angela Enright lecturers and lecture titles

Year	Lecturer	Title
2012	Angela Enright	Global Challenges in Anesthesia.
2013	*Cancelled*	
2014	Alan Merry	The road to patient safety.
2015	Joanne Douglas	General anesthesia, obstetrics and the brain: conundrums and challenges.
2016	Frances Chung	Sleep apnea, obesity hypoventilation syndrome, overlap syndrome: are we sleepwalking into disaster?
2017	Jason Frank	Is there a better way to build expert anesthesiologists? The myths and magic of the new Canadian system of training.
2018	Franco Carli	Enhanced recovery Canada: from soloed provider to team player.
2019	Patricia Houston	We all belong – advancing diversity, equality and inclusion in anesthesiology.

Further reading

Enright A, Wilson IH, Moyers JR. The World Federation of Societies of Anaesthesiologists: supporting education in the developing world. *Anaesthesia* 2007; **62** (Suppl. 1): 67-71.

Funk LM, Weiser TG, Berry WR, Lipsitz SR, Merry AF, Enright AC, *et al*. Global operating theatre distribution and pulse oximetry supply: an estimation from reported data. *The Lancet* 2010; **376** (9746): 1055-61.

Enright A. A friend in need: evaluating the impact of Lifebox in Burkino Faso. *Canadian Journal of Anaesthesia* 2019; **66**: 139-42.

ENTONOX

Michael Eric Tunstall (1928-2011)

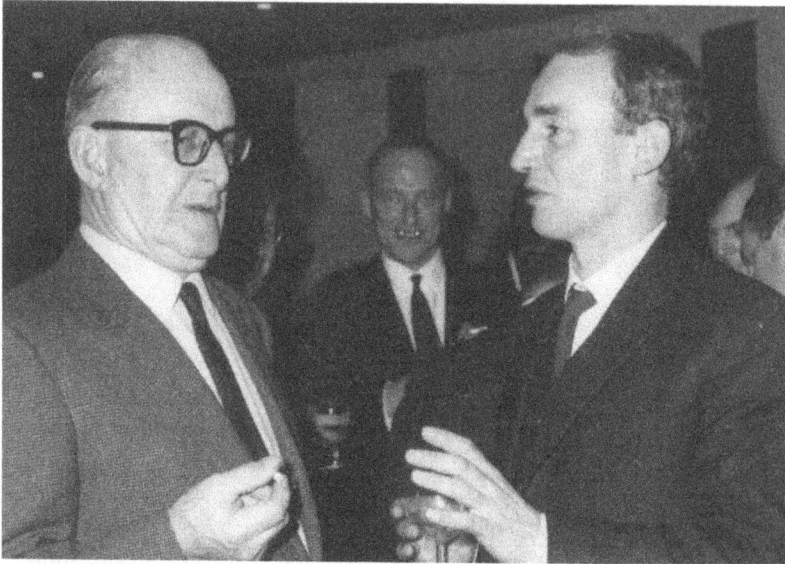

Michael Tunstall (R) with Sir Ivan Magill (L). Photograph from Dr Fiona Knox.

Entonox is known internationally as the name of a 50:50 gas mixture of nitrous oxide and oxygen in a single cylinder, used in maternity units to provide analgesia in labour. The invention of this stable mixture came from the anaesthetist Michael Tunstall, but this was just one of several important advances he made for the care of obstetric patients and newborn babies.

Michael Tunstall was born in Assam, India in 1928 and was brought by his parents to the UK when aged 8 years for schooling in Sheffield. Due to the travel restrictions of the Second World he was unable to see them again until aged 16. During that time, he won a scholarship to Monmouth School, next attended the Chelsea Polytechnic and finally entered Medical School at University College Hospital, London. He qualified in 1952 and did house jobs followed by two years of National Service as a Regimental Medical Officer in Germany. On return to England, he spent the year 1955 as a senior house officer at Leicester Royal Infirmary – achieving two diplomas: obstetrics and anaesthetics.

In 1956 he entered general practice in Ventnor, Isle of Wight, but soon realised that the National Health Service would not enable him to combine work in all his three areas of interest. He was impressed by Robert James ('Jim') Hamer Hodges, a Consultant Anaesthetist at the Portsmouth group of hospitals, who had sessions on the Isle of Wight and anesthetized one of his patients. So, a year later Tunstall began anaesthetic specialist training in Portsmouth, followed by London and Oxford. He passed the examinations for Fellowship of the Faculty of Anaesthetists, Royal College of Surgeons in 1959.

Working in obstetric operating theatres as a senior registrar in St Mary's Hospital, Portsmouth in 1960, he was required to resuscitate neonates and, with Hamer Hodges, he promoted tracheal intubation for this.

Entonox

In 1961 Tunstall persuaded the British Oxygen Company (BOC) to apply the solvent action of compressed gases (Poynting effect) to prepare a stable mixture of 50% nitrous oxide and 50% oxygen v/v, contained in one cylinder – despite initial resistance from the company. He successfully used this product to provide obstetric analgesia at St Mary's Hospital and had a preliminary communication on this published in the *Lancet*. After his publication of the invention, BOC patented the process and called the mixture Entonox. In 1962 Tunstall used it in dental anaesthetic practice.

A concern was that if the temperature of a cylinder of Entonox fell below -6°C. (e.g. during transport or if stored outside in winter), the gases may separate. Therefore, instructions were provided that ideally, after delivery, the cylinders should be marked with the date and then stored for at least 24 hours in a room kept at about 10°C. Alternatively, the cylinder could be gently warmed and inverted several times to remix the gases. In 1965 the Central Midwives Board approved Entonox for unsupervised use by midwives.

Neonatal resuscitation and ventilation

In 1962 Tunstall was appointed as a Consultant Anaesthetist at the Royal Infirmary in Aberdeen. There he continued his innovative work on neonatal resuscitation and showed the benefit of positive pressure ventilation, at a time when the prevailing view was that it was unsuitable for neonates. Ventilation of neonates soon became accepted and he earned the respect of the paediatricians.

Failed intubation drill

Through the 1960s to 1970s rapid sequence induction of general anaesthesia (using thiopentone and suxamethonium) and intubation became adopted for obstetrics in the UK; the maternal deaths from aspiration of gastric contents fell but there was a rise in deaths due to difficulties with intubation. In response, Tunstall devised a failed intubation drill, which he presented at a meeting of the Obstetric Anaesthetists Association (OAA) in 1976. This was further developed and promoted by the OAA and the reports of subsequent confidential enquiries into maternal deaths (CEMD).

Isolated forearm technique (IFT)

Tunstall next tackled the risk of awareness under the light general anaesthesia with neuromuscular blockade (NMB) used for obstetrics. He devised the isolated forearm technique (IFT) of detecting wakefulness under general anaesthesia for caesarean section in 1977. A standard blood pressure cuff on the right upper arm was inflated to 200-250 mm Hg before dosage of suxamethonium, so that the right hand was excluded from the consequent muscular paralysis. Movements of the hand in response to verbal instructions would then indicate the patient's wakefulness – to which the anaesthetist could respond by deepening the anaesthetic until wakefulness was no longer indicated. If, after the operation, such a patient had no recall of the intraoperative events, Tunstall called the condition "amnestic wakefulness" (which could also be traumatic).

Tunstall was the President of the OAA for 1987-90 and was awarded its Gold Medal in 1990. He officially retired in 1992, but continued to innovate premixed 0.25% isoflurane in 50% nitrous oxide and 50% oxygen for analgesia in labour. This was facilitated by his appointment as Honorary Research Fellow in the Department of Environmental and Occupational Medicine at the University of Aberdeen, where he worked with Dr John A.S. Ross. The mixture was given the name 'Isoxane' and patented. For this achievement, in 1994 Tunstall and Ross were awarded the Auris Prize sponsored by Aberdeen University Research Industrial Services.

The IFT was modified for use with non-depolarising NMB, but although regarded by some as the gold standard of consciousness monitoring, it received much unfair criticism from many. So, it came to be accepted as a research tool, but was never widely adopted in clinical practice.

In retirement Tunstall continued his leisure activities of sailing, wind surfing and beach running as well as hill walking. Above all he enjoyed his family. He was a quiet, unassuming man with a good sense of humour. In 1994 the Association of Anaesthetists of Great Britain and Ireland awarded him Honorary Membership. In 2006 he was awarded a DSc by the University of Aberdeen – its highest academic accolade. Sadly, his last years were tormented by leukaemia and head and neck cancer.

Further reading

Reynolds F. Obituary M.E. Tunstall (1928-2011). *International Journal of Obstetric Anesthesia* 2011; **20**: 206-7.

Tunstall ME. Obstetric Analgesia. The Use of a Fixed Nitrous Oxide and Oxygen Mixture from One Cylinder. *Lancet* 1961; **2**: 964.

Tunstall ME, Hamer Hodges RJ. A sterile disposable neonatal tracheal tube. *Lancet* 1961; **1**: 146.

Tunstall ME. Neonatal Resuscitation. *British Journal of Anaesthesia* 1964; **36**: 591-9.

Ross JAS, Marr IL, Tunstall ME. Entonox and its Development. In: Smith EB, Daniels S (Eds.) *Gases in Medicine -Anaesthesia*. Cambridge: The Royal Society of Chemistry, 1998; 27-41.

News and Notices: the OAA Meeting at Nottingham 26 March 1976. *Anaesthesia* 1976; **31**: 850 (Failed intubation drill).

Tunstall ME. Detecting wakefulness during general anaesthesia for caesarean section. *British Medical Journal* 1977; **1**: 1321.

FEATHERSTONE PROFESSORSHIP AND ORATION

Henry Walter Featherstone (1894-1967)

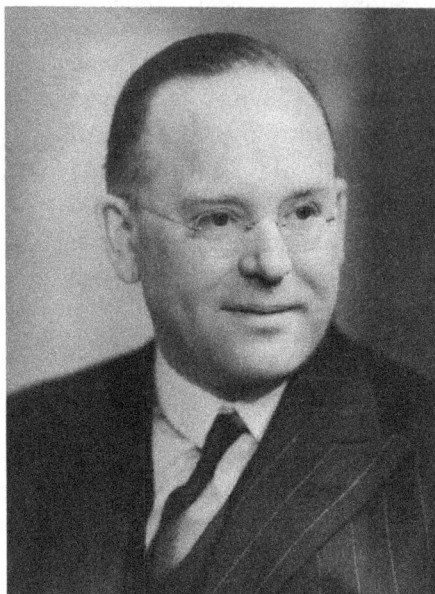

Henry W. Featherstone. Image courtesy of The Anaesthesia Heritage Centre, AAGBI.

The Association of Anaesthetists of Great Britain and Ireland (AAGBI) began its award of Featherstone Professorship in 2014 – in honour of Henry Featherstone, who was the founder of the AAGBI in 1932. The call for nominations has specified "practising clinicians and scientists who have made a substantial contribution to anaesthesia and its related subspecialties in the fields of safety, education, research, innovation, international development, leadership, or combination of these." The Professorship is held for two years, during which the holder may be required to deliver a Featherstone Oration (Table 1) at a major Association meeting – usually the Winter Scientific Meeting.

Henry ('Harry') Walter Featherstone was born in the Erdington area of Birmingham, England in 1894. He was educated there at King Edward's School, followed by Trinity College, Cambridge and the University of Birmingham. He obtained the Conjoint diploma in 1916 and did house jobs before graduating MB, BChir the following year. Then he joined the Royal Army Medical Corps (RAMC) and served at Salonica and on the Western Front at Passchendaele. After the Great War he returned to Birmingham where, influenced by the first British provincial full-time anaesthetist Dr W.J. McCardie, he chose an appointment as anaesthetist to the General Hospital.

Featherstone was academically minded and in 1924 he successfully defended his MD thesis on pulmonary complications of anaesthesia. Appointments at other hospitals and private practice came his way, but being blessed with a financially sound family background, he was able to confine himself to anaesthesia and he published many papers and chapters on anaesthetics in books. Appointment as clinical lecturer in anaesthetics to the University of

Birmingham came in 1928. He travelled to observe clinical practice at the Mayo Clinic and hospitals in Canada and was active in the Royal Society of Medicine (RSM), becoming President of its Anaesthetic Section in 1930.

In January 1932 Featherstone met informally with active members of the Section of Anaesthetics, RSM to discuss the perceived need for forming an association of anaesthetists to improve the terms and conditions of service of anaesthetists in Great Britain and Ireland. Encouraged by their support he wrote to 100 anaesthetists inviting them to a preliminary meeting, which he set up the following April. The response was enthusiastic and the AAGBI was born at its inaugural formal meeting on 1 July 1932, Featherstone becoming the first President.

Notably Featherstone successfully negotiated the regulations for an examination for a Diploma in Anaesthetics (DA) to be awarded jointly by the Conjoint Examining Board in England, the Royal College of Physicians of London and the Royal College of Surgeons of England. The first examination was held in November 1935, by which time he had just stepped down as President of the AAGBI. However, owing to the tragic suicide of the Honorary Secretary, William Howard Jones in July 1935, he nobly took on this mantle for four years.

Throughout the Second World War, Featherstone again served in the RAMC: first in the 14th General Hospital, which was sent to France in 1940, then attached to a US Army hospital and finally in command of hospital ships. He was demobilised in 1945 as a Lieutenant-Colonel, having been awarded the OBE (Military). On return to England he resumed his Birmingham General Hospital post and teaching at the University, but he had much reduced private practice. When the NHS started in 1948, he was contracted for four sessions. He continued to travel and notably in October 1948, he delivered an excellent lecture to a meeting of the International Anesthesia Research Society held in Montreal – on the history of the specialty of anaesthesia in the UK, detailing the origin and purpose of the Faculty of Anaesthetists of the Royal College of Surgeons of England.

Featherstone was justifiably honoured with the AAGBI's John Snow Medal in 1946. Further awards he received were: Honorary LLD by the University of Edinburgh in 1947, Honorary Membership of the AAGBI in 1957, and Honorary Fellowship of the Faculty of Anaesthetists of the Royal College of Surgeons of England in 1962.

Table 1. Winners of Featherstone Professorship and oration titles

Year	Professor	Oration Title
2014	Steve Yentis	Research not research
2015	Andrew Bodenham	Safer interventional procedures in anaesthesia and critical care
2016	Cyprian Mendonca	Airway training: past, present and future
2017	Richard Griffiths	Hip fractures, challenges, solutions and looming problems
2018	William Fawcett	Surgery, anaesthesia and stress
2019	Rachel Collis	Nil Oration
2019	Matt Wilson	Nil Oration

Further reading

Boulton TB. *The Association of Anaesthetists of Great Britain and Ireland 1932-1992 and the Development of the Specialty of Anaesthesia*. London: AAGBI, 1999; 16-28, 47-51, 704-9.

Obituary. H.W. Featherstone, OBE, TD, MA, MD, LLD, FFARCS. *British Medical Journal* 1967; I: 380.

Featherstone HW. The Faculty of Anesthetists of the Royal College of Surgeons of England. (A Note on Its Origin and Purpose). *Anesthesia and Analgesia* 1949; **28**: 269-72.

FICK PRINCIPLE

Adolf Eugen Fick (1829-1901)

Adolf E. Fick was born in 1829 in Kassel, Germany. He was educated at the gymnasium there, followed by the University of Marburg where he was greatly influenced by his teacher, Carl F.W. Ludwig. In 1849 Fick had a sojourn in Berlin, studying under some of the great physicians and physiologists of the time. He then returned to Marburg and obtained his MD in 1851 with a dissertation on visual errors due to astigmatism. After a few months he followed Ludwig to Zurich where he was prosector in anatomy from 1852 until 1855, when he was appointed associate professor.

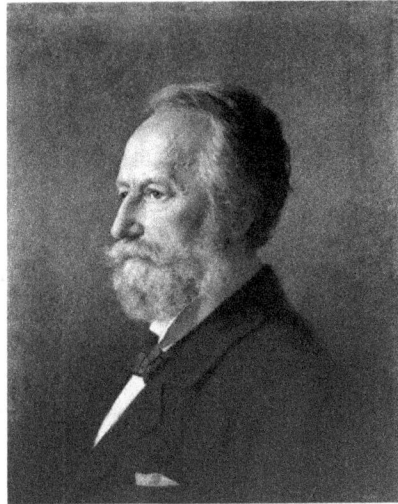

Adolf Eugen Fick. Credit: Photograph by Friedrich Dolezalek of an original painting by Anton Klamroth. Wikimedia Commons.

At Zurich in 1855 Fick published his landmark laws of diffusion. The Scottish chemist, Thomas Graham had presented his law of diffusion of gases some twenty years earlier. Fick used a molecular approach to describe the diffusion of solutes in solution, showing that the flux was down a concentration gradient. Diffusion is a fundamental concept in understanding the movement of respiratory gases and the uptake and distribution of inhalation anaesthetic agents.

In 1862 Fick was appointed full professor of physiology at Zurich. Six years later he moved to be the chair at the Physiological Institute, University of Würzburg. There in 1870 he enunciated the principle of calculating cardiac output:

Cardiac output (l/min) = $\dfrac{\text{Oxygen } (O_2) \text{ consumption (ml/min)}}{\text{Arteriovenous } O_2 \text{ difference in mixed blood (ml/l)}}$

Alternatively, this **Fick principle** could be applied to calculate the cardiac output from the pulmonary carbon dioxide (CO_2) excretion and

CO_2 concentrations in arterial and mixed venous blood samples. Initially this equation became known as the 'indirect' Fick principle, because at that time it was not possible to directly measure the components. To determine the O_2 content of mixed venous blood indirectly, expired air had to be equilibrated with alveolar gas. The indirect method of assaying the O_2 consumed was to measure inspired and expired volumes and their O_2 contents.

Although arterial puncture was known in 1870, it was not until the 1930s that Werner T.O. Forssmann showed how to thread a catheter through a vein into the human heart and Donald Van Slyke provided a method of measuring O_2 and CO_2 in blood. Then the term 'direct' Fick method was introduced, although use of the Van Slyke apparatus was laborious. Forssmann was a student of Adolf Fick's son, Rudolf. In 1956 Forssmann, André F. Cournand and Dickinson W. Richards won the Nobel Prize for Medicine. The arrival of the pulmonary artery catheter (Swan-Ganz) in 1970 enabled sampling of true mixed venous blood. Further convenience followed with the commercial provision of automated blood gas analysers.

The Fick principle can be extended to dilution methods of measuring cardiac output: indicator (e.g. indocyanine green) or thermal. The provision of a thermistor at the tip of the Swan-Ganz catheter facilitated the thermodilution method. At the proximal part of the catheter (in right atrium) a bolus of cold glucose solution is injected, mixes in the circulation and the change in temperature of the blood is measured at the pulmonary artery by the thermistor. Software in the apparatus associated with the catheter deduces the cardiac output. The direct Fick method of measuring cardiac output is considered the most accurate and the standard by which other methods are judged.

Measurement of cardiac output began to be mentioned in textbooks of anaesthesia in the 1960s. Anaesthetists and intensivists have appreciated its use as an important adjunct during and after surgery in many critically ill patients. In addition, the Fick principle underpins all methods of measuring blood flow to an organ where there is a steady flow of a substance to or from the organ, the concentration of which can be assayed. The equation is:

Blood flow to the organ = $\dfrac{\text{Rate of arrival or departure of a substance X}}{\text{Arteriovenous difference in concentration of X.}}$

This has been applied to cerebral, hepatic, renal, pulmonary and uterine blood flow.

An Adolf Fick Fund was established in 1929 by two of his sons. From this the Adolf Fick Prize is awarded by the Physics and Medical Society Würzburg once every five years for outstanding contributions to physiology.

Further reading

Vandam LD, Fox JA. Adolf Fick (1829-1901), Physiologist. *Anesthesiology* 1998; **88**: 514-8.

Fick A.Ueber die Messung des Blutquantums in der Herzenventrikeln. *Sitzung der PhysMed Gesell zu Würzburg* 1870; **16**: 36.

Magee P, Tooley M. Intraoperative monitoring. In: Hardman JG, Hopkins PM, Struys MMRF (Eds.) *Oxford Textbook of Anaesthesia*. Oxford: Oxford University Press, 2017; 709.

GILLIES LECTURE

John Gillies (1895-1976)

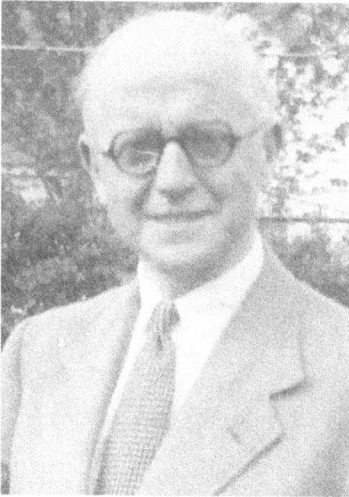

John Gillies. Image courtesy of Mr John Gillies (grandson).

John Gillies was born in Edinburgh, Scotland where he was educated at Broughton School and admitted to the University of Edinburgh Medical School in 1913. From the following year he had a four-year break in his studies because of the Great War, serving in the Highland Light Infantry. He spent a long time up to the Armistice as a prisoner of war and was awarded the Military Cross. Back in Edinburgh he qualified MB, ChB in 1923 and then went to a house physician post in Carlisle, England. He entered general practice in Halifax, Yorkshire in 1924. This work entailed a significant amount of anaesthetics, which captured his interest. In 1931, realising that to specialise he needed more training, he moved to London, where he worked under some great anaesthetists including Ivan Magill.

Gillies returned to Edinburgh in 1932 to be an anaesthetist at the Royal Hospital for Sick Children for an honorarium of £50 per annum. Soon he took up work in the professorial surgical unit at the Royal Infirmary of Edinburgh, where in 1940 he founded the Department of Anaesthetics. In those days the hospital pay for anaesthetists in the UK was inadequate, so that they had to supplement it by private practice. He designed a new anaesthetic machine, a prototype being built on site about 1941, after which it was produced commercially. In 1944 he co-authored with R.J. Minnitt the sixth edition of *Textbook of Anaesthetics*. After the Second World War in 1946 he was invited to be Director of Anaesthesia to the Royal Infirmary and lecturer to the University of Edinburgh (later Simpson Reader).

In 1948 H.W.C. Griffiths and Gillies published a landmark paper on high spinal anaesthesia to induce hypotension and produce a 'bloodless' operating field. The following year a theatre team from the Royal Infirmary of Edinburgh answered a call to perform a lumbar sympathectomy (to relieve leg pain) under anaesthesia on HM King George VI at Buckingham Palace. Gillies was the anaesthetist and duly received the Companion of the Victorian Order (CVO). In 1950 he delivered the Joseph Clover Lecture of the Faculty of Anaesthetists, Royal College of Surgeons of England. His lecture was titled "Anaesthetic factors in the causation and prevention of excessive bleeding during surgical operations" and in it he coined the term 'physiological trespass'.

Gillies served on the Editorial Board of the *British Journal of Anaesthesia* until 1948. From 1947-50 he was President of the Association of Anaesthetists of Great Britain and Ireland (AAGBI), completing ongoing negotiations with the Royal College of Surgeons of England to form the Faculty of Anaesthetists and in 1948 he was a founder member of the Board. Crucially the negotiations resulted in upgrading of the examination system for the anaesthetists and consequent consultant status equal to other specialists in the newly formed National Health Service (NHS). In 1950 he and H.H. Pinkerton of Glasgow, re-established the Scottish Society of Anaesthetists (SSA), Gillies serving as President until 1951. The SSA encompassed the regional societies in Scotland and Gillies instigated an annual Scientific Meeting and Registrars' meeting. He was also President of the Section of Anaesthetics, Royal Society of Medicine (RSM) 1951-52. Internationally he served on the Interim Committee whereby the World Federation of Societies of Anaesthesiologists (WFSA) was established in 1955.

The high academic standard of Gillies' Department attracted medical graduates from the UK and North America. No less than seven of his protégés, including his first-born son, became professors of anaesthesiology. Gillies received many awards in recognition of his services to anaesthesia: Clover Lecturer, Faculty of Anaesthetists 1950, Liston Victoria Jubilee Prize (Royal College of Surgeons of Edinburgh) 1951, Hickman Medal (RSM) 1953, John Snow Medal (AAGBI) 1958, Canadian Anaesthetists' Society Gold Medal 1969. He was elected FRCPEd, FFARACS and FFARCSI.

After retiring in 1960 Gillies enjoyed many recreational activities, but he was unhappy after the death of his wife in 1975, and he passed away the following year. Three of his four children had become highly respected anaesthetists: Alastair J. Gillies (Rochester, New York, USA), Deidre M.M. Gillies (Montreal, Canada) and Ian D.S. Gillies (London, England). In 1978 the SSA instituted an annual John Gillies Memorial Lecture at its Annual Scientific Meeting. Each lecturer has been given a crystal glass bowl bearing the crest of the SSA. Long after his death, anaesthetists who knew John Gillies continued to remark that he was a very kind man and a consummate gentleman.

Table 1. The John Gillies lecturers and lecture titles

Year	Lecturer	Title
1978	Gordon Robson	Physiological Trespass
1979	G Jackson Rees	On the scientific basis for the development of paediatric anaesthesia
1980	O P Dinnick	In Somno Securitas – a sermon in safety
1981	J D Robertson	Anaesthesia for Royalty
1982	T Cecil Gray	Safety – a mirage?
1983	James P Payne	The quality of care
1984	H W C Griffiths	Clinical anaesthesia, retrospective and prospective
1985	M Keith Sykes	Safety in anaesthesia – simplicity versus surveillance
1986	Alastair H B Masson	Inter Pares
1987	J I M Lawson	Relaxation – a historical perspective
1988	D Bruce Scott	A little knowledge
1989	William R MacRae	Forty years on
1990	Alastair A Spence	Whither breathing
1991	Iain A Davidson	Trespass with care
1992	W D A Smith	An open mind
1993	Michael E Tunstall	Isonox
1994	J A W Wildsmith	Neurological Trespass
1995	G Kenny	Technology – friend or foe
1996	William C Bowman	Pharmacological manipulation of neuromuscular transmission
1997	J Thorburn	From here to here
1998	Alan Aitkenhead	Safety in anaesthesia
1999	Douglas Arthur	Thou Grim Mischief Making Chiel
2000	J E Charlton	Safe practice
2001	S Ingram	Quality and anaesthesia – how do we judge?
2002	Ian Calder	Low, High, Low
2003	C Howie	Making it better
2004	David H T Scott	Safety in anaesthesia – the introduction of new technology
2005	John H McClure	Standards of care in obstetric anaesthesia
2006	W A Chambers	Do you want to get better?
2008	B Cowan	Things that go bump – the mistakes are out there just waiting to be made
2009	R Glavin	I wish I hadn't done that
2010	B Toft	Nobody's perfect
2011	M Daniel	Crossing the chasm
2012	R Sneyd	What kind of doctor, what kind of health service?
2014	Neil Morton	Developmental harm and anaesthesia
2015	A Longmate	Quality, Safety and Improvement in Healthcare
2016	Kathleen Ferguson	Making safety sense
2017	Ellen O'Sullivan	History and advancement in airway management
2018	Nancy Redfern	Making anaesthesia safer by looking after ourselves
2019	Neil Jeffers	Non technical skills in high stakes environments

Further reading

Gillies J. Retrospect. *Scottish Society of Anaesthetists News Letter* 1972; **13**: 19-24.

Gillies J. Anaesthetic factors in the causation and prevention of excessive bleeding during surgical operations. *Annals of the Royal College of Surgeons of England* 1950; **7**: 204-21.

Helliwell PJ. Obituary John Gillies, CVO, MC, MB,ChB, FRCP(Ed), FRCS Ed), FFARCS (Hon), FFARACS, FFARCSI. *Anaesthesia* 1976; **31**: 1311-12.

McKenzie AG. The Gillies anaesthetic machine. *Anaesthesia* 2008; **63**: 771-7.

McKenzie AG. John Gillies (1895-1976). *Journal of the Royal College of Physicians of Edinburgh* 2019; **49**: 260-1.

GLOSTAVENT ANAESTHESIA MACHINE

Roger J. Eltringham (1939 -)

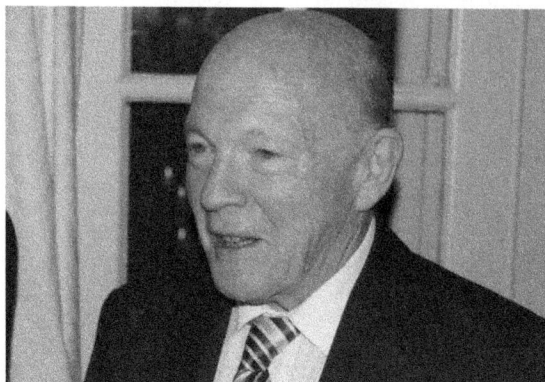

Roger Eltringham was born in London, England in 1939 and educated at Cranbrook School in Kent, followed by St Andrews University Medical School, from which he graduated MB, ChB in 1964. He passed the FFARCS in 1971, trained in anaesthesia in Bristol, and in 1974 was appointed to a Consultant post at the Gloucestershire Royal Hospital. The following year he also became the medical officer for Gloucester Rugby Club.

In 1988 he became a member of the Education Committee of the World Federation of Societies of Anaesthesiologists (WFSA), which was formed in 1955 to `make available the highest standards of anaesthesia for all peoples of the world`. Although this has been achieved in some countries, in many others this aim has still not been realised. One of the reasons for this has been the lack of an anaesthetic machine which is both affordable and can meet the specific needs of those practising in isolated, difficult or dangerous situations.

Modern anaesthetic machines have become so sophisticated that the administration of general anaesthesia can now be virtually risk free. This is a great achievement, but unfortunately such machines are not suitable for use in many parts of the world for the following reasons:

(1) they are very expensive and therefore unaffordable in low income countries;
(2) even if they have been donated, and cost nothing initially, the running costs are substantial;
(3) their function is dependent on uninterrupted supplies of both oxygen and electricity;
(4) they require regular attention from skilled engineers for servicing and maintenance.

The many attempts to introduce the latest and most sophisticated machines into isolated hospitals in low income countries have not proved successful. The vast sums of money invested have been largely wasted, because the same mistakes are repeated over and over again. The essential point is that the needs of those practising under difficult conditions, in isolated hospitals in developing countries cannot be met by the donation of conventional anaesthetic machines, however sophisticated and expensive. A completely different type of anaesthetic machine is required that is specifically designed to overcome the additional difficulties confronting them.

In 1997, Eltringham discussed the problem with Dr Andrei Varvinski, a trainee who had previously served in the Russian navy and had valuable experience of anaesthesia in difficult situations. He pointed out that the use of an oxygen concentrator would eliminate the problem of supplying oxygen cylinders to remote locations. Eltringham's group therefore purchased an oxygen concentrator and combined it with a gas driven ventilator and a draw over breathing system. When the three components were mounted on a standard nursing trolley, together with a reserve oxygen cylinder, they realised they had an anaesthetic machine which was not only inexpensive but could continue to function if the oxygen failed, or the electricity failed or even if they both failed. Although it fulfilled exactly the requirements of those anaesthetists working in isolated hospitals in low income countries, its appearance did not inspire confidence among potential users and no commercial enterprise was willing to develop it.

Just as they were contemplating abandoning the concept altogether, Eltringham was surprised to receive an invitation to speak to the Institute of Engineers in London. He accepted the invitation although he was half expecting it was really meant for someone else and that it was a case of mistaken identity. His fears seemed justified as the audience did not seem particularly interested in the subject and there were no questions or discussion. He was therefore very surprised when, just as leaving the building, a member of the audience rushed over and intercepted. He apparently liked the concept and wanted to know who was manufacturing it. When Eltringham explained that several manufacturers had been approached but no-one seemed interested, he was invited to visit his engineering company in Devon to discuss its potential.

It was here that he first met Robert Neighbour, a brilliant engineer who immediately appreciated the potential of this innovation. Although he had no previous experience of anaesthetic machines, he was convinced it could be developed successfully.

Over the next few years Neighbour made weekly visits to the Gloucestershire Royal Hospital where he was able to witness conventional anaesthetic machines in action, meet anaesthetists from developing countries and hear about the additional problems they faced. Back in his workshop he was able to utilize his engineering expertise to improve various aspects of the 'Glostavent' – so named after Gloucester Rugby Club, because it was initially hoped the then amateur club might contribute to the cost of its development. However, the club then turned professional and all its funds went on financing players. Gradually Neighbour developed the machine to the extent that It could fulfil all the requirements of anaesthetists working in isolated hospitals in developing countries. It consists of three key components:

(1) an oxygen concentrator so that oxygen can be produced locally on site and is therefore not dependent on the delivery of oxygen cylinders;
(2) a draw over breathing system, which has the advantage of enabling the carrier gas to pass through a low resistance vaporizer by the sub-atmospheric pressure generated by inspiration – therefore It does not require gases to be delivered under pressure as in the standard plenum system used in most anaesthetic machines;
(3) a mechanical ventilator which is driven by pressurised oxygen rather than electricity.

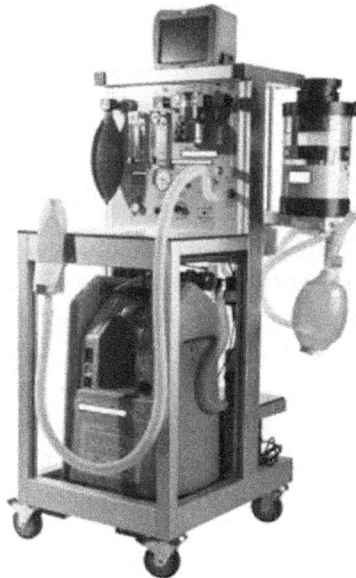

Figure 1. Glostavent Anaesthetic Machine. Image from Dr R.J. Eltringham.

The three components have been combined to form a versatile anaesthetic machine, known as the Glostavent (Figure 1). It is reliable, effective and inexpensive and is suitable for use in both adults and children, using either controlled or spontaneous respiration. It is particularly suited for difficult environments as it can continue to function, without interruption if the supply of oxygen fails or the electricity fails or even if they both fail simultaneously. Compared to the latest and most sophisticated machines which can cost £70,000 and more, it is extremely inexpensive at £13,500.

In difficult and dangerous situations, especially in war zones or following natural catastrophes, emergency anaesthesia may be required under field conditions, that is, outside a hospital environment. A portable version of the Glostavent, costing £3500, is available for use in such situations (Figure 2). It is presented in a small case, weighs just 10 Kg and can be assembled, ready for use, in less than 5 minutes. A battery driven portable ventilator weighing 10 Kg and costing £1500 is also available for use in these circumstances (Figure 3).

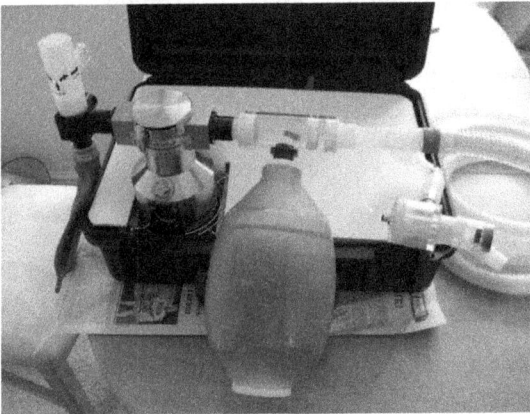

Figure 2. Portable model of Glostavent. Image from Dr R.J. Eltringham.

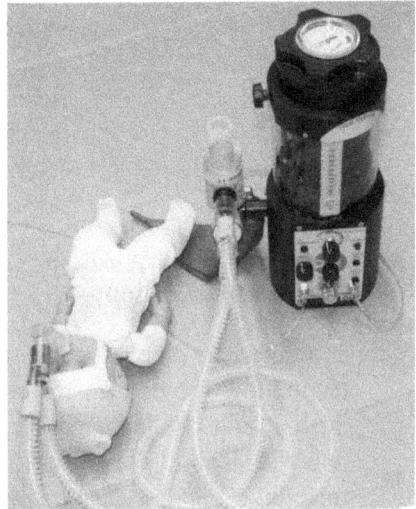

Figure 3. Battery driven portable ventilator. Image from Dr R.J. Eltringham.

Honours awarded to Eltringham include: from the AAGBI, the Pask Certificate of Honour in 1995 and Honorary Membership in 2004; from the Royal College of Anaesthetists, the Humphry Davy Award (q.v. page 47) in 2005; from the Society for Education in Anesthesiology, the McLesky Lectureship in 2004; and from the ASA, the Lewis Wright Memorial Lectureship in 2010. He served as Vice President of the WFSA 2004-8. Next he became Chairman and founder member of the charity 'Safe Anaesthesia Worldwide' in 2010 and continues in this role.

Further reading

Eltringham RJ, Neighbour RC. The environmental impact of the Glostavent anesthetic machine. *Anesthesia and Analgesia* 2015; **120**: 1264-70.

NICHOLAS GREENE AWARD

Nicholas Misplee Greene (1922-2004)

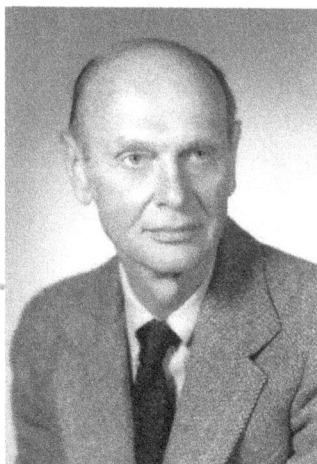

Nicholas Greene was born in Milford, Connecticut and his early years were spent there as well as in New York, Michigan, Massachusetts, California and Alabama, USA. As his parents were divorced, he was shuttled between relatives and went to boarding school from age 8. After graduating from Phillips Academy in Andover MA, he attended Yale College, qualifying BS in 1944 and then MD from Columbia University, New York City in 1946. After a house officer post at Columbia's Presbyterian Hospital (where he admired Dr Virginia Apgar), he served two years as a general medical officer in the US Navy. Then he became a Resident in Anesthesiology at the Massachusetts General Hospital (MGH) under Henry Beecher.

Nicholas M. Greene. Image reproduced with permission from Bulletin of Anesthesia History.

Soon after he arrived at MGH, there was a visit by John Gillies of Edinburgh (Scotland), who demonstrated his method of inducing hypotension to reduce intra-operative bleeding by means of high spinal anaesthesia. Beecher was impressed and in late 1950 he sent Greene to Edinburgh to learn the technique under Gillies' supervision. Gillies (q.v. page 76) inspired Greene and fuelled his enthusiasm to investigate the physiological effects of spinal anaesthesia, which would come to define his academic career. Duly taught, Greene returned to MGH to successfully employ hypotensive spinal anaesthesia for the surgeons Meigs and Linton and he eventually published on this in 1954.

On invitation in 1952, Greene served as Director of Anesthesia at Strong Memorial Hospital, University of Rochester NY. He returned to Yale in 1955 to be the School of Medicine's first Professor of Anesthesiology. In 1958 he published a monograph on the physiology of spinal anaesthesia, which would run to many editions.

Through Greene's guidance, anesthesiology at Yale achieved excellence and became an independent Department in the Medical school in 1971. He served as Editor-in-Chief of both *Anesthesiology* 1973-76 and of *Anesthesia and Analgesia* 1977-91. While in the latter role, he published a book *Key Words in Anesthesiology* (1980). The New England Society of

Anesthesiologists elected him President for 1978-79. He retired from Yale University in 1987, becoming Professor Emeritus.

At this time, he indulged his interest in ornithology by taking safaris in East Africa. Appalled by the lack of resources there for anaesthesia practice, he volunteered to teach, and founded the Overseas Teaching Programme (OTP) with funding agreed by the American Society of Anesthesiologists (ASA) in October 1989. In June 1990 it was agreed that the OTP would aim to set up an anaesthesia residency training programme at the University Teaching Hospital in Lusaka, Zambia. Volunteer teachers were recruited from the USA and Canada to begin the programme there in February 1991. Then in May 1991 agreement was secured to have a second OTP affiliation with the non-sectarian Kilimanjaro Christian Medical Centre in Moshi, Tanzania for a programme starting in February 1992. During this period, Greene accepted an invitation from Dr Ruth Hutchinson to be the Guest Lecturer at the annual Refresher Course of the Zimbabwe Anaesthetic Association, held in Harare in August 1991. He retired from being Director of the OTP after five years in 1994; that year at the ASA Annual Meeting in San Francisco he was awarded a President's Citation for his "tireless devotion" to improving anaesthesia in low and middle income countries. Sadly, in 1997 a change in policy by the Zambian authorities caused the programme there to be terminated and it was therefore re-established in Accra, Ghana. In the following years, the activities of the OTP waned.

Having become a Trustee of the Wood Library-Museum (WLM) in 1987, Greene set up a Publications Committee which developed the WLM into a scholarly press. Seminal books were reprinted, and some texts written in German, French and Russian were translated into English. In 1996 Greene inaugurated the WLM Laureate of the History of Anesthesia, a quadrennial award made on the decision of a Laureate Committee after deliberating on internationally submitted nominations.

Greene received many honours in recognition of his services to anaesthesia. Locally, in 1960 he won the Horace Wells Club Award (q.v. page 243). The ASA conferred on him their highest honour, the Distinguished Service Award, in 1989. In the field of regional anaesthesia, he delivered the Gaston Labat Lecture in 1987, the T.H. Seldon Lecture in 1991 and was awarded the Carl Koller Gold Medal in 1992. He also delivered the Emery A. Rovenstine Lecture in 1992. His other medals were the silver medal of Columbia University's College of Physicians and Surgeons at its bicentennial, and medals from the Swedish Society of Anaesthetists. The Royal College of Anaesthetists awarded him Honorary Fellowship, and he was elected to Honorary Membership of the Association of Anaesthesiologists of Uganda and of the Japanese Society of Anaesthesiologists.

Seven years after his death, the ASA established the Nicholas Greene, M.D. Award for Outstanding Humanitarian Contribution, which since 2011 has been presented each year at its annual meeting.

Table 1. Nicholas Greene, M.D. Award winners

Year	Recipient	Year	Recipient
2011	Phillip O. Bridenbaugh	2016	Mark W. Newton
2012	Angela Enright	2017	Kelly McQueen
2013	George A. Gregory	2018	Patrick M. McQuillan
2014	Lena E. Dohlman	2019	Elizabeth Frost
2015	Medge D. Owen	2020	Elizabeth T. Drum

Acknowledgement

The Anesthesia History Association kindly gave permission to reproduce the portrait photograph from the *Bulletin of Anesthesia History*.

Further reading

Greene NM, Bunker JP, Kerr WS, Von Felsinger JM, Keller JW, Beecher HK. Hypotensive spinal anaesthesia: respiratory, metabolic, hepatic, renal and cerebral effects. *Annals of Surgery* 1954; **140**: 641-51.

Greene NM. *Physiology of Spinal Anesthesia*. London: Baillière, Tindall & Cox Ltd., 1958.

Greene NM. Anaesthesia in Underdeveloped Countries: A Teaching Program. *The Yale Journal of Biology and Medicine* 1991; **64**: 403-7.

Greene NM. The pleasures of anesthesiology. In: Fink BR, McGoldrick KE (Eds). *Careers in Anesthesiology*. Volume IV. Park Ridge, Illinois: Wood Library-Museum of Anesthesiology, 2000.

McGoldrick KE. Nicholas M. Greene: Visionary Educator, Clinician, Editor, and Humanitarian. *Anesthesia and Analgesia* 2012; **115**: 1423-30.

FRED HEHRE LECTURE

Frederick W. Hehre Jr. (1923-1980)

Frederick W. Hehre was born in Harrison, New Jersey and was educated at the high school in Kearny. In 1941 he went to Columbia College followed by Columbia University, New York where he graduated MD in 1947. He then did a year as an intern at St Clare's Hospital, New York City, followed by residency in anaesthesia over 1948-50 at the Columbia Presbyterian Hospital. He was one of Virginia Apgar's last residents. After remaining there for a further six years' experience, he moved to Yale University where in 1958 he was appointed Director of Obstetric Anaesthesia, working under Nicholas Greene (q.v. page 84).

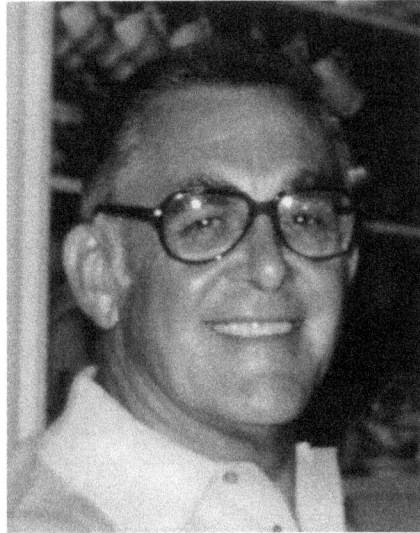

Frederick W. Hehre. Image courtesy of Dr William Camann.

From 1960 Hehre published much on continuous lumbar epidural analgesia in obstetrics. In 1969 he was a founder member of the Society for Obstetric Anesthesia and Perinatology (SOAP). Notably in 1970 he and his colleagues at Yale reported 50537 consecutive obstetric anaesthetics with zero mortality. He was also involved in the development of electronic fetal monitoring. By 1974 he had published over forty papers on obstetric anaesthesia in peer reviewed journals. At this time, he contributed a chapter to *Clinical Anesthesia* which drew attention to the shortage of 'out of hours' staffing in obstetric anaesthesia and the need for supervisors to cover residents in this area. Then in 1975 he was appointed chair of the Department of Anesthesiology at the Boston University Medical Centre.

Hehre was highly regarded for his clinical acumen and revered as a teacher. He participated in most of the SOAP meetings where he was a lively character sporting a bow tie and holding a glass of wine. Sadly, he died unexpectedly in April 1980 of a massive myocardial infarction. Within a month the Board of Directors of SOAP agreed to establish an annual memorial lectureship in his name. The first Frederick W. Hehre Jr. Memorial Lecture was given at the 1981 SOAP meeting in San Diego.

Table 1. Fred Hehre lecturers and lecture titles

Year	Lecturer	Title
1981	Gertie Marx	Monitoring the Mother During Labor.
1982	L. Stanley James	Record lost
1983	Edward Hon	Whose Distress – Mother?, Fetus?, Doctor?
1984	Philip R. Bromage	Evolution and Revolution in Obstetrical Anesthesia.
1985	Sol M. Shnider	The Fellows Made Me Do It.
1986	Frank C. Greiss Jr.	The Evolution of the Placental Circulation with Comments on Clinical Implications.
1987	John J. Bonica	Mechanisms and Pathways of the Pain of Childbirth.
1988	Tony Yaksh	New Horizons in the Control of the Spinal Cord Level of the Sensory and Autonomic Response to Pain.
1989	Francis M. James	Lessons Learned from Obstetric Anesthesia.
1991	Milton H.Alper	History of Anesthesia at the 'Old Boston Lying-In' Hospital.
1992	Bradley E. Smith	Frederick W. Hehre, MD: Visionary of the Past, Example for the Future of Obstetric Anesthesia.
1993	Frederick P. Zuspan	New Thoughts on an Old Disease: Preeclampsia/Eclampsia.
1994	Felicity Reynolds	In Defence of Bupivacaine.
1995	Ronald Melzack	Current Concepts of Pain.
1996	Charles P. Gibbs	Obstetric Anesthesia – USA.
1997	Mieczslaw Finster	Abandoned Techniques and Drugs in Obstetrics and Obstetric Anesthesia.
1998	Gershon Levinson	Controversies During a Career in Obstetric Anesthesia.
1999	Sheila E. Cohen	What's New, What's Hot? A 25 Year Retrospective of Obstetric Anesthesia: Lessons for the New Millenium
2000	Michael J. Cousins	Persistent Pain: A Disease Entity?
2001	M. Joanne Douglas	Looking to the Past to Find a Vision for the Future.
2002	David M. Dewan	Obstetric Anesthesia 1977 - 2002 A Personal Perspective – from Consilience to Victory.
2003	Donald Caton	Medical Science and Social Values.
2004	Samuel C. Hughes	Maternal Mortality: What have we learned and how do we use it?
2005	James C. Eisenach	Pain and Delivery – Why, What and When?
2006	David Chestnut	Lessons learned from obstetric anesthesia.
2007	David J. Birnbach	Malpractice or Miscommunication? The importance of Improved Communication between Anesthesiologists, Patients and our Colleagues.
2008	Alan C. Santos	See One, Do One, Teach One: Is This What Women Really Want?
2009	Joy L. Hawkins	Meant to honor someone for his/her substantial contribution to the subspecialty.

2010	Susan K. Palmer	The use of human albumin for obstetric patients.
2011	William Camann	The Blunt End of the Needle.
2012	Gordon Lyons	A Critical Exam of Regional Technique.
2013	Richard Smiley	Passion.
2014	David J. Wlody	Mentorship in career development.
2015	Warwick Ngan Kee	Reflections on the Evolution of the Management of Hypotension During Spinal Anesthesia for Cesarean Delivery.
2016	Lawrence C. Tsen	From Music to Medicine – A Meditation
2017	Cynthia A. Wong	Two Steps Forward and One Step Forward.
2018	Robert A. Dyer	From Queen Victoria to Duchess Kate
2019	Jose C.A. Carvalho	Dogmas in Obstetric Anesthesia – The Balance Between Evidence, Common Sense, Habit and Fear.

Acknowledgement

Judith Robins, Registrar of the Wood Library-Museum of Anesthesiology, kindly assisted with the list of Fred Hehre lectures.

Further reading

Kalas DB, Hehre FW. Departmental evolution of obstetric anesthesia. A 12-year survey. *Obstetrics and Gynecology* 1970; **36**: 156-61.

Hehre FW. Observations, Philosophic and Opinionated on Obstetric Anesthesia Coverage. *Clinical Anesthesia* 1974; **10**: 323-33.

Ostheimer GW. In Memoriam: Fred Hehre. *SOAP Newsletter* 1981; **12**: 1.

HEIDBRINK VALVE

Jay Albion Heidbrink (1875-1957)

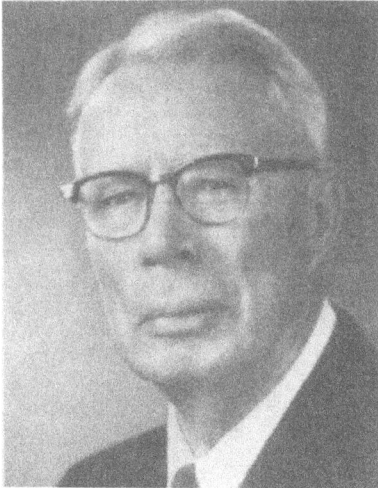

Jay Albion Heidbrink was born in Boaz, Richland County, Wisconsin, USA in 1875. He went to the University of Michigan 1898-1901 and qualified DDS, returning to Wisconsin to set up a dental practice. Shortly after the Cleveland dentist Charles K. Teter brought out his nitrous oxide/oxygen machine in 1903, Heidbrink purchased the first one he saw. However, he noticed several problems with this apparatus, and when he moved to practise in Minneapolis in 1906, he began his own modifications.

Jay A. Heidbrink. Image courtesy of the ADSA.

In 1912-13 Heidbrink produced his first commercial anaesthesia machine: his 'Model A'. Then he was able to combine his dental practice with a manufacturing business by engaging in a financial partnership with Dr Thomas Hartzell, who was the head of oral surgery at the University of Minnesota Dental School. He was joined by a salesman, Walter McGillivra and they began to make their own pressure reducing valves. From 1918 Heidbrink taught dentists singly in the use of the gas machine and in the 1920s he extended this to teaching clinics.

Heidbrink had filed US patents (No. 1,265,910) in 1918 and (No. 1,309,686) in 1919 for his machines administering a mixture of nitrous oxide and oxygen, the proportions of the mixture being automatically maintained despite an increase in volume of flow to the patient. He and his Company brought legal suits on alleged patents infringement against Elmer I. McKesson, which were unsuccessful in the District Court. An appeal against the judgement was arranged in the Supreme Court in 1924, but it was again unsuccessful.

Heidbrink filed a patent for a ventilator in 1929 and this was passed (US Patent 1,917,940) in 1933. It included an adjustable expiratory valve, with the purpose of allowing the escape of exhaled and surplus gas but preventing the entry of outside air; additionally, it allowed gas to escape if the pressure exceeded a set level on the valve. This came to be known as the 'Heidbrink valve' and it was copied for use in many anaesthesia breathing systems. It is still described in the latest textbooks on anaesthesia, although often accompanied by the term 'adjustable pressure limiting (APL) valve' – see Figure 1. The valve disc was made as light as possible and had a stem which was set into a guide to ensure correct positioning on the seating. Circling the stem and guide was a lightweight coiled spring, which pushed the disc against the seating for closure. The contact between disc and seating was 'knife edge' so that the area of contact was small – to reduce any adhesion.

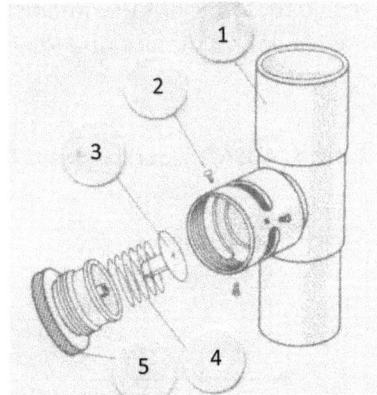

Figure 1. The Heidbrink valve: 1- taper; 2- retaining screws; 3- disc; 4- spring; 5- valve top.

The other inventions by Heidbrink were not as long lasting as the 'Heidbrink valve'. By the late 1930s he had marketed on both sides of the Atlantic two further popular items.

- Heidbrink dry flowmeter, called "kinetometer": gas flow was indicated by the height of a metal rod against a graduated scale in a glass tube. There were fine adjustment controls at the top of the apparatus with emergency large-volume valves worked by levers below the meters.
- Heidbrink oxygen tent: had a vogue for about two decades. It was used when oxygen therapy was indicated for delirious patients or those who would not tolerate a mask or nasal catheter. Heidbrink's model efficiently provided thorough ventilation by a motor blower. The temperature and humidity were regulated by blowing the oxygen through ice. The percentage of carbon dioxide was regulated by means of a soda-lime canister.

Heidbrink's anaesthetic machine progressed to 'Model T' and then in 1938 came his Simplex Dental Model. His apparatus was used by the American military in the Second World War. He retired from clinical practice in 1946.

In 1954 the American Dental Society of Anesthesiology (ADSA) presented jointly to Heidbrink and Charles K. Teter, their inaugural annual award for most significant contribution to the advancement of anaesthesiology in dentistry. Just a few months before his death in 1957, Heidbrink provided the ADSA with his memoirs, which were published in three consecutive issues of their *Newsmonthly*. The Heidbrink Company endowed the ADSA for the purpose of recognizing other achievers, and subsequently the annual award was called the Heidbrink Award. While most recipients have been dentists, the list has included some notable medical graduates: Frederick W. Clement, Francis F. Foldes, John J. Bonica and Philip O. Bridenbaugh.

Table 1. ADSA/Heidbrink Award winners

Year	Recipient	Year	Recipient
1954	Jay A. Heidbrink, DDS Charles K. Teeter, DDS	1989	Harry Lange, DDS
1955	Edward C. Thompson, DDS	1990	Harold Panuska, DDS
1956	Daniel F. Lynch, DDS	1991	Peter Sykes, LDS Yasuya Kubota, Dr
1957	Leonard M. Monheim, DDS	1992	Alvin Salomo, DDS
1958	William B. Kirmey, DDS Sterling V. Mead, DDS	1993	Herbert Berquist, DMD
1959	Harry Seldin, DDS	1994	Peter Jacobsohn, DDS
1960	Neils Jorgensen, DDS	1995	John Lytle, MD DDS FACD
1961	B. H. Harms, DDS	1996	Stanley F. Malamed, DDS
1962	Mendal Nevin, DDS Cloyd C. Schultz, DDS	1997	C. Richard Bennett, DDS PhD
1963	Morgan L. Allison, DDS	1998	Joel M. Weaver, DDS PhD
1966	Morris Fierstein, DDS	1999	Robert Campbell, DDS
1968	S.L. Drummond-Jackson, DDS	2000	John A. Yagiela, DDS PhD
1969	Hillel Feldman, DDS	2001	Raymond A .Dionne, DDS PhD
1970	W. Harry Archer, DDS	2002	J. Theodore Jastak, DDS PhD
1971	Edward J. Driscoll, DDS	2003	Kenneth Hargreaves, DDS PhD
1972	Joseph P. Osterloh, DDS	2004	Gerald Allen, MD
1973	Frederick W. Clement, MD	2005	Philip O. Bridenbaugh, MD
1974	Seymour Alpert, MD Charles Coakley, MD	2006	Morton B. Rosenberg, DMD
1975	Francis F. Foldes, MD	2007	Daniel A. Haas, DDS PhD
1976	William Greenfield, DDS	2008	Wolfgang Jakobs, MD DDS PhD
1977	Frank M. McCarthy, MD DDS	2009	Yuzuru Kaneko, Prof
1978	N. Wayne Hiatt, DDS	2010	Harcourt M. Stebbins, DDS
1979	Norman Trieger, DMD MD	2011	James P. Phero, DMD
1980	Milton Jaffe, DDS MA	2012	Ralph Epstein, DDS
1981	William R. Wallace, DDS	2013	Paul A. Moore, DMD PhD
1982	Adrian Hubbel, DDS	2014	O. Ross Beirne, DMD PhD
1983	Daniel M. Laskin, DDS MS	2015	Daniel E. Becker, DDS
1985	L. Lawrence Kerr, DDS	2016	Karen E. Crowley, DDS
1986	Sylvan M. Shane, DDS	2017	Christine L. Quinn, DDS MS
1987	Thomas Jones, DDS Thomas Quinn, DMD	2018	Jeffrey B. Dembo, DDS
1988	George A.E. Gow-Gates, MDS	2019	Joseph A. Giovannitti Jr, DMD

Jay Albion Heidbrink was posthumously awarded the Horace Wells Club of Connecticut annual award of merit (q.v. page 243) in 1958. He was the third person thus honoured and the certificate was presented to his son, Robert Heidbrink of Orlando, Florida.

Further reading

Heidbrink JA. Memoirs. *Newsmonthly of the American Dental Society of Anesthesiology* 1957; **4(3)**: 5-11.

Heidbrink JA. Memoirs. *Newsmonthly of the American Dental Society of Anesthesiology* 1957; **4(4)**: 16-19.

Heidbrink JA. Memoirs. *Newsmonthly of the American Dental Society of Anesthesiology* 1957; **4(5)**: 16-17.

Davey AJ. Adjustable Pressure Limiting (APL) valves. In: Davey AJ, Diba A (Eds.) *Ward's Anaesthetic Equipment* (Fifth Edn.). Philadelphia: Elsevier Saunders, 2005; 155-6.

MOML. Heidbrink v. McKesson U.S. Supreme Court Transcript of Record with Supporting Pleadings. Farmington Hills (Michigan): Gale, 2011.

HOFMANN ELIMINATION OF ATRACURIUM

August Wilhelm von Hofmann (1818-1892)

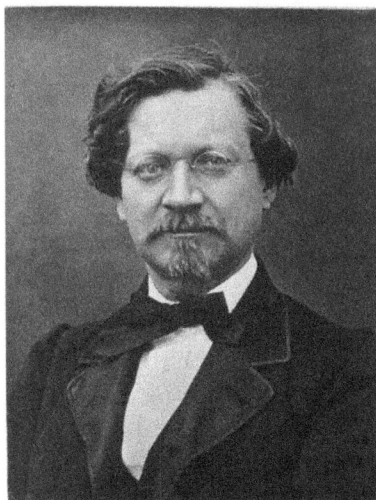

Students of anaesthesia are expected to know that the non-depolarising neuromuscular blocking drug (NDNMBD), atracurium, undergoes spontaneous degradation in plasma by ester hydrolysis and Hofmann elimination. The eponym belongs to August Wilhelm von Hofmann.

Thanks to Prince Albert, the Consort to Queen Victoria, in 1845 August Wilhelm von Hofmann was offered and accepted the Directorship of the new Royal College of Chemistry (RCC) in London, England. Recruited from Bonn in Germany, Hofmann had a PhD in chemistry and had been assistant to the great Justus von Liebig. Hofmann successfully established laboratory style teaching at the RCC.

August W. von Hofmann. Image reproduced courtesy of the Royal Society of Chemistry Library.

In 1851 Hofmann was the first chemist to synthesize quaternary amines and he showed that when quaternary tetraethylammonium hydroxide is heated, an alkene is formed by elimination of tertiary triethylamine vapour and water:

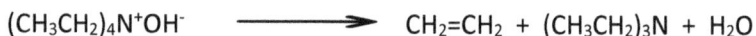

$$(CH_3CH_2)_4N^+OH^- \longrightarrow CH_2=CH_2 + (CH_3CH_2)_3N + H_2O$$

Note that three bond changes have occurred: a hydrogen-carbon bond is broken as the hydroxide ion removes a proton, an electron pair moves to form a carbon-carbon double bond, and the electron pair of the carbon-nitrogen bond becomes the lone pair of the eliminated amine. This reaction, a way of converting a quaternary amine into a tertiary amine, became known as **Hofmann's elimination**.

Most famously while in London, Hofmann considered whether coal tar could be used as a basis to synthesize quinine, which had to be imported in the form of cinchona bark from Peru at great expense. Put to this task in 1856 his student, William Henry Perkin instead produced the synthetic dye, mauve (aniline purple) – the start of a burgeoning synthetic dye industry.

Hofmann returned to Germany in 1865 to a position at the University of Berlin. There he founded the German Chemical Society. He was honoured by many awards: Fellow of the Royal Society in 1851, that Society's Royal Medal in 1854 and Copley Medal in 1875, and the Albert Medal of the Royal Society of Chemistry in 1881.

In the 1960s there was much research into the pharmaceutical development of improved NDNMBDs. At the University of Strathclyde, John Stenlake noted that petaline from the Lebanese plant *Leontice leontopetalum* had a structure resembling half of the tubocurarine molecule, but also underwent spontaneous degradation in mild alkali by the Hofmann elimination pathway. Several series of compounds were therefore synthesised over the next twenty years, culminating in atracurium besylate. This was found to be a potent NDNMBD and in human plasma underwent both ester hydrolysis and Hofmann elimination (see Figure 1).

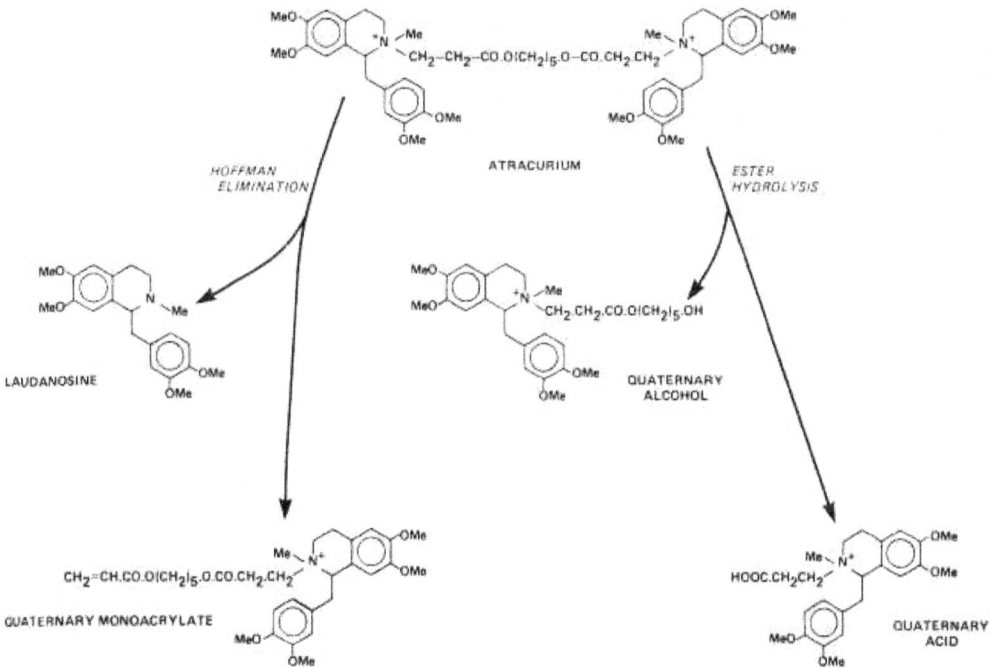

Figure 1. Routes of breakdown of atracurium.

Atracurium was patented in 1977 by Wellcome Research Laboratories and a clinical evaluation by James Payne (q.v. page 174, Professor of Anaesthesia at the Royal College of Surgeons of England) and Roy Hughes was published in 1981. Although it caused some histamine release, this was usually small.

Stability in the ampoule was achieved by the low pH of the solution (3.5) and storage at 5° C. In the plasma its muscle relaxant effect was terminated non-enzymatically after about 35 minutes by Hofmann elimination and ester hydrolysis. It was released for clinical use in the UK in 1982. For the first time there was a NDNMBD with a duration of effect independent of the level of plasma cholinesterase, renal and hepatic function. This clearly was an advantage for patients with renal or hepatic impairment and those critically ill.

The histamine release caused by atracurium limited its marketing in the USA. Chemically it consists of a mixture of three groups of geometric isomers, totalling ten stereoisomers in the *cis* and *trans* configurations. These could be separated by high pressure liquid chromatography. In 1995 Wellcome plc largely sold up to Glaxo plc, which developed the 15% of the atracurium mixture constituted by the 1R *cis* 1R' *cis* isomer (51W89) as this did not cause histamine release and was a more potent NDNMBD. The product cisatracurium was found to be predominantly broken down by Hofmann elimination with minimal ester hydrolysis. It became established in clinical practice in both the UK and the USA.

Further reading

Encyclopaedia Britannica.

Alston TA. The Contributions of A.W. Hofmann. *Anesthesia and Analgesia* 2003; **96**: 622-5.

Stenlake JB, Waigh RD, Urwin J, Dewar GH, Coker GG. Atracurium: conception and inception. *British Journal of Anaesthesia* 1983; **55**: 3S-10S.

Boyd AH, Eastwood NB, Parker CJR, Hunter JM. Pharmacodynamics of the 1R *cis* 1'R *cis* isomer of atracurium (51W89) in health and chronic renal failure. *British Journal of Anaesthesia* 1995; **74**: 400-4.

MAURICE P HUDSON PRIZE

Maurice William Petre Hudson (1901-1992)

Maurice W.P. Hudson was born in London, England in 1901 and educated at Sherborne School. He went to St Thomas's Hospital Medical School, London and qualified MRCS LRCP in 1924, proceeding to MBBS (London) the following year. After being resident house surgeon, casualty officer, resident anaesthetist and clinical assistant in ENT at St Thomas's Hospital, he passed the Diploma in Anaesthetics (RCP&S) in 1936. Hudson then set up a dental practice at 15 Harley Street, London – equipped with full facilities for dental surgery and anaesthesia. Here was a place to which the dentist could bring his patient and Hudson could provide the anaesthesia. And so, he became a highly skilled dental anaesthetist.

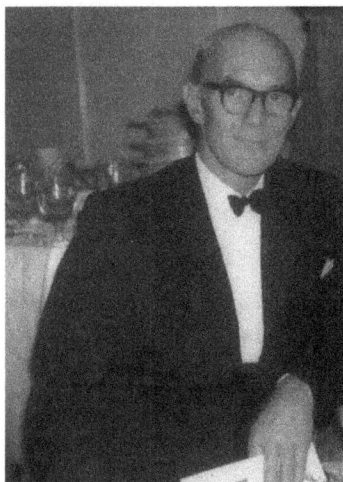

Maurice W. P. Hudson. Image courtesy of Lindsay Hudson (granddaughter).

Hudson developed a special interest also in anaesthesia for facio-maxillary surgery, and by 1941 he provided this service at Queen Mary's Ministry of Pensions Hospital, Roehampton. In 1943 he published on the head-strap harness he designed for securing nasotracheal tubes. This harness became well known, being mentioned in Noel A. Gillespie's book *Endotracheal Anaesthesia* and illustrated in the first and second editions of C.S. Ward's *Anaesthetic Equipment*. In 1948 Hudson was elected FFARCS and on the birth of the NHS, he was appointed Consultant anaesthetist to the Westminster Hospital, the Royal Free Hospital and the University College Hospital Dental Department, where he became senior anaesthetist and lecturer to dental students.

On the invitation of Stanley Drummond-Jackson (q.v. page 59) Hudson became a founder member of the Society for the Advancement of Anaesthesia in Dentistry (SAAD) in 1957. The following year he published on the remote control he devised for closing the Heidbrink valve (q.v. page 91) on a Magill (Mapleson A) circuit. This was achieved by replacing the disc and spring with a rubber tambour, connected by tubing to an air-filled balloon which on squeezing would cause the tambour to close the valve completely. This apparatus was useful in cases of head and neck surgery where the expiratory valve was inaccessible under sterile drapes – facilitating lung ventilation.

Hudson was President of SAAD from 1960 to 1963. In 1965 he published a comprehensive article on methohexitone in the Current Therapeutics section of *The Practitioner*. He opined that it was a valuable addition for those who had adequate practice in venepuncture and noted that dental surgeons were taking advantage of its property of rapid recovery, by intermittent use for conservative dental procedures lasting one to two hours. Observing that one or two very experienced dental surgeons used suxamethonium for endotracheal intubation in the dental chair, he declared that this should *not* be attempted until very experienced. This pre-empted the report from the Joint Subcommittee of the Central Health Services Council on outpatient dental anaesthesia (1967) and subsequent Drummond-Jackson libel case.

Hudson taught on all the instructional courses of SAAD until the mid-1970s, when he was compelled by arthritis to retire from practising. In 1975 he contributed to the correspondence section of the *British Medical Journal*. Therein he described his use in over 500 cases of intravenous diazepam combined with methohexitone to facilitate endotracheal intubation without suxamethonium – avoiding muscle pains; he pointed out the need for adequate oxygenation.

On Hudson's death in 1992 his Will revealed a bequest to SAAD of £1000. The SAAD Council decided to use this to establish a Maurice Hudson Archive of videotape transcriptions of the early SAAD training films. About five years later Hudson's daughter, Miss Dorothy Betty Hudson, made a generous donation to the Royal College of Anaesthetists and asked that the interest on the capital sum be used for an annual 'Maurice Hudson Prize' for the best paper on his favourite subject - resuscitation. The paper for the first award in 1998 was selected by Dr David Zideman. In the following year, advertisement in the College *Newsletter* invited competition from an "anaesthetic trainee who is the principal author of the best paper relating to resuscitation published, or accepted for publication, in a peer reviewed journal". From 2011 the criteria for the prize were extended to papers relating to the management of acutely ill patients (Table 1).

Table 1. Maurice P Hudson Prize winners

Year	Recipient	Article
1998	Rhiannon Lewis	The teaching of cardiopulmonary resuscitation in schools in Hampshire.
1999	Charles Deakin	Effects of positive end-expiratory pressure on trans-thoracic impedance – implications for defibrillation. The effects of respiratory gas composition on transthoracic impedance. A comparison of transthoracic impedance using standard defibrillation paddles and self-adhesive defibrillation pads.

2000	Simon Whyte	Neonatal resuscitation – a practical assessment.
2007	Scott Bird	Defibrillation during renal dialysis: a survey of UK practice and procedural recommendations.
2008	J Rechner	A comparison of the laryngeal mask airway with facemask and oropharyngeal airway for manual ventilation by critical care nurses in children.
2009	Lesley Green	Can't intubate, can't ventilate! A survey of knowledge skills in a large teaching hospital.
2010	Fiona Kelly	Effect of mild induced hypothermia on the myocardium.
2011	Andrew Conway Morris	Reducing ventilator-associated pneumonia in intensive care: impact of implementing a care bundle.
2012	Tariq Husain	Strategies to prevent airway complications: a survey of adult intensive care units in Australia and New Zealand.
2013	Joyce Yeung	Factors affecting team leadership skills and their relationship with quality of cardio-pulmonary resuscitation.
2015	David Hunt	Transfer of the critically ill adult patient.
2016	Annemarie Docherty	The impact of restrictive versus liberal transfusion strategies on patient outcomes in patients with cardiovascular disease excluding those undergoing cardiac surgery: a systematic review and meta-analysis.
2017	Michael Charlesworth	An observational study of critical care physicians' assessment and decision-making practices in response to patient referrals.
2018	Vasileios Zochios	The effect of high-flow nasal oxygen on hospital length of stay in cardiac surgical patients at high-risk for respiratory complications: a randomised controlled trial.

Acknowledgement

Lindsay Hudson, granddaughter of Maurice Hudson, kindly assisted with information and the photograph.

Further reading

Hudson MWP. An endotracheal harness. *British Medical Journal* 1943; **II**: 647.

Hudson MWP. Remote control for expiratory valve. *Anaesthesia* 1958; **13**: 90-91.

Hudson MW. Methohexitone. *The Practitioner* 1965; **194**: 421-5.

Hudson MW. Drug combinations for anaesthesia. *British Medical Journal* 1975; **I**: 194-5.

Sykes P. Obituary Maurice Hudson President of SAAD 1960-1963. *SAAD Digest* 1993; **10 (4)**: 69-70.

HUMPHREY ADE AND ADE-CIRCLE BREATHING SYSTEMS

David Humphrey (1947-)

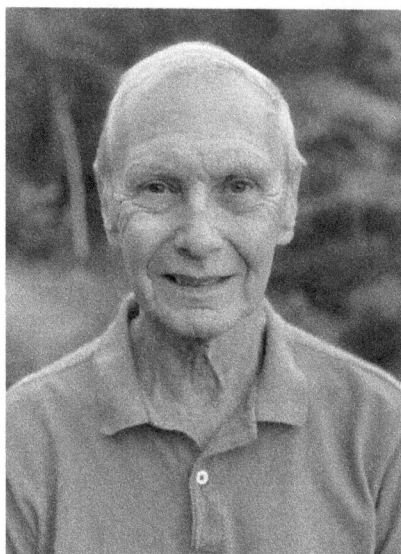

David Humphrey was born in London and educated at Winchester College. He studied medicine at University College Hospital, London and graduated MB BS in 1970. House jobs included medicine at UCH London, and surgery at North Middlesex Hospital London. In 1973 he worked as a doctor at a mission hospital in Zululand, South Africa which had few facilities and a very limited budget. Having been taught to use fresh gas flow (FGF) of 8 l/min with a Magill system and 4 l/min with a circle, he realised that the oxygen cylinders ran out very fast and were not easily refilled as this entailed an 80 km return journey over treacherous African muddy roads often unpassable for weeks. This motivated his future research in designing a breathing system which used as little fresh gas as possible, was versatile and easy to use.

After four years in Zululand, Humphrey became a trainee anaesthetist in 1978 at King Edward VIII Hospital in Durban and in 1980 graduated with a DA (SA). Within his first three months there, his attention was drawn by Prof John Downing to papers on the Bain and Lack coaxial breathing systems, published in *Anaesthesia* 1976. The thought occurred to him that the two could be combined by some sort of switch mechanism at the fresh gas flow input, to achieve the advantages of both. With Prof Downing's stimulation and help, he submitted a protocol for approval, and built a crude working device, called an ADE system as it combined the principles of Mapleson A, D and E systems.

In 1979 Humphrey used a crude capnograph to test his ADE device against the Magill and Bain systems. During spontaneous ventilation in adult anaesthetized patients, he found differences in the efficient elimination of CO_2 between all three systems. The Bain was very much less efficient as expected, the Magill much less so but there was evidence of some rebreathing. The ADE eliminated CO_2 better than the Magill which was reputed to function with maximum efficiency. Humphrey then repeated the trial with a new inline capnograph and obtained the same results. In 1980 he presented his work for the Registrar's research prize at the South African Anaesthetists' congress –

and won. The following year he presented it to the Section of Anaesthetics, Royal Society of Medicine in London – and won the Registrar's Prize essay.

Humphrey's first design of the ADE breathing system was published in *Anaesthesia* in 1983. Next this ADE system was compared with the Magill at the Royal Postgraduate Medical School, Hammersmith. The authors (J. Dixon *et al*) confirmed that in spontaneously breathing anaesthetised patients, rebreathing occurred at a significantly lower fresh gas flow with the ADE system than the Magill – published in the *Anaesthesia* in 1984.

Next Humphrey proceeded to test the ADE system in its Mapleson D/E controlled ventilation mode. This involved switching a lever on the inspiratory limb to exclude the reservoir bag, and a second lever on the expiratory limb to exclude the exhaust valve and, at the same time, open a port to connect a tube to the ventilator. The system was now just two tubes to and from the patient and connected to the ventilator, exactly the same as the Bain and T-piece systems. As expected, the results recorded for the ADE system when used with a ventilator showed no differences in function. This confirmed the ADE as a multipurpose system for adults for both spontaneous and controlled ventilation at the flick of two levers. Later in 1984 Humphrey modified the ADE to a *simpler single lever* system. He negotiated commercial production by a firm in Shrewsbury, England.

By this time Humphrey was Lecturer in the Department of Physiology, University of Natal in Durban and he turned his attention to the use of the ADE system in paediatric anaesthesia. As the resistance through the ADE system had been shown to be half that of the Magill (Dixon *et al*, 1984) Humphrey claimed that the system could be used for spontaneous respiration in children in the A mode and controlled ventilation in the E mode. This was evaluated in paediatric use (< 20 kg) at the Hospital for Sick Children, Great Ormond Street, London in 1991. The authors reported that when breathing spontaneously in the A mode, no patient experienced rebreathing at FGF 3 litre min^{-1}; rebreathing started at 124 ml kg^{-1} min^{-1}. The authors also commented that the ADE was extremely efficient in this mode. Humphrey observed that this flow was the same in his studies being 123 ml kg^{-1} min^{-1}, both studies being about three times lower than the flow 300-500 ml kg^{-1} min^{-1} recommended for the T-piece.

Humphrey then redesigned the APL valve to offer four significant advantages. It was engineered to save *all* dead space gas and only expel alveolar gas. The disc (valve seat) had to rise up a chimney (funnel) against a light spring coiled around the central spindle before it would open. The pressure generated by the spring (about 1 cm H_2O) was sufficient to force dead space gas to be saved up the inspiratory limb. The valve would then only open once the reservoir was full, which would occur if a fresh gas flow equal to alveolar ventilation was added to the bag. At this point the pressure in the bag would increase and open the valve to eliminate alveolar gas. A second benefit when recycling through a soda lime canister, was that this valve remained *closed* during most of the expiratory phase; expired gas would first flow through the canister to be saved in the reservoir bag on the inspiratory limb. Again, only once the reservoir bag was full would the valve open *automatically* to release any remaining expired gas. At no time did the valve need to be closed by the anaesthetist, a safety against barotrauma if the valve was accidentally closed too much. A third advantage was that for manual ventilation, the anaesthetist simply placed a finger on the spindle protruding above the screw cap, pushing down to close the valve (without screwing the valve down) and squeezed the bag. The last benefit was that the spring provided a small amount of positive end expiratory pressure (PEEP), which Humphrey thought would be beneficial in preventing alveolar collapse in supine anaesthetized patients, especially in the elderly and the young.

In 1999 Humphrey designed an add-on soda lime canister to make the ADE system into a recycling system as well as a semi-closed system. He positioned the reservoir bag on the inspiratory limb to conserve fresh gas and reduce circuit resistance during inspiration. To achieve this configuration with the ADE system, all that was required was to attach a specially designed canister (with built-in one-way valves) to the ADE main body, locked and sealed with just two lock nuts; it could be attached in seconds.

With P. Dobromylskyj, Humphrey presented research on the use of the ADE-circle for anaesthesia in cats and dogs at the British Small Animal Veterinary Association (BSAVA) congress at Birmingham UK in 2000. The ADE-circle was well received and soon introduced into veterinary anaesthesia – see Figure 1. By 2009 the system had been bought by over 1000 veterinary practices. In 2015 the very low fresh gas flows required of the Humphrey (semi-closed) system in Mapleson A mode were again confirmed in cats and dogs by Gale *et al* from the University of Sydney. Unfortunately, medico-legal liability regulations made it too expensive for an independent researcher to insure it for human use in the EU, but it remained useful for human use elsewhere.

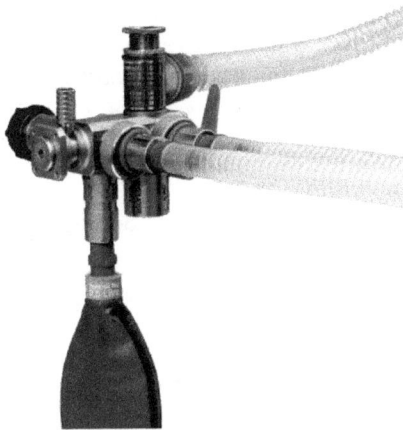
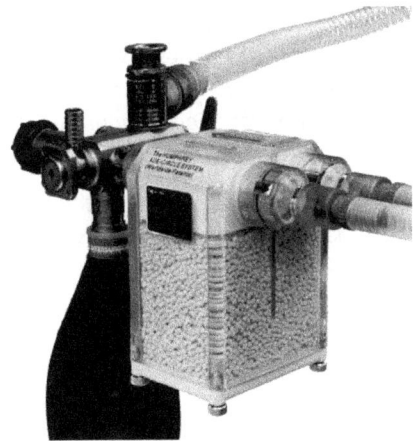

(a)	(b)

Figure 1. The Humphrey ADE anaesthetic breathing system for human and veterinary use: (a) semi-closed, (b) circle (with soda lime canister attached).

Humphrey achieved his aim of making a universal multipurpose anaesthetic breathing system that was simple and safe to use. He received two prestigious awards for the ADE breathing system: the Shell Design Award in 1985 and the SABS Design Institute Award for Engineering in 1999. Although retired from university teaching, he has continued to research and teach its use in veterinary practice, having anaesthetized among others, lions, pandas, pelicans, cats, dogs and green mambas! He retains an interest in human anaesthesia in such projects as "Operation Smile" in Madagascar and on Mercy ships where his equipment is being used.

Further reading

Humphrey D. A new anaesthetic breathing system combining Mapleson A, D and E principles. A simple apparatus for low flow universal use without carbon dioxide absorption. *Anaesthesia* 1983; **38**: 361-72.

Dixon J, Chakrabarti MK, Morgan M. An assessment of the Humphrey ADE anaesthetic system in the Mapleson A mode during spontaneous ventilation. *Anaesthesia* 1984; **39**: 593-6.

Humphrey D. The ADE anaesthetic breathing system. *Anaesthesia* 1984; **39**: 715-7.

Humphrey D, Brock-Utne JG, Downing JW. Single lever Humphrey ADE low flow universal anaesthetic breathing system. Part I: comparison with dual lever ADE, Magill and Bain systems in anaesthetized spontaneously breathing adults. *Canadian Anaesthetists' Society Journal* 1986; **33**; 698-709.

Humphrey D, Brock-Utne JG, Downing JW. Single lever Humphrey ADE low flow universal anaesthetic breathing system. Part II: Comparison with Bain system in anaesthetized adults during controlled ventilation. *Canadian Anaesthetists' Society Journal* 1986; **33**; 710-718.

Orlikowski CEP, Ewart MC, Bingham RM. The Humphrey ADE system: evaluation in paediatric use. *British Journal of Anaesthesia* 1991; 66: 253-7.

Stanway G, Magee A. Chapter 12: Anaesthesia and Analgesia. In: Mullineaux E, Jones M, Pearson AJ (Eds) *BSAVA Manual of Practical Veterinary Nursing*. Gloucester: BSAVA, 2007.

Gale E, Ticehurst KE, Zaki S. An evaluation of fresh gas flow rates for spontaneously breathing cats and small dogs on the Humphrey ADE semi-closed breathing system. *Veterinary Anaesthesia and Analgesia* 2015; 42: 292-8.

Anaequip- Vet UK, 2 Millstream Bank, Worthen, Shrewsbury S5 9EY, UK; www.anaequip.com (Accessed 5 May 2020).

BJORN IBSEN LECTURE

Bjorn Aage Ibsen (1915-2007)

Bjorn Aage Ibsen was born in 1915 in Copenhagen. He graduated MD from the University of Copenhagen in 1940 and proceeded to a post at a provincial hospital in Jutland, followed by service in several medical departments. Becoming interested in anaesthesiology, he went to do an anaesthesia residency from 1949-1950 at the Massachusetts General Hospital under Henry K. Beecher. At that time Beecher was studying blood carbon dioxide levels and acid-base balance in patients undergoing thoracic surgery. Ibsen returned in 1950 to work at the Rigshospitalet (University Hospital) in Copenhagen as a free-lance anaesthetist. In those days, anaesthesiology was not recognised as a specialty in Denmark and anaesthesia was directed by the surgeons.

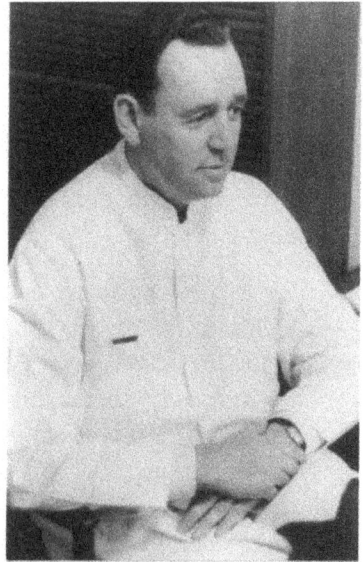

Bjorn A. Ibsen. Image provided by Dr Preben Berthelsen.

In the autumn of 1952, a severe epidemic of paralytic poliomyelitis (bulbar) struck Copenhagen. The Blegdam Hospital had just one tank ventilator and six cuirass ventilators, but 50-60 new patients were being admitted daily! The chief physician (Professor of Epidemiology), H.C.A. Lassen reluctantly consulted Ibsen. Review of the records of four children who had been ventilated but died from the disease, revealed that they had very high serum bicarbonate levels; shortly before death they had been noted to have high blood pressure and sweating. The physicians had interpreted the blood chemistry as metabolic alkalosis, but Ibsen realised that this was incorrect. The clinical picture indicated carbon dioxide accumulation caused by under-ventilation and non-clearance of secretions; biochemically there was respiratory acidosis with some metabolic compensation. The solution he proposed was insertion of a cuffed tracheostomy tube (under local anaesthesia) and intermittent positive pressure ventilation by squeezing the bag of a 'to-and-fro' system with carbon dioxide absorption (Waters). A clinical trial on one patient (a girl aged 12) was successful and then the method was employed on all the patients needing it, by relays of medical students squeezing the bags. The result was a dramatic fall in mortality. The epidemic subsided in the spring of 1953.

Ibsen was then appointed at the Kommunehospitalet in Copenhagen to organize the anaesthetic service and there he opened the first intensive care unit in the world. This was a *general* intensive therapy unit, providing 24 hours a day monitoring and treatment of all types of medical and surgical cases with respiratory or circulatory problems. The first publication on intensive therapy was by Bjorn Ibsen and Norwegian anaesthetist Tone Dahl Kvittingen in *Nordisk Medicin*, 18 September 1958. Although written in Danish, there was a resume in English and by this time Copenhagen had achieved international status in anaesthesia through the Anaesthesiology Centre Copenhagen, which had begun in 1950. The idea was gradually taken up worldwide.

Ibsen produced two textbooks on anaesthetics and intensive care in the 1950s (in Danish). In 1961 he was appointed to the inaugural editorial board of the journal *Acta Anaesthesiologica Scandinavica*; issues began in 1967 and he remained on the board until 1971. He published about 50 papers on various aspects of intensive therapy in peer reviewed journals. Due to restructuring of health care in Copenhagen, acute care was discontinued at the Kommunehospitalet in about 1975 and, to avoid transferring to another unit, Ibsen began a new chapter in his life – developing a major interest in pain clinics and chronic pain. Honours he received include: the Danish poliomyelitis medal and anaesthetic medal, the Purkinje medal from Czechoslovakia, and honorary membership of the European Resuscitation Council.

From 1990 the Danish Society of Anaesthesiology and Intensive Care Medicine arranged the Bjorn Ibsen Lecture to be held in Denmark. Initially it alternated with the Ole Secher Lecture (q.v. page 212), but since 2006 it has occurred triennially due to the addition of the Henning Ruben lecture to the series.

Acknowledgement

Dr Preben Berthelsen kindly provided the list of Bjorn Ibsen lectures.

Table 1. Bjorn Ibsen lecturers and lecture titles

Year	Lecturer	Title
1990	Lis Dragsted	Utility value studies of intensive therapy.
1992	Dag Lundberg	The development of modern shock therapy.
1994	Bent Juhl	From IPPV to LTMV. From intensive care unit to respiratory centre.
1996	Lars Heslet	The balance between pro- and anti-inflammatory mechanisms of systemic inflammation.
1998	Hans Flaatten	Evidence based intensive medicine.
2000	Anders Larsson	Intensive therapy – from revolution to evolution.
2002	Luciano Gattinoni	Pathophysiology of acute respiratory distress: implications for mechanical ventilation.
2004	Graham Ramsay	Surviving sepsis campaign guidelines.
2006	Jukka Takala	Intensive care 10 years in the future.
2009	Anders Larsson	NOT HELD
2011	Else Tonnesen	Intensive therapy – what have we learned since the polio epidemic?
2014	Bodil Steen Rasmussen	Oxygen treatment and the intensive patient: "too much of a good thing?"
2017	Lone Nikolajsen	Pain – an anaesthesiological challenge?

Further reading

Berthelsen PG, Cronqvist M. The first intensive care unit in the world: Copenhagen 1953. *Acta Anaesthesiologica Scandinavica* 2003; **47**: 1190-5.

Zorab J. Bjorn Ibsen. In: Baskett JF, Baskett TF (Eds.) *Resuscitation Greats*. Bristol: Clinical Press Ltd., 2007; 293-9.

Berthelsen PG. Bjorn Aage Ibsen (1915-2007). in Memoriam. *Acta Anaesthesiologica Scandinavica* 2007; **51**: 1292-3.

Obituary. Bjorn Ibsen. *British Medical Journal* 2007; **335**:674.

Bernard Richard Miller Johnson (1905-1959)

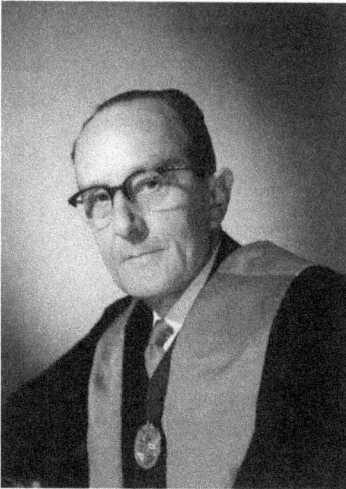

Bernard R.M. Johnson. Image by kind permission of the Royal College of Anaesthetists.

Bernard Johnson was born in London, England in 1905 and educated at Brighton College. At the age of seventeen he began Medical School at the Middlesex Hospital and qualified in 1927. After house jobs he had a year abroad, where he was interested in tropical medicine, but returned to the Middlesex to begin training in anaesthesia. He proved to be adept in this specialty: by 1933 he was appointed anaesthetist to St Peter's Hospital and to the dental department of University College Hospital. Appointment to the full staff of the Middlesex Hospital followed in 1936. He was highly proficient in the use of the new intravenous anaesthetic drugs and endotracheal anaesthesia, building up an extensive private practice. This included working with R.R. Macintosh and W.S. O'Connell in the 'Mayfair Gas Company' based in Harley Street, London – they carried their apparatus in a car to the various dental surgeries and nursing homes. Early in 1939 he was awarded the Diploma in Anaesthetics (DA) without examination.

Soon after the outbreak of the Second World War he joined the Royal Army Medical Corps where his service was exemplary, rising to the rank of Lieutenant-Colonel and Advisor in Anaesthetics to the Central Mediterranean Force. During this period (1943) he joined the Council of the Association of Anaesthetists of Great Britain and Ireland (AAGBI).

Johnson returned to his civilian practice in 1946 and served as Honorary Treasurer of the AAGBI 1947-50. In 1949 he contributed the chapter on intravenous anaesthesia in Frankis T. Evans' textbook *Modern Practice in Anaesthesia*. He was appointed civilian Consultant in Anaesthesia to the War Office in 1952. Motivated to improve the academic standing of anaesthesia, he was much involved in the AAGBI's petition for a Faculty of Anaesthetists within the Royal College of Surgeons. This came into being in 1948 with Archibald Marston as Dean and Johnson as Vice Dean; Johnson served as the second Dean from 1952 until 1955, in which year he was appointed Senior Consultant Anaesthetist at the Middlesex Hospital. As Dean of the Faculty, Johnson was involved in the initiation of the diploma of the Fellow of the Faculty of Anaesthetists of the Royal College of Surgeons (FFARCS) examination in

November 1953 and continued to be an examiner himself. He travelled in Europe and to Australia on invitation to give lectures and demonstrations. After his term as Dean he continued as chairman of the Research Committee of the Faculty, securing funding from the British Oxygen Company (BOC) for a professorial chair. Dr Ronald F. Woolmer was the first appointed to this BOC Chair of Anaesthesia in January 1959.

Johnson was awarded Honorary Fellowship of the Association of Greek Surgeons and of the Royal Australian College of Surgeons. On home soil he was President of the anaesthetic section of the Royal Society of Medicine 1955-56 and was elected FRCS in 1956. Sadly, he died suddenly in May 1959. Before his death he contributed the chapter on anaesthesia in genito-urinary surgery in the textbook *General Anaesthesia* edited by Frankis Evans and Cecil Gray, which was published that year.

In June 1961 a memorial plaque to Bernard Johnson was unveiled in the main laboratory of the Research Department of Anaesthetics of the Royal College of Surgeons of England. Collections for a Bernard Johnson Memorial Fund realised £4500, the plan being to establish the Bernard Johnson Anaesthetic Tutorship for Postgraduate Students. The Faculty of Anaesthetists then provided the Bernard Johnson Postgraduate Advisor. Gradually this post evolved from one to three Advisors.

One Advisor

Initially the role of the Advisor was concentrated on supporting the Overseas Doctors Training Scheme (ODTS). From the 1980s, increasing numbers of women were appointed to training posts in anaesthesia and thus the need for part-time or flexible training. By 1992 the Faculty became the Royal College of Anaesthetists.

Two Advisors

From 1997 the post of Bernard Johnson Advisor was upgraded to *two* positions: (1) the ODTS; (2) guidance for unsuccessful candidates at the FRCA examinations *and* giving advice about flexible training.

(1) The medical training initiative (MTI) was launched by the Department of Health UK in 2009, and the ODTS became rebranded under the MTI from 2011: to the International Programmes (IP).
(2) In the new millennium, interviewing of candidates who were unsuccessful in the FRCA examinations, was taken over by the Examinations Committee. By 2006 flexible training began to be termed 'less than full-time training' (LTFT).

Three Advisors

By 2013 a *third* post of Bernard Johnson Advisor was added:

(3) Bernard Johnson Advisor for Academic Training in recognition of the importance of academia within training. The role was to facilitate academic careers especially when blended with dual training in anaesthetics and intensive care medicine or pain medicine.

Regarding the other two posts:

(1) IP: the College continued the MTI scheme to support trainees coming to the UK for up to 24 months. In addition, it developed fellowships for UK trainees wishing to undertake 'out of programme experience' (OOPE). Placements in Low to Middle Income Countries (LMIC) were arranged, in which up to six months of OOPE would be recognised as part of the UK training programme. By 2016 this post was renamed 'Global Partnerships'.
(2) LTFT continued.

The term of office of the three Bernard Johnson Advisors is currently three years, renewable for a further 3-year term.

Further reading

Obituary Dr Bernard Johnson. *Anaesthesia* 1959; **14**: 419-21.

Royal College of Anaesthetists Report 1996/97: Bernard Johnson Advisers in Postgraduate Anaesthesia Studies.

Jones M. Flexible training in anaesthesia. *The Royal College of Anaesthetists Bulletin* 2006; **40**: 2022-5.

Evans C. Bernard Johnson Advisor – less than full-time training. *The Royal College of Anaesthetists Bulletin* 2011; **66**: 6-8.

Wark K. Report from the Bernard Johnson Advisor on the International Programme. *The Royal College of Anaesthetists Bulletin* 2011; **68**: 6-8.

James J. The role of the Bernard Johnson Adviser for the International Programmes. *The Royal College of Anaesthetists Bulletin* 2014; **83**: 33-35.

Langton J, James J, Burke M. RCoA Global Partnerships – the legacy of Bernard Johnson. *The Royal College of Anaesthetists Bulletin* 2016; **100**: 52-54.

JORGENSEN TECHNIQUE

Niels Bjorn Jorgensen (1894-1974)

The Jorgensen technique of intravenous sedation was introduced by Niels Bjorn Jorgensen in 1945 at Loma Linda University, California. It was promoted for use in conjunction with local anaesthesia in dentistry.

Niels B. Jorgensen was born on the island of Fyn, Denmark. Brought up in the tradition of helping work on his father's farm, he was initially not a promising scholar. But at the age of 17 an illness instigated his attention to study, and he proceeded to pass the exams for entrance to Copenhagen University. In 1919 he enrolled in the School of Dentistry at the University of California (Berkeley). He graduated DDS in 1923 and obtained a post as resident in oral surgery at the Southern California Edison Company hospitals. There he encountered strong men who would faint at the sight of a needle and dental chair, prompting his interest in sedation.

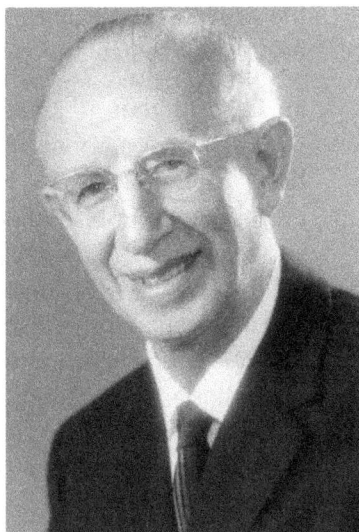

Niels Bjorn Jorgensen. Image courtesy of the School of Dentistry, Loma Linda University.

Next Jorgensen became friendly with the Chairman of Stomatology at the College of Medical Evangelists, Richard H. Riethmuller who was Professor of Anesthesia at the University of Southern California School of Dentistry, and who in 1912 had produced *Local Anesthesia in dentistry*, the English translation of Guido Fischer's textbook in German. Riethmuller's Assistant Professor of Stomatology was Herbert Childs, who engaged Jorgensen from 1942 to give lectures on sedation and local anaesthesia at the White Memorial Hospital in Los Angeles, the site of the training programmes for the clinical students, interns and residents of the Schools of Medicine and Dentistry, Loma Linda University. There Jorgensen undertook a course on surgical anatomy of the head and neck. He then expanded his University involvement, attending the Loma Linda campus. From 1945 he was assisted by Dr Forrest Leffingwell (who became Professor of Anesthesiology at the College of Medical Evangelists) in developing intravenous sedation. They started with administration of pentobarital sodium and later added pethidine (meperidine) and scopolamine (hyoscine).

Jorgensen did important anatomical work on measurement of skulls to improve the performance of local anaesthetic blocks of the maxillary nerve and the inferior alveolar nerve, publishing these in the *Journal of Oral Surgery* in 1948 and 1952 respectively. During this time, he also facilitated a film on the advantage to children of combining oral sedation with local anaesthetic nerve block to achieve painless dentistry.

In 1953 Jorgensen joined the new School of Dentistry at Loma Linda University as Professor of Oral Surgery. He lectured and exhibited a film at the Royal Dental College in Copenhagen, Denmark in 1956 where there was much interest in his intravenous sedation technique. The American Dental Society of Anesthesiology presented him with its Heidbrink Award (q.v. page 92) in 1960. In 1961 Jorgensen and Leffingwell published a landmark paper "Premedication in Dentistry" in *Dental Clinics of North America*. Therein was described their method of intravenous sedation when required with local anaesthesia, emphasising *slow* injection of small increments of pentobarbital sodium, followed if desired by small dosage of pethidine with scopolamine – and having a vasopressor ready in case of hypotension, as well as oxygen and equipment for instant resuscitation.

Jorgensen put much energy into producing teaching films. Notably, his film "Inferior Alveolar, Lingual and Buccal Nerve Block" won the 1965 Grand Prix Award in Paris. The Society for the Advancement of Anaesthesia in Dentistry (SAAD) awarded him the John Mordaunt Prize in 1966. A total of nine films were produced.

The book *Premedication, Local and General Anaesthesia in Dentistry* by Jorgensen and Jess Hayden, Jr. (Associate Professor of Anatomy) was published in 1967. In this the "Jorgensen technique" was described.

1. Pentobarbitone in 10 mg doses injected every 30 seconds, engaging the patient in casual conversation – until relaxed and lightly sedated;
2. Supplementation by a mixture of pethidine 25 mg and hyoscine 0.32 mg diluted in 5 ml to optimize;
3. Local blockade performed and dental treatment performed.

This book was sold throughout the USA and Europe, translated into Spanish for distribution in South America, and ran to three editions.

Jorgensen retired at Loma Linda University in 1969, but he continued to teach as Emeritus Professor of Oral Surgery. The Jorgensen technique was described in standard anaesthetic textbooks well into the 1980s. Since then, more suitable drugs have arrived, in comparison to which the original

Jorgensen technique, though safe, had long induction and recovery times with drowsiness and 'hangover' effects. However, the principles which he espoused were years ahead of the guidelines on intravenous sedation eventually produced by various anaesthetic associations. These concepts – keeping the patient relaxed but conscious with all protective reflexes intact and responding rationally to verbal commands – have remained key to intravenous sedation while pain is controlled by excellent local anaesthesia.

Further reading

Jorgensen NB, Leffingwell F. Premedication in Dentistry. *Dental Clinics of North America* 1961; **5**: 299-308.

Jorgensen NB, Hayden J. *Premedication, Local and General Anaesthesia in Dentistry*. London: Henry Kimpton, 1967.

Drummond-Jackson SL. "The Jorgensen Technique" a tribute to Niels Bjorn Jorgensen. *Anesthesia Progress* 1969; **16**: 119-22.

Hayden J. The Limits of Excellence: What One Man Can Do. *Anesthesia Progress* 1978; **25**: 75-84.

JOULE – ENERGY SETTING FOR DEFIBRILLATOR

James Prescott Joule (1818-1889)

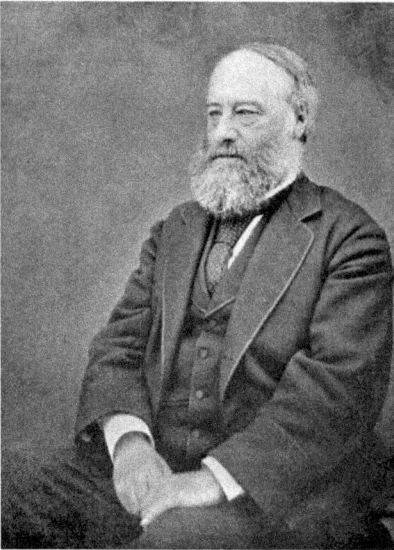

James Prescott Joule. Image in Public Domain. Credit: Wikimedia Commons.

In the event of a cardiac arrest in the operating theatre, it is usually the anaesthetist who will lead the resuscitation including the application of defibrillator pads and the discharge of an electric shock (biphasic direct current) by a defibrillator. The energy of the shock is measured in **joules** (J) – usually set at 150 J. In cardiothoracic surgery when the chest is open, internal defibrillation is performed with paddles applied directly across the ventricles; this requires considerably less energy than external defibrillation: 10-20 J is used. Following cardiac surgery, patients are commonly nursed in a cardiac intensive care unit, with a defibrillator on standby. In outreach, anaesthetists are key members of resuscitation teams and often lead the resuscitation algorithm in accordance with Advanced Life Support guidelines, including biphasic shock if indicated. Anaesthetists may also need to perform cardioversion (synchronized shock) with a biphasic defibrillator in theatre or critical care settings – to treat certain tachyarrhythmias; the energy required for this is up to 200 J. For defibrillation in paediatrics (child < 8 years), special paediatric electrodes are applied and far less shock energy is discharged, e.g. 4 J/kg.

James Prescott Joule was born on 24 December 1818 in Salford, Lancashire, England into a wealthy family, owners of the largest brewery in Manchester. He had a spinal weakness resulting in a degree of kyphosis, which contributed to him having a shy and retiring personality. From the age of fifteen, he was tutored in chemistry privately by John Dalton, the propounder of atomic theory. Joule began his own research from the age of nineteen, by which time he worked in the management of the brewery. He was interested in the production of heat by mechanical work and electricity and he could afford to pay an instrument maker to produce a highly accurate thermometer. In 1840 he determined that the heat generated in a wire by an electric current was proportional to the resistance and the square of the current (Joule's Law). Although his abstract on this was rejected for publication in the *Transactions of* the *Royal Society*, it was printed in their *Proceedings*. In 1842 he was elected to the Manchester Literary & Philosophical Society.

Comparing the steam engine and the electric motor, Joule was interested in determining and improving the efficiency of machines, which dissipated much energy as unwanted heat. In 1843, he designed an experiment to determine the amount of mechanical work required to produce a given amount of heat: 'the mechanical equivalent of heat'. He went on to design further experiments for this measurement. Oft-told is his apparatus of 1845: within an insulated copper cylinder (calorimeter) of water, a paddle wheel was rotated via a coupling to a drum which was rotated by cords attached via two pulleys to falling weights – the work done on the water caused a rise in temperature, which was measured. Baffles in the cylinder prevented the water from whirling around. Sixteen rewinds to repeat the fall of weights was required to generate enough heat for a small rise in temperature. By 1847 he had acquired much experience with this apparatus, and stated that the mechanical equivalent of heat was a physical constant of about 782 ft.lb.wt./B.Th.U. (in the units of the day). So began the establishment of the equivalence of heat and other forms of energy. This work was the basis on which Hermann von Helmholtz stated the Law of Conservation of Energy in 1847 (later called the First Law of Thermodynamics).

Joule presented the results of his measurements in June 1847 at the annual meeting of the British Association for the Advancement of Science held in Oxford. Most of his audience were sceptical – Joule was not given recognition by the scientific community. Reasoning that the expenditure of mechanical energy should render water at the bottom of a waterfall warmer than at the top, he challenged the sceptics to measure this temperature difference: 1° F. for a fall of 778 feet.

Two months later, Joule married and took his bride on honeymoon to the French Alps, aiming to measure the temperature difference in the water falling the height of the Cascade de Sallanches at Chamonix. There he met William Thomson (later to be Lord Kelvin), who joined in, but they failed to get a good measurement because of the spray. Thomson befriended Joule and gave due credit to his work. The two collaborated and in 1852 they discovered the 'Joule-Thomson effect': when a real gas is forced through a plug or valve and is kept insulated, it does work in expanding and cools itself.

By this time Joule had begun to receive honours. He was made a Fellow of the Royal Society in 1850 and in 1852 he received the Royal Medal for his 1850 paper "On the Mechanical Equivalent of Heat" published in the *Philosophical Transactions of the Royal Society of London*.

After just seven years of marriage, Joule's wife died in 1854 and he remained a widower for the rest of his life. He was elected President of the Manchester Literary and Philosophical Society in 1860 and again in 1868. From 1863 he was a member of the British Association for the Advancement of Science's Committee on electrical units.

From 1875 to 1877 Joule devoted himself to the improved measurement of the mechanical equivalent of heat, for which he received a grant from the Royal Society. In the cellar of his house in Salford, he set up a refined paddle wheel apparatus. The calorimeter was not fixed but was held in balance against the frictional drag of water as the paddle wheel was rotated by cranks – this was the method of Gustave-Adolphe Hirn of Colmar, France. Joule suspended the cylinder on a wire and kept it in equilibrium by an opposing couple applied by cord passing round a groove in the calorimeter and over a pulley to a weight at each end. With this he obtained his final value for the mechanical equivalent of heat: 772.55 ft.lb.wt./B.Th.U. This was published in *Philosophical Transactions* in 1878.

Numerous honours were bestowed on Joule: he was awarded the Copley Medal by the Royal Society in 1870 "for his experimental researches on the dynamical theory of heat" and by 1871 he had received three honorary degrees. He was elected President of the British Association for the Advancement of Science in 1872 and again in 1887. The Royal Society of Arts awarded him the Albert Medal in 1880 " for having established, after most laborious research, the true relation between heat, electricity and mechanical work, thus affording to the engineer a sure guide in the application of science to industrial pursuits".

From 1886 Joule's health seriously declined. He died in 1889 and was buried in Sale, Greater Manchester. The head of his gravestone is inscribed with the number "772.55". A statue of Joule was commissioned and placed in the Manchester Town Hall, where it stands opposite that of John Dalton. In his honour, there is a white marble tablet in the north choir aisle of Westminster Abbey, London; it is inscribed "James Prescott Joule F.R.S., of Manchester, in recognition of services to science, in establishing The Law of the Conservation of Energy and determining The Mechanical Equivalent of Heat". The Joule's family brewery is still operating, but it has relocated to Market Drayton in Shropshire. There is a public house named "The J.P. Joule" in Sale.

In 1895, Carl von Linde and William Hampson independently exploited the Joule-Thomson effect to use air as a refrigerant. This idea has continued in modern refrigeration processes. Anaesthetists came to realise that the Joule-Thomson effect contributed to the cooling of nitrous oxide cylinders when in use, but that the main cause was the latent heat of vaporization.

The **joule** was adopted as the unit of electrical work, heat, mechanical energy and work in 1948 at the 9th General Conference on Weights and Measures, avoiding the calorie as far as possible. This unit was also formally approved in 1960 in the International System of Units (SI). It is now defined as:

- the work done when the point of application of a force of one newton is displaced through a distance of 1 metre in the direction of the force
- the work done per second by a current of 1 ampere flowing through a resistance of 1 ohm.

A postage stamp of Joule, in a set of five commemorating Grand Physics, was issued by Guinea-Bissau in 2009 – see Figure 1.

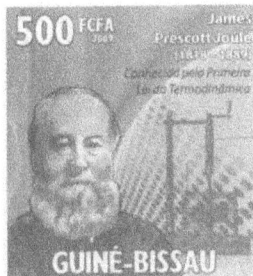

Figure 1. James Prescott Joule on postage stamp of Guinea-Bissau. The background illustration is Joule's apparatus for measuring the mechanical equivalent of heat.

Further reading

Defibrillation (Chapter 9). In: *Advanced Life Support* (6th Ed.). Resuscitation Council (UK), 2011.

Cardwell DSL. *James Joule: A Biography*. Manchester: Manchester University Press, 1989.

FOSTER KENNEDY REVIEW

Robert Foster Kennedy (1884-1952)

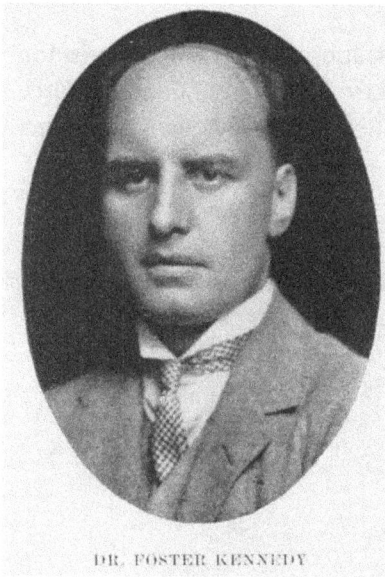

Image credit: Wikimedia Commons

The 'Foster Kennedy review' was a high impact paper, condemning the use of spinal anaesthesia, which was published in the October 1950 issue of *Surgery, Gynecology and Obstetrics*. The first author of the paper was R. Foster Kennedy, the Professor of Neurology at Cornell University and head of the neurological service at Bellevue Hospital, New York, USA. Titled "The grave spinal cord paralyses caused by spinal anesthesia", the paper reported 12 cases from the literature and another 3 from Kennedy in 1945. It pointed out that often spinal cord symptoms appeared long after the patient had been discharged from surgical care, so that the association between progressive paralysis of the legs and the previous spinal anaesthetic was not noted. The review was widely read by surgeons and enthusiastically reported in the lay press in the USA, intimidating some anaesthetists to desist from subarachnoid block. This was despite a major weakness in the paper, viz. the lack of detail concerning the conditions and level of competence in the spinal anaesthesia. Furthermore, there was no denominator data, as pointed out in a response to the journal by Henry K. Beecher, Professor in Anaesthesia at the Massachusetts General Hospital.

In the UK, the 'Foster Kennedy review' was not even mentioned in the two main anaesthetic journals for over two years. However, in October 1953 the Woolley and Roe case came to Court and attracted much publicity. Indeed, following this case, spinal anaesthesia in the UK went into decline for some 25 years.

By 1954, Robert Dripps and Leroy Vandam of the University of Pennsylvania published a long-term follow-up of 10098 spinal anaesthetics, finding no major neurological sequelae; minor sequelae occurred in 0.8% of the series: residual signs or symptoms of numbness, which were mostly transient. This study seemed to vindicate the technique in the USA.

Robert Foster Kennedy was born in Belfast and was educated at Royal School, Dungannon in Northern Ireland. He studied medicine at Queens University, Belfast and passed his final examinations at the Royal University of Ireland, Dublin in 1906. Soon after, he obtained a resident medical post at the National Hospital for Nervous Diseases at Queens Square in London. There he was influenced by Victor Horsley and others, advancing to become a respected neurologist with publications on syringomyelia. He obtained the MD of Queens University, Belfast "with high commendation" in 1910, in which year he moved to a post at the Neurological Institute in New York.

In 1911 Foster Kennedy published perhaps his most famous paper on the diagnosis of frontal lobe tumours by the signs of ipsilateral optic atrophy and contralateral disk oedema (papilloedema), which came to be known as "Foster Kennedy syndrome". He was elected Fellow of the Royal Society of Edinburgh in 1912.

During the First World War he served in France: initially for the French Army, then the British (Royal Army Medical Corps) and finally the American Army (Harvard Surgical Unit, under Harvey Cushing) until the end of the war. He made a study of shell shock and attained the rank of Captain.

Returning to the USA, he was appointed Professor of Neurology at Cornell University and head of the neurological service at Bellevue Hospital in 1919. His reputation spread – as a neurologist, teacher and speaker. In 1938 he was president of the Association for Research in Nervous and Mental Diseases, and in 1940 he became president of the American Neurologic Association.

From the late 1930s Kennedy expressed his controversial views on eugenics. He supported castration of some "defectives": limiting this to the feebleminded. Early in 1939 he was briefly the president of the Euthanasia Society of America. He stated his support for euthanasia "for creatures born defective", but not voluntary euthanasia for those seeking an end to pain.

Foster Kennedy was considered an excellent British ambassador to the USA. Despite declining health, he travelled to Queens University, Belfast in 1951 to receive the honorary degree of D.Sc. Later in the year he became terminally ill with polyarteritis nodosa.

Further reading

Kennedy F, Effron AS, Perry G. The grave spinal cord paralyses caused by spinal anesthesia. *Surgery, Gynecology and Obstetrics* 1950; **91**: 385-98.

Dripps RD, Vandam LD. Long-term follow-up of patients who received 10,098 spinal anesthetics. I: Failure to discover major neurological sequelae. *Journal of the American Medical Association* 1954; **156**: 1486-91.

Obituary R. Foster Kennedy, M.D., F.R.S.Ed. *British Medical Journal* 1952; **I**: 165-6.

Dictionary of Ulster Biography. Robert Foster Kennedy (1884-1952): Physician; Neurologist. http://www.newulsterbiography.co.uk (accessed 26 November 2019).

Offen ML. Dealing with "defectives" – Foster Kennedy and William Lennox on eugenics. *Neurology* 2003; **61**: 668-73.

DAVID M. LITTLE, JR. PRIZE

David Mason Little, Jr. (1920-1981)

David M. Little was born in Boston MA and educated at Middlesex School and Princeton University NJ, USA. He then studied medicine at Harvard Medical School, graduating in 1944, and proceeded to internship at Hartford Hospital, Connecticut. This was followed by military service in the US Navy. In 1947 he returned to Hartford Hospital to do a residency in anaesthesiology under Dr Ralph M. Tovell. Next, he took up private practice in Stamford, Connecticut until 1951, when he was appointed Assistant Professor of Anesthesiology at Yale University School of Medicine in New Haven CT. He served again in the US Navy during the Korean War from 1953 to 1955. On his return in 1955, he moved back to Hartford Hospital to be a Senior Staff Anesthesiologist.

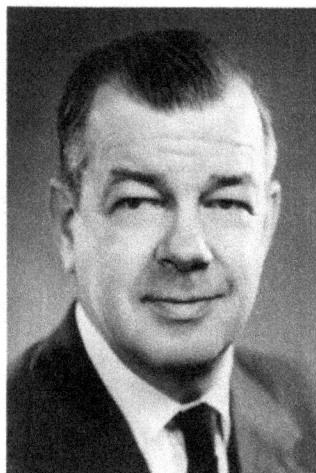

David M. Little. Image courtesy of the Wood Library-Museum of Anesthesiology.

Little was highly respected as a teacher in the art and science of anaesthesia. He published much on diverse aspects of anaesthesiology in peer reviewed journals over a period of 33 years. In 1957 he began a bimonthly "Classical File" in the *Survey of Anesthesiology* (edited by C. Ronald Stephen, q.v. page 221), collecting seminal papers from the 1700s through to the 1960s. Early letters and scientific papers were reprinted, all preceded by Little's excellent introductory comments, which provided the background information and captured all the salient points of the article. He was co-author to Stephen of the book *Halothane (Fluothane)* in 1961. The New England Society of Anesthesiologists elected him President for 1962-63.

In 1968 Little co-edited with T.K. Burnap a book *The flying death*, a compilation of classic papers and commentary on curare: volume 6 (2) in the International Anesthesia Clinics series. He served the American Society of Anesthesiologists (ASA) in several capacities: Chairman of the Section on Education, General Chairman of the Annual Meeting, Secretary of the Board of Trustees of the Wood Library-Museum (WLM), and Chairman of the Board of Directors' Committee on Scientific Affairs. A Diplomate of the American Board of Anesthesiology, he advanced in that body to be Director, Secretary-Treasurer and President. He was honoured by the Horace Wells Club Award (q.v. page 243) in 1972 and elected President of the ASA for 1974, followed by the Distinguished Service Award of the ASA in 1979.

Little continued the Classical File series for 25 years, right up to his untimely demise in 1981. No doubt he had hoped to attend the First International Symposium on the History of Anaesthesia in the spring of 1982 – this in turn led to the formation of the Anesthesia History Association (AHA) the following year. The AHA founders, Roderick Calverley and Selma Calmes were also WLM Trustees, and they supported the editing of Little's Classical Files by C. Ronald Stephen and colleagues into one book. This was published by the WLM in 1985: while many historical letters were provided in full, most papers were reduced to summaries; but Little's acclaimed introductions were unaltered. In the same year, the AHA announced that it was establishing a David M. Little, Jr. Prize for outstanding studies in the history of anaesthesiology. It was proposed that this would be an annual award at the Annual Meeting of the AHA (Table 1).

Table 1. David M. Little, Jr. Prize winners (1998-2011)

Year	Recipient	Article
1997	Leroy D. Vandam	The Last Days of William Green Morton.
1998	Emanuel M. Papper	Anaesthesia and the Surgical Experience.
1999	Norman Bergman	The Genesis of Surgical Anesthesia.
2000	Donald Caton	What a Blessing She had Chloroform: the Medical and Social Response to the Pain of Childbirth from 1800 to the Present.
2001	M.S. Albin	The use of anesthetics during the Civil War, 1861-1865.
2002	David B. Waisel	The role of World War II and the European theatre of operations in the development of anesthesiology as a physician specialty in the U.S.A.
2003	Maltby J.R. (Ed.)	Notable Names in Anaesthesia.
2004	P. Vinten-Johansen, H. Brody, N. Paneth, S. Rachman, M. Rip	Cholera, Chloroform, and the Science of Medicine: A Life of John Snow.
2005	Lucien E.Morris, M.E. Schroeder, M.E. Warner (Eds.)	A Celebration of 75 Years Honoring Ralph Milton Waters, M.D., Mentor to a Profession.
2006	D.R. Bacon, M.J. Lema, K.E. McGoldrick, (Eds.) David C. Lai	The American Society of Anesthesiologists: A Century of Challenges and Progress. Pentothal Postcards.
2007	E. Kalliardou, A.G. Tsiotou, D. Velegrakis, A. Avgerinopoulou, E. Poulakou, L. Papadimitriou	Historical aspects of inhalation anesthesia in children: ether and chloroform.
2008	M. Keith Sykes, John Bunker	Anaesthesia and the Practice of Medicine: Historical Perspectives.
2009	J. Thirlwell, R.J. Bailey (Eds.) E. Lowenstein, B. McPeek (Eds.)	Supplement 1 of *Anesthesia and Intensive Care* 2008, Vol.36. Enduring Contributions of Henry K. Beecher Medicine, Science and Society.
2010	David Shephard	From Craft to Specialty: A Medical and Social History of Anesthesia and its Changing Role in Health Care.
2011	Rajesh P. Haridas	Photographs of Early Ether Anesthesia in Boston: The Daguerreotypes of Albert Southworth & Josiah Hawes.

Table 2. David M. Little, Jr. Prize winners (2012-2018)

Year	Book	Journal Article	Other Media
2012	Gerald L. Zeitlin. Laughing and Crying about Anesthesia: A Memoir of Risk and Safety.	G.S. Bause, C.C. Tandy. Remembering Patrick P. Sim, MLS (1939-2010): Our "Tiger Amongst the Tomes" at WLM.	-
2013	P. Sim, D. Caton, K.E. McGoldrick, P. Snider, F.A. Reilly. The Heritage of Anesthesia: P. Sim's Annotated Bibliography of Rare Book Collection of the WLM.	S. Shafer, G. Bause, D. Bacon, S. Calmes, J. Edmonson, K.McGoldrick, *et al.* The Giants Behind the Journal.	B.E. Smith. Videotaped interviews for 2012 for J.W. Pender Collection of Living History.
2014	E.I. Eger II, L.J. Saidman, R.N. Westhorpe (Eds.). The Wondrous Story of Anesthesia.	Christine M. Ball. The Foregger Midget: A Machine that Travelled.	C.L. Mai, M. Yaster, P.G. Firth, A. Zulfiqar, S. Rodriguez, L. Chu, *et al.* The History of Pediatric Anesthesia Timeline Project.
2015	-	George S. Bause. "Masters of Anaesthesia" MSA Degrees During the 1893 World's Fair	Peter J. Featherstone. History of Anaesthesia Society Website.
2016	Alistair G. McKenzie. The Centenary of the Scottish Society of Anaesthetists 1914-2014.	Anne L. Craig, Sukumar K. Desai. Human Medical Experimentation with Extreme Prejudice: Lessons from the Doctors' Trial at Nuremberg.	M. Cronin, C. Ball. Trailblazers & Peacekeepers: Honouring the ANZAC Spirit. G. Kaye Museum Anaesthetic History Online Exhibition.
2017	M.G. Cooper, C.M. Ball, J.R. Thirlwell. Proceedings of the 8th International Symposium on the History of Anaesthesia.	M.L. Edwards, D.B. Waisel. Geoffrey Kaye's Center of Excellence for the Australian Society of Anaesthetists.	D. Drzymalski, A. Miller, W. Camann. From the Mayflower to the Maternity Ward: Obstetric Anesthesia & Mt. Auburn Cemetery. SOAP & Youtube video.
2018	Akitomo Matsuki. The Origin and Evolution of Anesthesia in Japan.	Adrian A. Matioc. An Anesthesiologist's Perspective on the History of Basic Airway Management: The "Artisanal Anesthetic" Era: 1846 to 1904.	-
2019	Manisha S. Desai and Sukumar P. Desai (Eds.). Proceedings of the 9th International Symposium on the History of Anesthesia.	Peter J. Featherstone. Improvised Anesthesia, Surgery, and Resuscitation in Far East Prisoner of War Camps, 1942 to 1945.	-

As shown in Table 1, there was a long delay in commencing the award. Initially there was just one prize each year for the best paper or book published in the preceding year. From 2012 the awards were expanded to include best journal article, best book and best 'other media' (Table 2); there have also been occasional "special awards".

Further reading

Little DM. *Classical Anesthesia Files*. Park Ridge, Illinois: Wood Library-Museum of Anesthesiology, 1985.

Organizational News. David M. Little, Jr. Prize. *Anesthesia History Association Newsletter* 1985; 3(3): 2.

Bacon DR, McGoldrick KE, Lema MJ (Eds.). *The American Society of Anesthesiologists – A Century of Challenges and Progress*. Park Ridge, Illinois: Wood Library-Museum of Anesthesiology, 2005; 61, 148.

LUER SYRINGE, LOCK, CONNECTIONS

Jeanne Luer (Wülfing) (1842-1909)

Jeanne Luer was the daughter of Amatus Luer, who was a surgical instrument maker in Paris, France. She joined his business and in 1867 married Hermann Wülfing from Westphalia. Then Hermann managed the business matters, while Jeanne developed production in the workshop.

Early syringes commonly comprised a plunger which moved by screw action within a barrel, which had a nozzle with a screw thread to join a needle. By 1869 the Luers produced a calibrated glass and metal syringe with a tapered nozzle for push-fit into a needle having a hub with the same taper; the plunger was driven directly with a snug fit inside the barrel. See Figure 1.

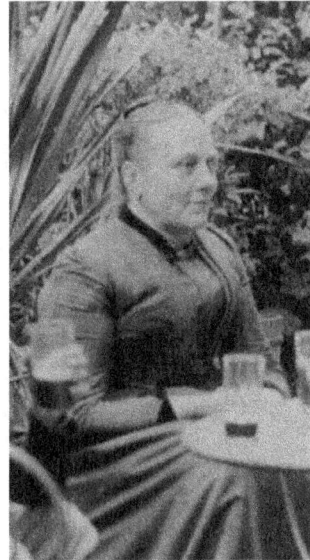

Jeanne Luer (Wülfing). Photograph courtesy of Pauline Roche (née Wulfing-Luer).

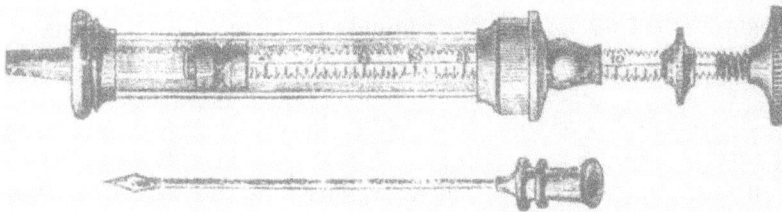

Figure 1. Luer syringe with conical nozzle and needle with taper hub for push-fit. Photograph from V. Von Bruns: *Arznei-Operationen oder Darstellung sämmtlicher Methoden der manuellen Application von Arzneistoflen*. Tübingen: H. Laupp, 1869

Wülfing was a member of the Society of German Physicians in Paris and from 1871, because of the war between Germany and France, he acted as custodian of the Society's excellent library for five years. The Luer all-glass syringe was produced about 1896 – initially it was not widely used. Between 1896 and 1903 several patents in the name of H.A. Wulfing-Luer were filed in

France, Austria and the USA. The American connection came from a visit to the Luers in Paris by Maxwell W. Becton and Fairleigh Dickinson in 1897. Later in that year, the Becton-Dickinson Company sold Luer syringes in Washington D.C. and in 1898 the Company bought exclusive rights to the syringe in North America.

Competition came around 1906 from the Record syringe made in Berlin by Dewitt and Herz. This glass and metal syringe had a very snug fitting piston, but it did not require lubricants. The problem was that the Luer and Record syringes had different sized nozzles so that care had to be taken that the needle fitted the syringe. It could be frustrating for the anaesthetist to discover that the syringe provided did not fit a carefully placed subarachnoid needle – and this persisted to the 1960s! About 1925 Col. F.S. Dickinson of Becton, Dickinson & Co. designed the Luer-Lok syringe. In this the nozzle had an inside thread which engaged the rim of the needle; a half-turn would lock the syringe onto the needle and a reverse half-turn would remove it.

In the late 1960s disposable plastic syringes with standard Luer connections were introduced, eliminating the problem of mis-matching fittings, as well as facilitating sterility. However, at that same time, Luer all-glass syringes were recommended for use with the Tuohy needle to locate the epidural space by the loss of resistance technique. It was advised that these reusable glass syringes be autoclaved with the plunger separate from the barrel, to avoid them sticking.

The Wülfing-Luers had their heydays in the early 1900s, the business passing to their son Guillaume and then grandson Paul Roussel. However, the family type business could not match the competition from large manufacturing companies, and it closed in 1995.

Disposable *Luer-lock* systems also came to be provided by several manufacturers. Luer-lock connectors in infusion sets became very important as total intravenous anaesthesia (TIVA) became more popular – to prevent disconnections or leaking with consequent awareness. In 1997 a new British standard was promulgated: BSEN1707 for conical fittings with a 6% Luer taper for syringes, needles and certain other medical equipment. This was harmonized with International Standard ISO594.

Conversely to the advantages stated for the 'universal' Luer connector in both intravenous and neuraxial use, in the new millennium there arose dissent. Well-publicised cases of intrathecal administration of cytotoxic and other 'wrong route' drugs led to demands in the press and some medical journals for new non-interchangeable (Non-Luer) connections on equipment designed for neuraxial administration. In 2014 it became mandatory in the UK for intrathecal chemotherapy equipment to be fitted with non-Luer connectors. Proposals to make neuraxial and regional anaesthesia needles non-Luer were postponed several times due to difficulties in manufacture of satisfactory products and the realisation that change in connector also introduced changes in flow of fluid in the needles. However, the multi-part ISO80369-6 standard has been developed for non-Luer connectors (also known as NRFit) and its acceptance is anticipated.

Acknowledgement

Prof. Andrea Sella kindly arranged contact with Pauline Roche, the great-granddaughter of Jeanne Wulfing-Luer.

Further reading

Sella A. Luer's syringe. http://www.rsc.org/chemistryworld/2012/08/luer-syringe (accessed 12 June 2015).

Schwidetzky, Rutherford NJ. History of Needles and Syringes. *Anesthesia and Analgesia* 1944; 23: 34-38.

Howard-Jones N. A Critical Study of the Origins and Early Development of Hypodermic Medication. *Journal of the History of Medicine and Allied Sciences* 1947; **2**: 201-49.

Cook TM, Wilkes A, Bickford Smith P, Dorn L et al. Multicentre clinical simulation evaluation of the ISO 80369-6 neuraxial non-Luer connector. *Anaesthesia* 2019; **74**: 619-29.

THE McCOY LARYNGOSCOPE

Éamon P. McCoy (1961 -)

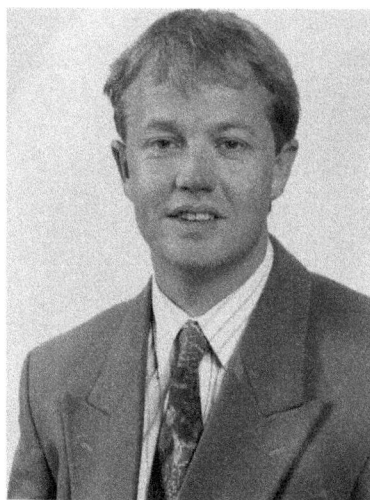

Éamon McCoy was born in Kisumu, Kenya in 1961 where his father was a missionary doctor. The family returned to Ireland in 1963 and lived in Bantry, Co. Cork. He attended medical school in University College Cork (UCC), graduating MB, BCh, BAO in 1986. After completing his pre-registration year in Cork University Hospital, he moved to the Royal Victoria Hospital (RVH), Belfast for anaesthetic training and became a fellow of the College of Anaesthetists of the Royal College of Surgeons in Ireland in 1990. He invented the McCoy levering laryngoscope in 1991 while training as an anaesthetic registrar. In 1992 he joined the academic anaesthetic department of the Queen's University of Belfast (QUB), mentored by Professor Rajinder Mirakhur. With an interest in pharmacokinetics this, and other research, resulted in more than 60 original scientific publications. He was awarded an MD on the pharmacology of neuromuscular blocking agents by QUB in July 1995.

McCoy spent a year as an anaesthetic overseas fellow with Professor John Russell in the Royal Adelaide Hospital, South Australia. This activity included clinical anaesthesia and air retrieval of the critically ill. He was involved in critical incident monitoring with Professor Bill Runciman and the Australian Patient Safety Foundation resulting in further scientific publication. In 1996 he was appointed Consultant Anaesthetist in the RVH, Belfast.

McCoy's levering laryngoscope was designed in 1991 to aid in the management of both the normal and difficult airway, and to mitigate many problems associated with endotracheal intubation. During an attachment to a maxillofacial unit as an anaesthetic registrar, McCoy noticed that in difficult situations during direct laryngoscopy, instead of the normal elevation of the structures in the same axis by moving the laryngoscope forwards and upwards parallel to the long axis of the handle, a levering movement of the blade may prove necessary. These situations could be caused by many anatomical peculiarities such as decreased mouth opening, enlarged tongue, recession of the mandible, protruding upper teeth or a fixed cervical spine. In such cases elevation of the epiglottis might prove difficult or impossible and the upper teeth could be damaged by using them as a fulcrum – without necessarily improving the view. This might happen with a standard curved or straight blade or any of their many modifications. The problem was that the fulcrum remained near the upper teeth and not at the epiglottis where it would be most effective.

The blades available at the time, once inserted, remained inflexible. Because there was no ability to adjust their shape during laryngoscopy there was no alteration allowed in the fulcrum which remained 8 to 14 cm proximal to the epiglottis, at the lips. Any degree of movement of the blade tip at the epiglottis depended on a much larger degree of movement at the handle. It was apparent that a blade designed to eliminate contact with the upper incisor teeth and also to have its fulcrum at a lower point within the pharynx might simplify elevation of the epiglottis and exposure of the larynx.

In order to design such a blade more than 50 lateral radiographs of the pharynx and sagittal-sectioned cadaver heads (Figure 1) were examined using medium and large size Macintosh blades in order to determine two measurements in question. Firstly, what degree of rotational movement of the blade tip was necessary in order to elevate the epiglottis? Secondly, at what proximal distance from the tip should a blade be hinged in order to achieve optimal elevation?

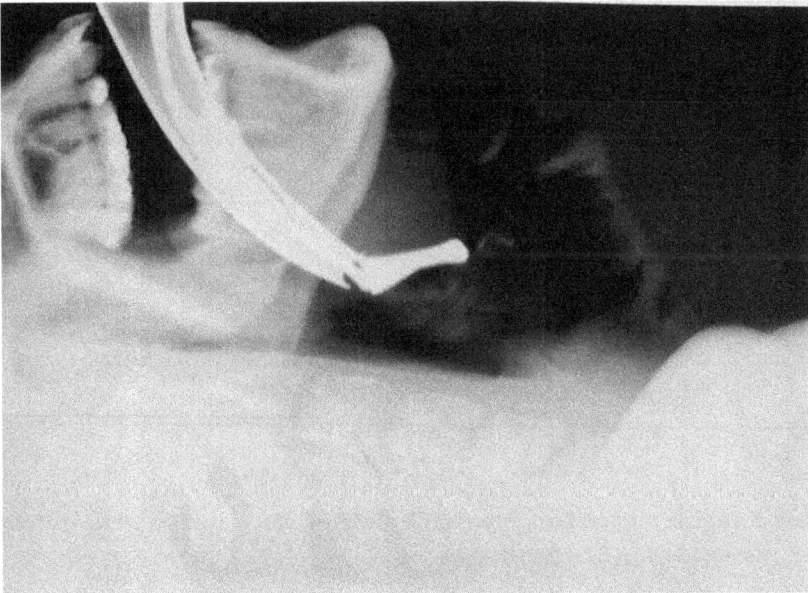

Figure 1. Lateral radiograph of neck showing prototype McCoy laryngoscope.

The necessary rotational tip movement proved to be between 45° and 60° and the hinged tip length 20-25 mm. Using these two measurements McCoy created the first design drawings.

A prototype was constructed based on the initial drawings and a patent was applied for in 1991, consisting of a background summary, a description and drawings of the modified instrument and a list of appropriate claims. McCoy then approached several medical equipment manufactures with a broad outline of the design and its advantages, suggesting that it would be easy for them to produce, would be commercially viable and would complement their existing product range. He was soon contacted by Rod Grundy the business manager of Penlon (UK) and, after a confidentiality agreement was signed, a full description of the device was forwarded to the company.

Under the direction of the Penlon's chief design draughtsman, David Byers, a second more sophisticated prototype was constructed which differed from the normal blade in four respects. It consisted of a hinged blade tip, a lever at the proximal end, a spring-loaded drum and a connecting shaft (Figure 2).

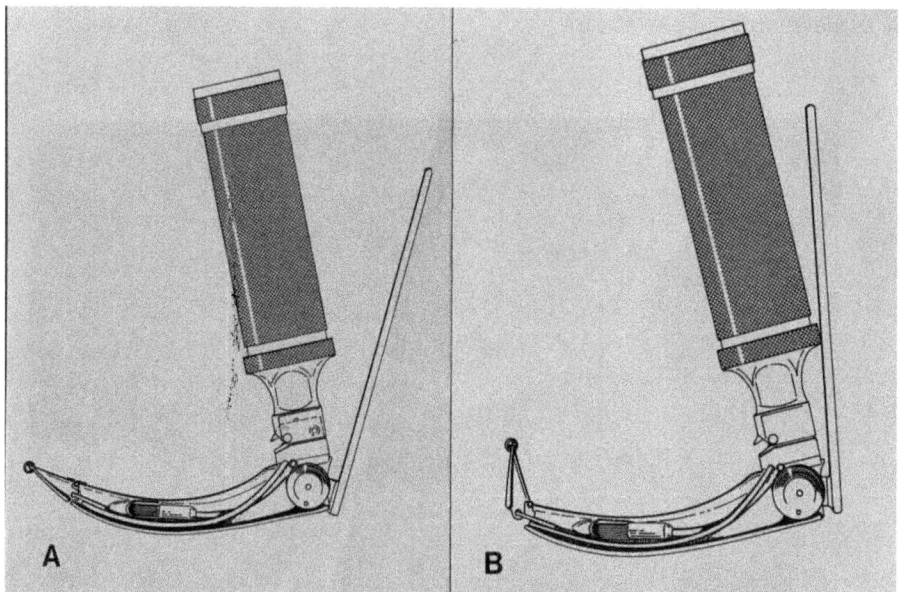

Figure 2. Drawing of the prototype McCoy levering laryngoscope blade with tip in (A) normal position, (B) elevated position.

Using this prototype further modifications were made to optimise the design in order to facilitate ease of use and efficiency in manufacture. Assessment of the final prototype showed that, with the adjustable tip inserted into the vallecula, gentle pressure on the proximal lever with approximately 20° movement caused the blade tip to elevate 70°, lifting the hyo-epiglottic ligament and exposing the larynx.

After further development, and with local and international independent clinical evaluation over the next 18 months, Penlon decided to proceed to manufacture and market the instrument as The McCoy Laryngoscope. An agreement to do so was signed in March 1993, proceeding to manufacture and marketing later in that year.

After the McCoy laryngoscope was placed on the market, the design was continually modified to facilitate both ease of manufacture and maintenance. It was subjected to many clinical evaluations by McCoy and others, particularly in comparison studies on the view obtained at laryngoscopy.

In Belfast by 1994 the McCoy laryngoscope was assessed with regard to the stress response to, and cervical spine movement during, laryngoscopy. These showed the benefits of this design in normal patients and suggested the advantages of the use of this instrument in difficult cases and in trauma.

To assess whether these advantages might be related to the requirement for the use of lower forces during laryngoscopy McCoy approached the Faculty of Mechanical and Manufacturing Engineering, QUB. A novel project was designed by engineers Professor Brendan Austin and his postgraduate research student K.C. Wong. The result of this collaboration was the design of a new device for measuring and recording offset load during laryngoscopy. Importantly this new instrument allowed the recording of many laryngoscopy parameters including the duration of laryngoscopy, the maximally applied forces, the mean force and the force-time integral. As the force measuring device was integrated into the laryngoscope handle the four parameters could be recorded and compared during laryngoscopy with many different blade designs. In 1995 a comparison of the forces exerted during laryngoscopy between the Macintosh versus the McCoy blade, showed that use of the McCoy blade required significantly reduced forces applied to the pharynx.

Since then the McCoy laryngoscope has been both a medical and commercial success, being the subject of multiple publications in the medical literature and cited widely. Chosen as a Millennium Product in the UK in 2000, It Is estimated that more than 100,000 have sold in more than 60 countries world-wide.

McCoy has received numerous awards: the Dr A. Harvey Granat Memorial Prize by the Neuroanaesthesia Society of Great Britain and Ireland (1993), the President's Medal by The Association of Anaesthetists of Great Britain and Ireland (1993), the Registrar's Prize by the Society for Computing and Technology in Anaesthesia (1994), the Purce Lectureship by the Royal Group of Hospitals, Belfast (1995). In March 1995 he was awarded the Cutler's Surgical Prize by the Royal College of Surgeons of England and in May of the same year he was named the United Kingdom Doctor of the Year. In October 1999 he was awarded the Alumnus Achievement Award by UCC.

McCoy co-founded, with John Beavis, an English orthopaedic surgeon, the medical aid charity International Disaster and Emergency Aid with Long Term Support (IDEALS) while working in the State Hospital, Sarajevo when that city was under siege during the Bosnian civil war (1993-95). He continued to deliver appropriate assistance in Sarajevo and Mostar after the war had ended (1995-2003). Since then he and other members of IDEALS have been active in areas which are both hazardous and challenging, using their experience to provide medical care and training as well as material aid. His special interests have continued in difficult airway and major trauma management, resuscitation and anaesthesia for head and neck surgery.

Further reading

McCoy EP, Mirakhur RK. The levering laryngoscope. *Anaesthesia* 1993; **48**: 516-19.

McCoy EP, Austin BA, Mirakhur RK, Wong KC. A new device for measuring and recording the forces applied during laryngoscopy. *Anaesthesia* 1995; **50**: 139-43.

McCoy EP, Mirakhur RK, McCloskey BV. A comparison of the stress response to laryngoscopy. The Macintosh versus the McCoy blade. *Anaesthesia* 1995; **50**: 943-6.

MACEWEN MEDAL

William Macewen (1848-1924)

William Macewen was born at Rothesay, Scotland in 1848. He had secondary education at the Collegiate School in Garnethill, Glasgow and in 1865 began medical studies at the University of Glasgow, graduating in 1869. After house jobs, he was appointed (1870) medical superintendent at the Glasgow Fever Hospital at Belvidere where he started to contemplate intubation of the larynx through the mouth instead of tracheostomy.

By the end of 1870 Macewen moved to private practice and found time to complete his MD in 1872. He also took on several civic appointments, then moving to the Glasgow Royal Infirmary in 1874 where he was promoted to full surgeon by 1876. He insisted on antiseptic practise and radically improved the hygiene of the wards and operating theatre allocated to him.

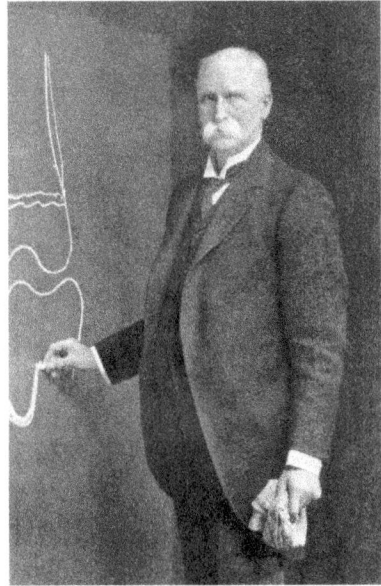

William Macewen. Credit: University of Glasgow Archives and Special Collections, Glasgow University Magazine, GB248 DC198.

In 1878 Macewen began definitive investigation of endotracheal intubation, initially on cadavers. He found that by passing the index finger into the mouth and depressing the epiglottis onto the tongue, he could then guide a tube over the back of the finger into the larynx. He tried rubber, flexible metal and gum-elastic tubes – and opted for gum-elastic. Next, he performed the technique on conscious patients, developing smoothness and was able to debunk the belief that this could not be tolerated. In July 1878 Macewen intubated a man before surgery for removal of epithelioma of the pharynx and back of the tongue: the tube was encircled with a gauze pack to prevent entrance of blood and secretions into the lungs; also, chloroform was easily given through the tube.

Macewen first mentioned this work at a meeting of the Glasgow Pathological and Clinical Society on 12 November 1878; he published it in the *Lancet* in 1880. His most quoted and epochal paper on four cases of successful orotracheal intubation appeared in the *British Medical Journal* in 1880 – two patients afflicted with tumour of the pharynx, one with burn and one with infection – all had resultant respiratory obstruction. This indeed was the introduction of endotracheal intubation in anaesthesia. Macewen went on to institute programmes for training and safe practice in anaesthesia.

In 1889 Macewen was offered the Professorship of Surgery in the Johns Hopkins Hospital in Baltimore, but he turned it down – the post went to William Stewart Halsted. Three years later he was appointed Regius Professor of Surgery at the University of Glasgow. His prowess in surgery was remarkable: renowned achievements in hernia repair, bone, cerebro-spinal and pulmonary surgery.

Macewen was elected an honorary Fellow of the Royal College of Surgeons of England in 1900, knighted in 1902 and later appointed surgeon to the King in Scotland. In the First World War he was Consultant Surgeon to the Royal Navy in Scotland; he organised pattern makers in the ship building industry to make excellent artificial limbs. Honorary degrees were awarded to Macewen by the Universities of Glasgow, Liverpool, Oxford and Trinity College, Dublin. He became President of the British Medical Association in 1922, in which year he received the freedom of Rothesay. The following year he was President of the International Surgical Congress in London.

The Difficult Airway Society (DAS) has awarded DAS Macewen Medals annually since 2009 to recognize members of that society who have distinguished themselves by service to airway management. This silver medal has the DAS emblem on one side and the head of Sir William Macewen on the obverse.

Table 1. DAS Macewen Medal winners

Year	Recipient	Year	Recipient
2009	Adrian Pearce	2014	Martin Bromley Mansukh Popat
2010	John Henderson Ralph Stephens Vaughan	2015	John A. Pacey Mohammed Nasir
2011	Ian Calder Archibald Brain Chandy Verghese	2016	Nicholas M. Woodall
2012	Ian Peter Latto William W. Mapleson	2017	Jairaj Rangasami Peter Charters
2013	Ronald S. Cormack John R. Lehane Sybill Storz		

Note that since 1926 the University of Glasgow has also awarded a Macewen Medal annually, on the recommendation of the Faculty of Medicine, to the student who has obtained the highest aggregate number of marks in Surgery in the Final Degree Examinations.

Further reading

Bowman AK. *Sir William Macewen*. London: William Hodge & Co. Ltd., 1942.

Report of meeting of Glasgow Pathological and Clinical Society on Nov. 12th, 1878. *Glasgow Medical Journal* 1879; **11**: 72-75.

Macewen W. Tracheal tubes introduced through the mouth for administration of chloroform during an operation for the removal of an epithelioma from the tongue and pharynx. *Lancet* 1880; **ii**: 906.

Macewen W. Clinical observations on the introduction of tracheal tubes by the mouth instead of performing tracheotomy or laryngotomy. *British Medical Journal* 1880; **2**: 122-4, 163-5.

Macewen W. Introduction to a discussion on anaesthetics. *Glasgow Medical Journal* 1890; **xxxiv**: 321.

SOAP GERTIE MARX LECTURE

Gertie Florentine Marx (1912-2004)

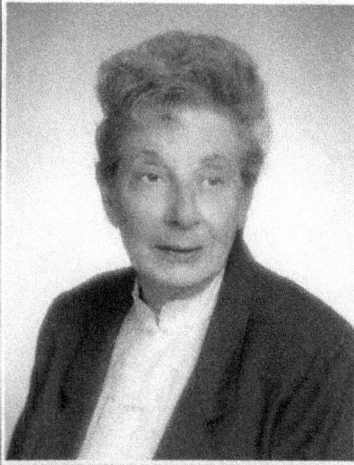

Gertie Marx was born in Frankfurt-am-Main, Germany in 1912. After schooling, she was admitted to the University of Frankfurt to study medicine. One of her mentors was the famous physician Franz Volhard. In 1936 she realised the Anti-Semitic policies of Adolf Hitler meant that as a Jew she should leave Germany. So, she moved to Bern to complete her medical course, qualifying in 1937. Later that year she immigrated into the USA where, after passing the proficiency in English test, the National Board examinations, and New York State Board examinations, she found an internship at the Beth Israel Hospital (New York City) in 1939.

Gertie F. Marx. Image reproduced with permission from *Bulletin of Anesthesia History*.

In contrast to Europe where about 40% of doctors were female, Gertie Marx found herself underprivileged as the only woman intern. She was pushed into anaesthesiology duties, which she began to like and next she enrolled as the first anaesthesiology resident at Beth Israel Hospital when a training program began there in 1940. She became interested in providing anaesthetic care for labouring women and developed skill at low spinal block. In 1943 she was appointed to the attending staff of the Beth Israel Medical Center (BIMC). Then she visited the obstetric hospital (US Marine Hospital) on Staten Island, NY to learn the technique of continuous caudal block from Robert Hingson. She duly introduced it to the BIMC where she was soon appointed Director of Obstetric Anaesthesia.

Marx moved to the new medical school at the Albert Einstein College of Medicine (AECM) in the Bronx, NY in 1955 to be Assistant Professor of Anaesthesiology. Once the obstetric service there had developed, she became Director of Obstetric Anaesthesia – practising and teaching epidural analgesia and spinal anaesthesia for over four decades. A notable paper by her and Stuart Wollman in 1968 was on the effect of fluid volume loading of the circulation before epidural block in the parturient. She emphasized the importance of knowledge of the physiological changes of pregnancy in establishing safe obstetric anaesthesia, and in 1969 she published *Physiology* of *Obstetric Anesthesia* (No.744 in the Bannerstone series of American lectures in anesthesiology). In 1973 she edited *Parturition and Perinatology* (Vol. 10/2 in the Clinical Anesthesia series). Importantly, in 1974 (with Girvice Archer) she measured the marked desaturation of pregnant women within 60 seconds of apnoea, compared with non-pregnant controls, thereby highlighting the importance of preoxygenation at induction of general anaesthesia and prompt re-oxygenation following intubation. In 1980 she edited with Gerard M. Bassell another book *Obstetric Analgesia and Anesthesia*. Her willingness and numerous articles, textbook chapters and the co-authoring of textbooks of obstetric anaesthesia, led to her becoming known (certainly in the USA) as "the mother of obstetric anaesthesia".

Although not a founder member in 1970 of the Society for Obstetric Anesthesia and Perinatology (SOAP), Marx became an avid attender of its meetings. In 1981 she was the founding editor of quarterly summaries of the latest world literature on obstetric anaesthesia: *Obstetric Anesthesia Digest*. She was honoured in 1988 by the American Society of Anesthesiologists with its Distinguished Service Award – the second woman to receive it (after Virginia Apgar). She travelled to London, England in 1993 to receive the College Medal of the Royal College of Anaesthetists. It was not until 1995 that she retired at the AECM as Emeritus Professor.

By the 1990s the award of Gertie Marx Prizes at the annual SOAP meeting was well established. First, second and third prizes have been presented in the competition for the best scientific paper by members in training, residents and fellows. From 2011-2017, SOAP offered a Gertie Marx Education and Research Grant, the goal being to provide initial funding for projects hoping to assist in applications later to bigger sources.

SOAP began the Gertie Marx Lecture at its annual meeting from 2010, initially coupled as the Foundation for Anesthesia Education and Research (FAER) Education Lecture.

As a tribute to Marx's work, the International Medical Development company developed a range of spinal needles specifically for obstetric anaesthesia, named after her. The design was pencil-point in line with the concept of the Whitacre and the further developed Sprotte needles (q.v. pages 217-19). However, it had a smaller side port than that (elongated) of the Sprotte and the standard length was longer (127 mm) than the Sprotte's (120 mm). The extra length promoted greater success when the needle was passed through a Tuohy epidural needle to achieve the spinal component of combined spinal-epidural (CSE) analgesia. The range included an extra-long size for use in obese women.

Table 1. Gertie Marx lecturers and lecture titles

Year	Lecturer	Title
2010	Michael R. Pinsky	Perioperative technology: use and limitations of non and minimally invasive hemodynamic monitoring.
2011	Sulpicio Soriano	Effects of anesthetics on neurodevelopment of fetus.
2012	Gordon Guyatt	Why bother with evidence-based obstetrical anesthesia.
2013	Ndola Prata	Maternal morality in resource-poor settings.
2014	Eleni Tsigas	Preeclampsia: what patients want you to know.
2015	Frederic W. Hafferty	Professionalism and the hidden curriculum.
2016	Mary E. D'Alton	Reducing maternal mortality and morbidity in New York and beyond.
2017	Ansgar Brambrink	Anesthetic neurotoxicity – an update.
2018	B. Carvalho, R.B. Clark, B. Smith, M.I. Zakowski	SOAP's 50th Anniversary.
2019	Lawrence C. Tsen	Obstetric anesthesia: are we there yet?

Acknowledgement

The Anesthesia History Association kindly gave permission to reproduce the portrait photograph from the *Bulletin of Anesthesia History*.

Further reading

Bassell GM. In Memoriam – Gertie F. Marx, MD (1912-2004). *International Journal of Obstetric Anesthesia* 2004; **13**: 141-3.

Wollman SB, Marx GF. Acute hydration for prevention of hypotension of spinal anesthesia in parturients. *Anesthesiology* 1968; **29**: 374-80.

Archer GW, Marx GF. Arterial oxygen tension during apnoea in parturient women. *British Journal of Anaesthesia* 1974; **46**: 358-60.

Marx GF, Hodgkinson R. Anaesthesia in the presence of complications of pregnancy. In: Obstetric Analgesia and Anaesthesia. *Clinics in Obstetrics and Gynaecology* 1975; **2:3**: 609

Riley ET, Hamilton CL, Ratner EF, Cohen SE. A comparison of the 24-gauge Sprotte and Gertie Marx spinal needles for combined spinal-epidural analgesia during labor. *Anesthesiology* 2002; **97**: 574-7.

MATSUKI PRIZE

Akitomo Matsuki (1939-)

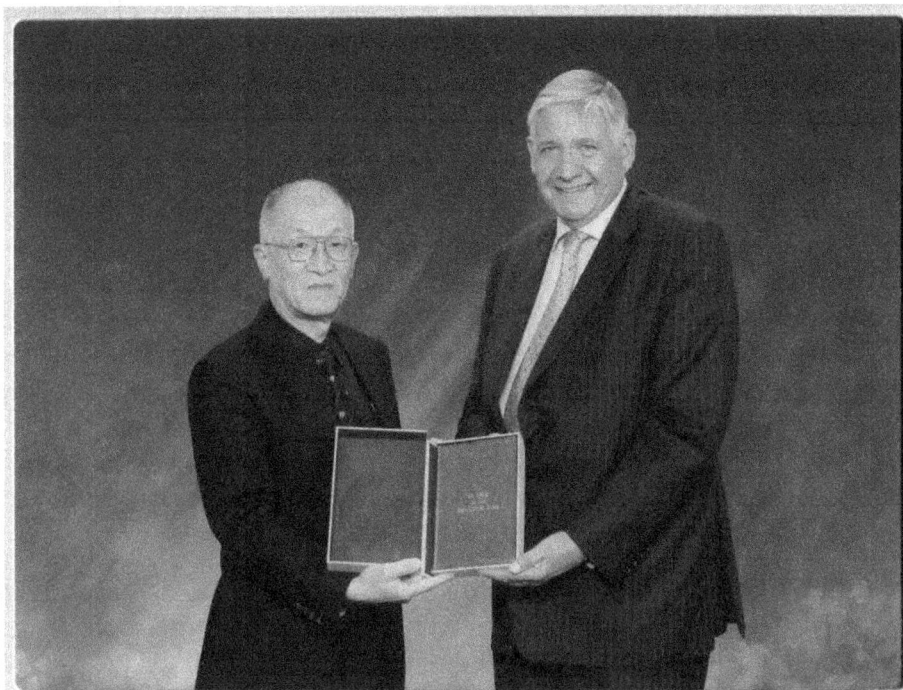

Akitomo Matsuki (L) presenting the 1847 book 'Dr. Snow On the Inhalation of Ether' to Dr David Wilkinson for the AAGBI Library: Hakodate, 2006. Image from A. Matsuki.

Akitomo Matsuki was born in Hirosaki, Japan in 1939. After education at Hirosaki Prefectural High School, he went to Medical School at Hirosaki University and graduated MD in 1966. He registered as an anaesthesiologist in 1968 and was appointed Assistant in the Department of Anesthesiology, Hirosaki University in 1970. The following year he was Board certified and obtained his PhD.

Matsuki worked as a research associate in the Department of Anesthesiology, University of Michigan in 1972, returning the following year to be Instructor in Anesthesiology at Hirosaki, where he was appointed Associate Professor in 1974.

In 1980 he went to the UK to study the history of anaesthesia, especially the transfer of information about ether anaesthesia from the USA. That September he attended the 7th World Congress of Anaesthesiologists held in Hamburg, Germany and was attracted to a panel discussion entitled 'Anaesthesiology: Past and Future'. During this he was very impressed by the presentation of Emeritus

Prof Sir Robert Macintosh (aged 80), who praised the achievements of John Snow, particularly his monograph 'On the inhalation of the vapour of ether in surgical operations' published in 1847. Macintosh stated that this classic book should be read at least once by every anaesthetist. Afterwards, as luck would have it, Matsuki ventured into an old medical bookshop in the congress hall and asked to see a book with no title on the spine and beyond his reach. On examination he was astonished to find it was the very book which Macintosh had been talking about! Furthermore, it had John Snow's handwriting on the front page to "The Editor of Zeitschrift für die gesammte Medicine".

Matsuki was visiting Fellow in the Department of Anaesthetics at the Radcliffe Infirmary, Oxford under Prof M.K. Sykes in September to October 1982. In 1987 he produced his own facsimile of John Snow's 1847 book, including the death certificate of John Snow and the review of the book in *Zeitschrift für die gesammte Medicine* by the Editor, Dr F.W. Oppenheim. This was published by the Iwanami Book Service Center in Tokyo, Japan. A copy was presented to every registrant at the 2nd International Symposium on the History of Anaesthesia held in London in July 1987. In a letter to Matsuki after the Symposium, Sir Robert Macintosh described the facsimile copy as "splendid".

From 1985 to 1990 Matsuki was Assistant Editor of the *Japanese Anaesthesia Journals' Review*, then becoming Editor for two years. In 1989 he was appointed Professor and Chairman of the Department of Anesthesiology at Hirosaki University School of Medicine. In 1997 he produced two more facsimiles using the same Tokyo publishers:

(1) James Young Simpson's 1849 (American) book 'Anaesthesia or the employment of chloroform and ether in surgery, midwifery, etc.';
(2) John Snow's 1858 book 'On chloroform and other anaesthetics: their action and administration'.

He attended the Chloroform Sesquicentenary meeting in Edinburgh, Scotland in September 1997, which included the annual meeting of the European Academy of Anaesthesiology. Fittingly, he presented a poster with J.W.R. McIntyre on the transmission of the news of chloroform anaesthesia from Edinburgh to Boston.

Matsuki retired from clinical practice in 2004, but became Emeritus Professor, Hirosaki University. He moved to Hakodate in northern Japan, where he continued to research and publish on medical history. He tried to establish a 'Museum Library of Anaesthesiology in Japan' but found support lacking. So, in 2006 he contacted Dr David Wilkinson, past Vice President of the Association of Anaesthetists of Great Britain and Ireland (AAGBI), to offer his copy of John Snow's 1847 book to the AAGBI's Library. Acceptance was authorised by the

Executive, which sponsored David Wilkinson to travel to Hakodate in December 2006 to collect the precious book. In recognition of Matsuki's extraordinary generosity, Wilkinson gave him in exchange the inaugural Charles King Award for contributions to heritage, from the AAGBI. The name came from the Charles King Collection of anaesthetic equipment which formed the nucleus of the AAGBI's Museum; however, this eponymous award was discontinued after 2013.

By this time Matsuki had received many other awards: the Yakazu Award of the Japanese Society for the History of Medicine (1999), Fellowship by election of the Royal College of Anaesthetists (2000), Distinguished Service Award of the Japan Medical Association (2001) and the Social Prize of the Japanese Society of Anesthesiologists (2006).

In 2009 the Matsuki Prize for research on anaesthesia history in Japan was instituted by the Japanese Society of Anesthesiologists and awarded at its annual meeting from 2011.

Matsuki published *A Short History of Anesthesia in Japan* in 2012 and this won the Publication Prize of Hirosaki University Press in 2013. His book *The Origin and Evolution of Anesthesia in Japan* was awarded the 2018 David M. Little, Jr. Prize from the Anesthesia History Association for best book published in 2017.

Table 1. Matsuki Prize winners

Year	Recipient	Work
2011	Kentaro Dote	Study on Gendai Kamada.
2013	Shigeru Saito	Study on the history of development of cardiotonics by Japanese.
2014	Toshiyuki Okutomi	Study on the history of painless delivery in Japan.
2017	Mitsugu Fujimori	Study on the history of anaesthesia in Kansai District (Osaka, Kyoto areas).
2018	Takashi Asai	Study on the history of tracheal intubation.
2019	Hirosato Kikuchi	Translation into Japanese of J Roger Maltby's *Notable Names in Anaesthesia* and other articles.
2020	Hiroshi Makino	Activities to promote study of the history of anaesthesia and JSA invitation of the 10th ISHA.

Further reading

Matsuki A. John Snow (1813-1858) and his book 'On the inhalation of the vapour of ether in surgical operations'. In: Atkinson RS, Boulton TB (Eds.) *The History of Anaesthesia*. London: Royal Society of Medicine Services, 1989; 498-500.

Wilkinson DJ. It's time the book came home. *Anaesthesia News* May 2007; No. 238: 3-5.

Matsuki A. *A Short History of Anesthesia in Japan*. Hirosaki: Hirosaki University Press, 2012.

MEYER-OVERTON HYPOTHESIS ON THE MODE OF ACTION OF GENERAL ANAESTHETICS

Most textbooks of anaesthesia have a chapter on the mechanisms of general anaesthesia in which it is mentioned that one of the earliest theories was the Meyer-Overton Lipoid Solubility Theory. In fact, this theory was propounded independently by the German chemist, Hans Meyer (1899) and the British botanist, Charles Overton (1901).

General anaesthetic drugs have a wide range of chemical structures, so Meyer and Overton focused on their non-specific physico-chemical properties. They deduced that anaesthetic drugs must be highly lipid soluble in order to reach the fatty material of the brain in contrast to their solubility in water. Meyer and his students found a strong correlation between the solubility of the drugs in olive oil (more specifically the olive oil: water partition coefficient) and their ability to immobilise tadpoles. Overton worked on algae and a variety of aquatic animals including tadpoles (mostly), fish, crustaceans and annelids, demonstrating that both liquid and gaseous anaesthetic drugs affected lipids in the brain. It was hypothesized that having reached the brain, these drugs modified the structural and dynamic properties of the nerve cell membrane and so altered the function of the neurones – including consciousness.

Some objections to the Meyer-Overton theory arose: water not really comparable to blood, and olive oil not comparable to body fat. Most notably, it was found that the Lipoid Solubility concept was only applicable to aliphatic compounds, excluding a large range of heterocyclic compounds and the inorganic substances, magnesium and bromide. Even within the aliphatic compounds there was a limitation of hydrocarbon chain length. Nevertheless, the Meyer-Overton hypothesis remained a major reference until after 1984 when Franks and Lieb published on the inhibition of the firefly's luciferase enzyme by a range of anaesthetics. This led to the concept of specific anaesthetic-receptor (protein) binding and studies on the ligand-gated ion channel family of receptors.

Hans Horst Meyer (1853-1939)

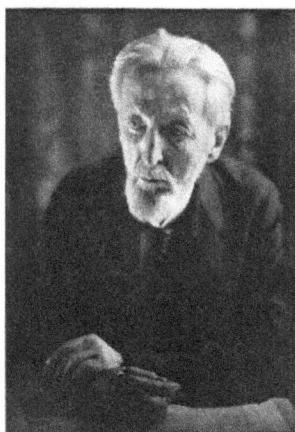

Hans Horst Meyer. Credit: Wikimedia Commons.

Hans Horst Meyer was born in Insterburg, East Prussia (now Chernyakhovsk in Russia). He studied medicine in Leipzig, Berlin and finally Königsberg, where he completed his doctorate in 1877. Next he worked in Strasbourg with Oswald Schmiedeberg, the founder of pharmacology. In 1881 he was appointed Professor of Pharmacology at Dorpat, now Tartu in Estonia, and in 1884 he moved to the Chair of Pharmacology at the University of Marburg. There in 1896 his interest was captured by Ernst von Bibra and Emil Harless' 1847 book *Die Wirkungen des Schwefeläthers in chemischer und physiologischer Beziehung*, which suggested that lipid solubility was key to the action of anaesthetics.

Meyer duly used tadpoles in aqueous solutions of different chemicals to investigate the mode of action of general anaesthetics, assisted by many students, including Fritz Baum. The first paper on the subject by Meyer in 1899 in *Archiv für experimentelle Pathologie und Pharmakologie* proposed three principles to explain the ability of a wide range of substances to produce narcosis or anaesthesia:

(1) lipid solubility and spread in living protoplasm;
(2) initial and predominant effects in fatty cells, especially nerve;
(3) relative potency must depend on the fat/water partition coefficient.

The second paper by Baum, which appeared on the very next page of the same issue of the journal, correlated minimum narcosis-inducing concentration in tadpoles with increasing olive oil: water partition coefficient. The third paper by Meyer in the same journal in 1901 further supported the Lipoid Solubility Theory by showing that for six different compounds, their narcosis in tadpoles and partition coefficient (olive oil: water) exhibited similar temperature dependence.

Meyer moved to the University of Vienna in 1904 to take up the inaugural Chair of the Department of Experimental Pharmacology.

In 1910 Meyer and Rudolf Gottlieb published an important pharmacology textbook, *Die Experimentelle Pharmakologie als Grundlage der Arzneibehandlung/ ein Lerbuch für Studierende und Ärzte*, which ran to nine editions.

In 1923, to mark his 70th birthday, the Hans Meyer Medal was founded by the Vienna Academy of Sciences. It was proposed to award this medal every fifth year for the most important contribution to pharmacology published in German. Meyer retired in 1924. Sadly in 1938 he was expelled from the German Academy of Sciences Leopoldina because he was considered "non-Aryan". He died in Vienna the following year.

Charles Ernest Overton (1865-1933)

Charles Ernest Overton was born in Stretton, Cheshire, England and he attended the Newport grammar school. In 1882, owing to his mother's chronic illness, the family moved to Zurich, Switzerland, where he completed his schooling and in 1884 he enrolled at the University of Zurich to study botany. He obtained his doctorate in 1889 and was then appointed as a lecturer in biology at the University of Zurich.

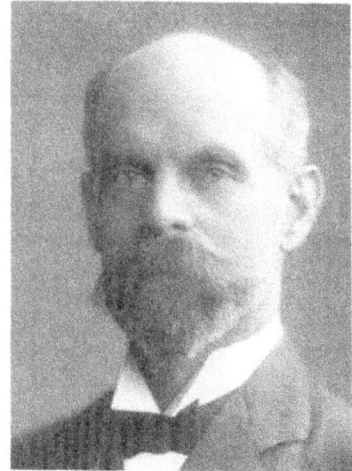

ERNEST OVERTON

From 1895 Overton's interest was captured by the permeability of plant and animal cells to various chemical compounds. In 1899 he noted that oily substances such as cholesterin (cholesterol) saturated the boundary between cell protoplasm and the exterior. This was crucial to developing further understanding of the cell membrane. 'Overton's rule' was stated as "the permeability coefficient of a solute is linearly related to its partition coefficient between oil and water".

Image, from Riksarkivet, is in the public domain.

In 1901 Overton published a book *Studien über die Narkose zugleich ein Beitrag zur allgemeinen Pharmakologie* (195 pages). At the same point he moved to Würzburg to become an assistant in physiology to Professor Maximilian von Frey. During his time in this post, Overton published on the role of sodium ions for the conduction of action potentials in nerve and muscle physiology, laying the foundation for the work of the future Nobel Prize winners J.C. Eccles, A.L. Hodgkin and A. F. Huxley.

Next in 1907 Overton moved to the University of Lund, Sweden to become its first Professor of Pharmacology. He remained there until his retirement in 1930.

Further reading

Meyer F. Zur Theorie der Alkoholnarkose. Erste Mittheilung. Welche Eigenschaft der Anästhetica bedingt ihre narkotische Wirkung? *Archiv für experimentelle Pathologie und Pharmakologie* 1899; **42**: 109-118.

Baum F. Zur Theorie der Alkoholnarkose. Ein physikalisch-chemischer Beitrag zur Theorie der Narcotica. *Archiv für experimentelle Pathologie und Pharmakologie* 1899; **42**: 119-137.

Overton CE. *Studies of narcosis and a Contribution to General Pharmacology* (1901). English translation, ed.by Lipnick RL. London: Chapman and Hall/ Wood Library-Museum of Anesthesiology, 1991.

Franks NP, Lieb WR. Do general anaesthetics act by competitive binding to specific receptors? *Nature* 1984; **310**: 599-601.

Lipnick RL. Hans Horst Meyer and the lipoid theory of narcosis. *Trends in Pharmacological Science* 1989; **10**: 265-9.

Perouansky M. The Overton in Meyer-Overton: a biographical sketch commemorating the 150th anniversary of Charles Ernest Overton's birth. *British Journal of Anaesthesia* 2015; **114**: 537-41.

MILLER'S 'ANESTHESIA'

Ronald Dean Miller (1939-)

Ronald D. Miller had his childhood and education in Indiana. He attended medical school at Indiana University in Bloomington, Indiana, graduating M.D. in 1964. He proceeded to residency in anaesthesia and a concurrent fellowship in pharmacology at the University of California in San Francisco, obtaining a master's degree in pharmacology. He won the ASA Residents' Essay Contest in 1968.

Miller served as a Staff Anesthesiologist in the US Navy from 1968. Stationed as a Lieutenant-Commander at Da Nang, South Vietnam in 1969 he was awarded the Bronze Star with a combat V for Meritorious Service, notably research into massive blood transfusion.

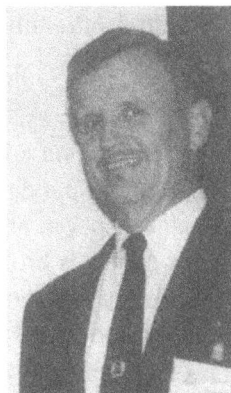

Ronald Dean Miller.
Photograph taken in 1997.

In 1970 Miller returned to San Francisco for appointment as Assistant Professor of Anesthesia and Pharmacology at the University of California. After four years he was promoted to Associate Professor and in 1978 he became full Professor of Pharmacology. From 1973 he served as an examiner for the American Board of Anesthesiology. He served on the Editorial Board of the journal *Anesthesiology* from 1978 to 1988.

Miller conceived the idea of a comprehensive textbook on anaesthesia and collaborated with 31 other contributors (all based in the USA), many of whom were internationally recognized experts in their fields of interest. The first edition of *Anesthesia*, which he edited, appeared in 1981, published by Churchill Livingstone. This work, comprising nearly 1600 pages in two volumes, had four main sections:

- Preparation of the patient and use of anaesthetic agents
- Physiological functions during anaesthesia
- Anaesthesia for various surgical subspecialties
- Consultant anaesthetic practice.

Inevitably the book was orientated to North American practice rather than British. It rapidly became established as the definitive text on anaesthesia all over the world, excepting where British anaesthetic practice prevailed.

Through 1981-1985 Miller was a member of the FDA Committee on Blood and Blood Products (when blood was discovered to transmit HIV). From 1982 he served as Vice Chairman of the Department of Anesthesia in San Francisco, becoming Chairman and Professor of Anesthesia in 1984. That year he co-edited with Robert K. Stoelting, M.D. another textbook *Basics of Anesthesia*.

The second edition of *Anesthesia*, edited by Miller, was published in 1986 as three volumes. There were now 70 contributors (all based in the USA), 11 new chapters and a further 890 pages. The section on intensive care medicine was greatly expanded and the new chapters included: anaesthetic history, medico-legal aspects, and basic sciences. This work was criticized for repetition (which of course is problematic with multiple authors), irritating mistakes and lack of cross-referencing. From the British point of view, although containing much that was not applicable to their practice, it was acknowledged as a useful resource because it was very comprehensive and well referenced.

The third edition of *Anesthesia* (1990) reverted to two volumes and involved more international contributors. In 1991 Miller was appointed Editor-in-Chief of the journal *Anesthesia and Analgesia*. He also served on the Editorial Board of the *British Journal of Anaesthesia* from 1993 to 1998. In January 1997 he delivered the Ohmeda Health Care Lecture at the Winter Scientific Meeting of the Association of Anaesthetists of Great Britain and Ireland, held in London. His title for the lecture was "Impact of health care reforms on the USA health service".

The textbook which Miller edited became famous and known as "Miller's *Anesthesia*". It remained up to date as new editions were released at approximately 5-year intervals. The fifth edition in 2000 had 135 authors, eight of whom were from outside the USA. For the first time, the book included the ASA practice guidelines. There were six sections:

- Introduction – the history of anaesthesia
- Basic science including physiology, pharmacology, intravenous anaesthetic delivery systems, statistics
- Clinical anaesthesia: general and regional, including monitoring and a new chapter on the use of transoesophageal echocardiography (TOE)
- Subspecialties including acute and chronic pain
- Intensive care including resuscitation, nutrition and brain death
- Miscellaneous including operating theatre management, quality improvement, simulation, Internet resources, ethics and medico-legal aspects.

It was issued with an accompanying compact disc (CD) of video clips of procedures. These included: insertion of a TOE probe, pulmonary artery catheter, brachial plexus and caudal block, insertion of double lumen tube, checking the anaesthetic machine, management of infusion pumps and intraoperative cell salvage.

The sixth edition in 2005 had the same six sections, but with major revision. The number of pages was now double that of the first edition. There were new chapters on implantable cardiac defibrillators, perioperative blindness, anaesthesia for robotic surgery, patient safety and implications of chemical and biological weapons. The accompanying CD had videos of patient positioning, tracheal intubation, thoracic epidurals, ultrasound-guided nerve blocks, needle cricothyrotomy and more. Purchasers were also given links to an associated website "e-dition" which would provide weekly updates from reputed specialists.

By the end of 2006, Miller retired from the position of Editor-in-Chief of *Anesthesia and Analgesia*, which he had conducted with distinction for sixteen years. In his career he published over 170 peer reviewed articles. In June 2009, aged 70, he retired from the Chair of Anesthesia and Perioperative Care at the University of California, San Francisco. That year saw the seventh edition of *Miller's Anesthesia*. There were now nine sections in the book and use was made of colour coding. A standard structure for each chapter was adopted: "Keypoints" at the beginning, followed by an introduction and then the main text with references.

For the eighth edition of *Miller's Anesthesia* in 2015, the Imprint Elsevier appeared, instead of Churchill Livingstone. There were more than 250 internationally reputed contributors, many from outside the USA. By this time, the textbook was translated into several languages. With ten new chapters, notable chapters in this edition were: "Anesthesia Business Models" including staffing and practice requirements in both North America and Europe, "Perioperative and Anesthesia Neurotoxicity", "Nonopioid Pain Medications", "Palliative Medicine", Non-Operating Room Anesthesia", "Anesthesia for Organ Procurement", "Anesthesia for Fetal Surgery" and "Evaluation and Classification of Evidence for the ASA Clinical Practice Guidelines". Again, purchasers were given access to a website, now called ExpertConsult.com.

In 2019 the ninth edition (current) of *Miller's Anesthesia* was the first to not have 'Ronald D. Miller' leading the list of editors. Instead the editors were listed as: M. Gropper, L. Eriksson, L. Fleisher, J. Wiener-Kronish, N. Cohen and K. Leslie. With a similar number of contributors to the eighth edition, over 80% were from the USA and only nine were based in the UK. Unsurprisingly therefore, much of the content is less applicable to UK anaesthetic practice. Inevitably with so many authors, there is variation in style of writing and some repetition. A strong point in this edition is the good cross-referencing. There is also an online version with 42 videos. Nearly 40 years on, *Miller's Anesthesia* has become arguably the most comprehensive and widely used textbook of anaesthesia in the world.

Miller has received numerous honours. He was elected Honorary Member of the Dutch Society of Anesthesiology in 1986 and of the German Society of Anaesthesia and Critical Care in 2005. He delivered the T.H. Seldon Memorial Lecture for the International Anesthesia Research Society in 2001, his title being "The role of publications in the future of anesthesia". In 2007 he was awarded the Distinguished Service Award of the American Society of Anesthesiologists (ASA). The following year he delivered the prestigious Emery A. Rovenstine Lecture at the annual meeting of the ASA: he spoke on "the pursuit of excellence".

Further reading

Tuman KJ. Ronald D. Miller: Tribute to a Past Editor-in-Chief. *Anesthesia and Analgesia* 2012; **115**: 1431-2.

American Society of Anesthesiologists, 20 October 2008. Ronald D. Miller, M.D., Honored with Distinguished Service Award. www.newswise.com/articles/ronald-d-miller-md-honored-with-distinguished-service-award (Accessed 22 May 2020).

Caldwell JE. Ronald D. Miller, M.D., M.S. The Pursuit of Excellence. *California Society of Anesthesiologists Bulletin* Spring 2009; 39-43.

THE MUSHIN MUSEUM

(HISTORY OF ANAESTHESIA MUSEUM/ AMGUEDDFA HANES ANESTHESIA)

William Woolf Mushin (1910-1993)

The Mushin Museum is a collection of historical artefacts which chronicle the use of anaesthesia and pain relief since the late 19th Century. Named after Professor William Mushin, who started the collection in 1947, the Mushin Museum has over 200 items and is a fascinating collection of historical objects reflecting the colourful and interesting history of anaesthesia.

William Woolf Mushin was born in East London, England in September 1910. Following his time at the Davenant School, he gained his medical education at the London Hospital Medical School, graduating in 1933 with several prizes. Resident jobs in London and wartime service followed and in 1942 Mushin was recruited by the first Professor

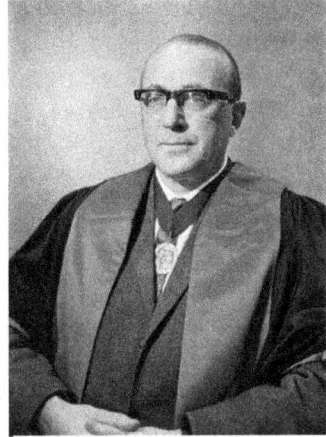

William W. Mushin. Image Credit: Mushin Museum.

of Anaesthetics in Europe, Professor Robert Reynolds Macintosh (1897-1989) at Oxford to be his First Assistant. Mushin's time in Oxford provided invaluable experience in teaching and research, giving Mushin the foundation for a prestigious career in anaesthesia. Macintosh and Mushin collaborated on the first edition of 'Physics for the Anaesthetist' (1946) and Mushin went on to edit future editions.

Mushin was appointed the first director of the Department of Anaesthetics, Welsh National School of Medicine in 1947, and gained oversight of anaesthesia in several hospitals in the Cardiff area. The appointment of Mushin to Cardiff was part of an urgent focus to improve the clinical service, and patient safety became a pervasive thread in the career of Mushin. He strove for improvements in anaesthesia data collection and together with John Lunn in 1982 published a seminal audit concerning mortality associated with anaesthesia; this later became the National Confidential Enquiry into Perioperative Deaths (NECPOD). In 1952 Mushin became the UK's third professor of anaesthesia to be appointed, following Macintosh (Oxford, 1937) and Pask (Newcastle, 1949). Under his leadership the anaesthetic department in Cardiff flourished and became a hub of clinical and research excellence with UK and worldwide standing. Mushin was an international expert on the mechanical ventilation of lungs, producing several authoritative textbooks on the subject including 'Automatic Ventilation of the Lungs' - known widely but not by him as 'the puffing bible', published in 1959. His ongoing curiosity about ventilation stemmed from his time as a teacher in Copenhagen in the 1950s during outbreaks of poliomyelitis. Mushin would certainly now be described as a perioperative physician and was involved in every aspect of patient care and was also a passionate educator, holding the position of Dean of the Faculty of Anaesthetists 1961-1964. Mushin retired in 1975 and was succeeded by Professor Michael Douglas Alan Vickers (1929-2007).

The Museum

The original museum pieces arrived in Cardiff with Professor Mushin when he moved from Oxford. From humble beginnings in a cardboard box, it rapidly expanded to be housed in a large glass fronted cupboard in the Main Laboratory of the Department of Anaesthesia in the Cardiff Royal Infirmary (CRI). Mushin was always committed to using the exhibits as a core part of teaching and would accordingly visit the museum during his weekly teaching rounds. When the Medical School moved from the CRI to the new University Hospital of Wales (opened 1971), the museum was also transferred and was housed in its present location in the Department's Seminar Room. In 2016, following a Cardiff University funded medical student programme, a new area of the Mushin Museum was designed by medical students and the Bill Mapleson Wing was opened. Housing some of the bigger museum items plus displays dedicated to military anaesthesia, this wing is named in honour of the late Professor William Wellesley Mapleson (1926-2017) who was instrumental in the advancement of research work generated by the academic department of anaesthesia in Cardiff. The Bill Mapleson Wing also houses the Lloyd Jones Library, named after retired anaesthetist Dr Peter Lloyd Jones who remains dedicated to the preservation of the department's history.

With a total floor space of nearly 60 square meters, over two sections, the Mushin Museum houses over 200 items that provide a colourful backdrop to the history of anaesthesia, both locally and internationally. Particular highlights include two Magill endotracheal apparatuses: one manufactured in 1927 and the next iteration manufactured in 1932 (Figure 1). These are displayed in the main museum section and feature in museum photographs of Mushin himself in the 1960s using these artefacts to teach medical students (Figure 2). Driven by Mushin, the academic department in Cardiff

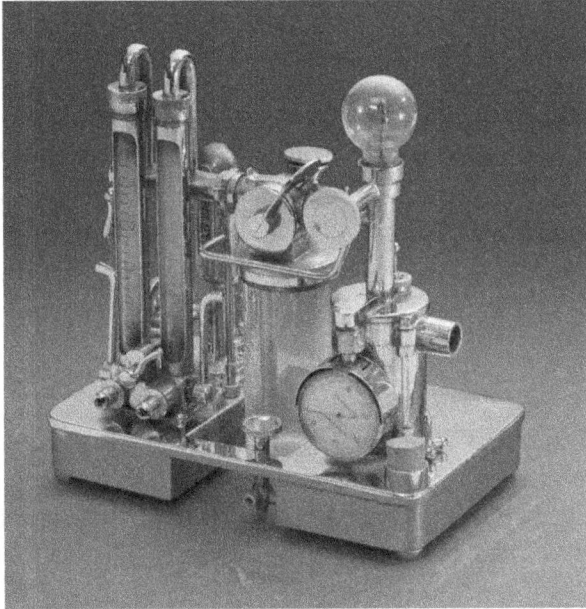

Figure 1. Magill endotracheal apparatus 1932. Image Credit: Mushin Museum.

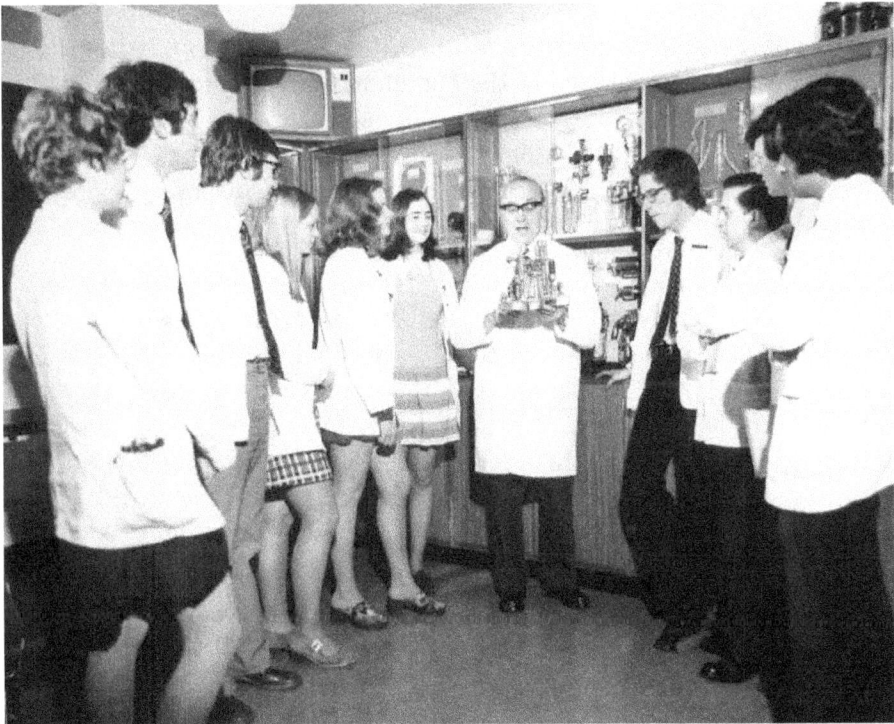

Figure 2. Professor Mushin using the historical collection to teach medical students c. late 1960s. Image Credit: Mushin Museum.

produced focused research on the mechanical ventilation of the lungs. Reflecting this heritage, the museum also has a large collection of ventilators from several manufacturers such as the British Oxygen Company and Blease Medical Equipment; all dwarfed however by the large Engström 150 artificial respirator manufactured by Mivab that sits proudly in the Bill Mapleson Wing. Furthermore, the Mushin Museum houses the first commercially available Patient Controlled Analgesia (PCA) machine, named the Cardiff Palliator. This apparatus was developed in Cardiff in the early 1970s by a team of medical engineers led by Professor Michel Rosen (1927-2018, former President of the College of Anaesthetists (1988-1991). Another interesting piece is one of the only complete curare tipped darts in the UK. It was mounted and presented to Mushin by the intrepid explorer, Richard Gill, in 1949. Sat amongst the many masks, vaporizers and ventilators, artefacts such as this dart remind us of the richness and diversity of anaesthesia history. The museum is housed in a busy anaesthesia department in Wales' largest hospital and can be viewed by appointment.

The Mushin Medal Lecture

Celebrating its 70th anniversary in 2018, the Society of Anaesthetists of Wales (SAW) was established in 1949 and honours Professor Mushin with a prestigious Mushin Medal Lecture. As a prelude to this keynote lecture, the SAW after dinner speeches became a regular stage for talks by many notable anaesthetists of the era; in 1950 Dr Edgar Stanley Rowbotham spoke on 'Continuous Spinal Anaesthesia' and in 1951 the after dinner speech was given by Professor Thomas Cecil Gray.

However, the first Mushin Medal Lecture was actually delivered at the Annual Meeting of the Association of Anaesthetists of Great Britain and Ireland (AAGBI) held in Cardiff in 1975. Professor E.S. Siker, the then Professor of Anesthesiology at the University of Pittsburgh, USA, delivered this inaugural Mushin Medal Lecture and spoke about 'the measure of competence', a subject much debated to this day. The second Mushin Medal Lecture was delivered on November 9th, 1977 in Cardiff at the SAW Annual Scientific Meeting by Sir George Godber GCB who was the Chief Medical Officer in England from 1960 to 1963. Recent notable Mushin Medal Lectures have been delivered by presidents of The Royal College of Anaesthetists, prominent figures in academic anaesthesia and Nobel Prize winners (for example, Sir Martin Evans, Nobel Prize in Medicine, 2007).

Mushin was bestowed with many prestigious honours including: the rank of Commander of the British Empire in 1971; the John Snow Medal in 1974 from the AAGBI; the Henry Hill Hickman Medal in 1978 from the Royal Society of Medicine; FFARACS (Hon) and FFASA (Hon) in 1959 and 1962, respectively; and in 1982 he was awarded a DSc (Hon).

Further reading

Lunn JN. William Woolf Mushin , CBE, DSc, FRCS, FRCA, FANZCA, FFA(SA), DA. *Anaesthesia* 1993; **48**: 461-2.

Mushin WW, Rendell-Baker L, Thompson PW. *Automatic Ventilation of the Lungs*. Oxford: Blackwell Scientific Publications, 1959.

ROBERT ORTON MEDAL

Robert Hamilton Orton (1906-1966)

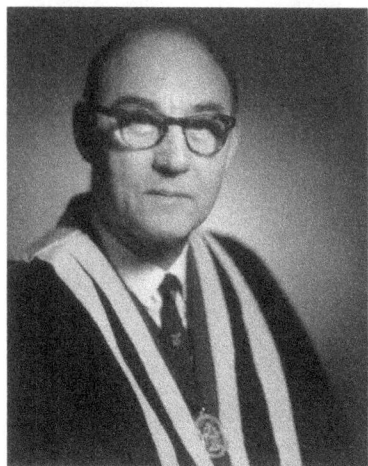

Robert Orton was born in Melbourne, Australia and educated at Wesley College in that city, showing prowess in mathematics. He was interested in technology: radio and electronics. On leaving school, he was admitted to the University of Melbourne. In his second year as a medical student (1926) he developed insulin dependent diabetes. He graduated MB BS in 1930 with many honours and prizes and obtaining an exhibition in medicine.

Robert H. Orton. Photograph by Athol Shmith, courtesy of Geoffrey Kaye Museum of Anaesthetic History, ANZCA.

From 1930 to 1934 Orton did resident medical jobs at the Alfred Hospital in Melbourne and then went into private practice until 1938, when he unfortunately contracted pulmonary tuberculosis. This was successfully treated with artificial pneumothorax, but the resultant fibrothorax reduced his respiratory function and this swayed his decision to choose anaesthesia for his further career. He became the honorary anaesthetist at the Alfred, Royal Melbourne and Royal Women's Hospitals. Becoming more interested in thoracic surgery, he also became honorary anaesthetist at the Austin Hospital.

In 1940 a thoracic surgery unit began at the Alfred Hospital and Orton was appointed full-time anaesthetist there. He went on to pioneer anaesthetic techniques in this specialty. During the restrictions of the Second World War he had his own workshop in which he made apparatus and instruments, thereby avoiding long delays in supplies from overseas. By 1946 he became the unit's whole-time *salaried* anaesthetist; he was pleased to be freed from private practice.

Orton was co-author to Kaye and Renton in the publication of the textbook *Anaesthetic Methods* in 1946. He was President of the Australian Society of Anaesthetists for 1946-47. By this time, he was known as a good teacher and relieving Lecturer in Anaesthetics at the University of Melbourne, which in 1948 introduced its Diploma in Anaesthetics (DA). That year he submitted an excellent thesis on thoracic anaesthesia, for which he was awarded the DA. He then became a member of the Examining Board. In 1949 he was elected a Fellow of the Faculty of Anaesthetists, Royal College of Surgeons of England (FFARCS).

Orton published some 15 papers between 1946 and 1954 mainly on cardiothoracic anaesthesia. In 1950 he was appointed Director of Anaesthetics at the Alfred Hospital; in 1953 this directorship was extended to resuscitation (not yet called intensive care). He was particularly interested in the assessment of new drugs and methods. With Geoffrey Kaye and Douglas Renton (q.v. page 188), he played a major role in the inauguration of the Faculty of Anaesthetists of the Royal Australasian College of Surgeons in 1952; a foundation Fellow, he served as its second Dean for 1955-59. Also, he was Director of the Examining Board for the Melbourne DA from 1956.

Ill health caused Orton to retire from clinical anaesthesia in 1957, but he continued to work in administration and education. He resigned as Director of Anaesthesia in 1966, but he was promptly made Director of Electronics at the Alfred Hospital and improved instrumentation in several departments. Sadly, he succumbed to diabetic atherosclerosis in December 1966.

Several honours were awarded to Orton in his lifetime. He was made an Honorary Member of the New Zealand Society of Anaesthetists in 1948, Embley Orator of the Victorian Branch of the British Medical Association in 1957, and an Honorary Fellow of the UK Faculty of Anaesthetists in 1961.

After his death, the Australasian Faculty introduced the Robert Orton Medal for distinguished service to anaesthesia – extended later by the ANZCA to perioperative medicine and/or pain medicine.

Table 1. Robert Orton Medal winners

Year	Recipient	Year	Recipient
1968	Margaret McClelland	1996	Geoffrey M. Clarke
1968	George F. Anson	1997	Jeanette R. Thirlwell Jones
1968	Harry John Daly	1999	Walter J. Russell
1973	John R. Ritchie	2004	John R.A. Rigg
1974	Geoffrey Kaye	2004	Graham C. Fisk
1975	Charles A. Sara	2004	Francis X. Moloney
1975	Ralph R. Clark	2005	Garry D. Phillips
1976	Kevin McCaul	2005	Pamela Macintyre
1983	Brian E. Dwyer	2005	Cindy Aun
1985	Maurice J.W. Sando	2007	Teik Ewe Oh
1987	Teresa R. Cramond	2008	Michael J. Cousins
1988	Douglas Joseph	2009	Peter Kam
1989	Robin W. Smallwood	2010	Paul S. Myles
1989	Gordon A. Harrison	2011	Duncan I. Campbell
1989	William M. Crosby	2012	Leona F. Wilson
1989	Noel M. Cass	2014	Kate Leslie
1990	Gwenifer C. Wilson	2014	William B. Runciman
1991	Thomas C.K. Brown	2016	David A. Story
1993	Ross B. Holland	2016	Stephen A. Schug
1994	Arthur B. Baker	2016	Alan F. Merry
1995	Peter D. Livingstone	2018	Richard G. Walsh
1995	Benedict J. Barry		

Further reading

Obituary Robert Hamilton Orton. *The Medical Journal of Australia* 6 May 1967; 935-8.

Orton RH. Anesthesia in Thoracic Surgery. *Anesthesia and Analgesia Current Researches* 1946; **25**: 96-109.

www.geoffreykayemuseum.org.au/fellows/deans-of-the-faculty-of-anaesthetists/robert-orton-anzca/ (accessed 15 February 2020).

GERARD W OSTHEIMER LECTURE

Gerard W. Ostheimer (1940-1995)

Gerard Ostheimer was born in Poughkeepsie, New York, USA in 1940 and educated at St Francis College in Pennsylvania. He went to the School of Medicine at the University of Pennsylvania, graduating in 1965 and then took an internship at Misericordia Hospital in Philadelphia. His training in anaesthesia included residency at the Hospital of the University of Pennsylvania, followed by a cardiovascular fellowship at the Mayo Clinic and a research fellowship at Massachusetts General Hospital. He qualified as a Diplomate of the American Board of Anesthesiology in 1971.

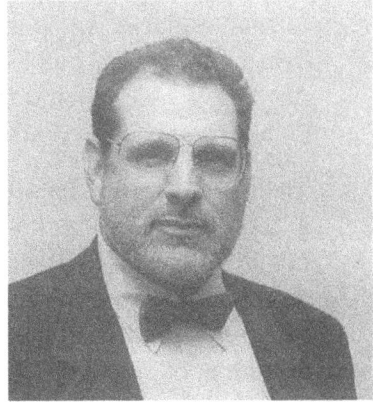

Gerard W. Ostheimer. Photograph courtesy of Prof. André Van Zundert.

Ostheimer became interested in obstetric anaesthesia and in 1972 was appointed anaesthesiologist at the old Boston Hospital for Women. In 1980 he was much involved in its union with the Peter Brent Brigham Hospital and the Robert Breck Brigham Hospital into the Brigham and Women's Hospital (BWH). That year he also became the President of the Society for Obstetric Anesthesia and Perinatology (SOAP). In 1981 he became the Director of Obstetrical Anesthesia at BWH, serving in this role until 1988. His textbook *Manual of Obstetric Anesthesia* was published by Churchill Livingstone in 1984 and there was a second edition in 1992.

Regional anaesthesia in obstetrics was strongly promoted by Gerard Ostheimer at the BWH – indeed it became known as "The House of Regional Anesthesia". From the late 1980s he assisted Benjamin G. Covino in setting up standards of practice in regional anaesthesia, obstetric anaesthesia and pain management for the USA.

In 1990 Ostheimer was appointed Editor-in-Chief of the journal *Regional Anesthesia*, the official publication of the American Society of Regional Anesthesia (ASRA) and the European Society of Regional Anaesthesia (ESRA). He immediately began to improve its status. While retaining Benjamin Covino and Philip O. Bridenbaugh as senior editors, he increased the editorial board to 31 members and within a year each issue had about ten original articles. He quickly published a Supplement containing all the issues of the first five volumes (1976-1980), as these had not been indexed. Above all he specified the "Uniform Requirements" for authors including structured abstracts and statements on ethics. Sadly, Covino died in 1991, but Ostheimer pushed on with the improvements. One of the first descriptions of ultrasonic guidance for nerve blocks was published in the 1992 volume. By 1994 the journal became the official publication also of the Asian Oceanic Society of Regional Anesthesia (AOSRA) and the Latin American Society of Regional Anesthesia (LASRA) and was truly international.

Ostheimer was appointed Professor of Anesthesia at Harvard Medical School in 1991. He served as President of ASRA for 1991-92. By this time, he had published over fifty articles in peer reviewed journals. On invitation he delivered several prestigious lectures, including the first Benjamin B. Covino Lecture at the Maimonides Medical Center in 1992 and the Henry S. Ruth Lecture at Hahnemann University, Philadelphia in 1993.

Ostheimer continued to serve as Editor-in-Chief of *Regional Anesthesia* until his untimely death in October 1995 suddenly of cardiac arrest. This was a shock to his many friends and colleagues. He was renowned for his clinical expertise in regional anaesthesia and as a lecturer, teacher and reviewer. Before his death he had co-edited with Andre Van Zundert another textbook *Pain Relief and Anesthesia in Obstetrics*. This was published the following year. Besides editing, Ostheimer personally contributed to the following chapters:

- Epidural needles and technique
- Spinal needles and technique
- Resuscitation and care of the newborn
- Organization of an anaesthetic service for obstetrics
- Standards for obstetric anaesthesia
- Financial considerations
- The labour and delivery suite.

Further editions of *Ostheimer's Manual of Obstetric Anesthesia* were also edited by David J. Birnbach.

From 1998 one of the lectures given at the annual meeting of SOAP, "What's New in Obstetric Anesthesia", was renamed the Gerard W. Ostheimer Lecture.

Table 1. Gerard W. Ostheimer lecturers

Year	Lecturer	Year	Lecturer
1998	David Campbell	2009	John T. Sullivan
1999	Hoyt McCallum	2010	Jill M. Mhyre
2000	Linda S. Polley	2011	Paloma Toledo
2001	B. Scott Segal	2012	Alexander Butwick
2002	David H. Wlody	2013	Arvind Palanisamy
2003	Audrey S. Alleyne	2014	Lisa R. Leffert
2004	Lawrence C. Tsen	2015	Katherine W. Arendt
2005	Brenda A. Bucklin	2016	Philip E. Hess
2006	Roshan Fernando	2017	Brian T. Bateman
2007	Alison Macarthur	2018	Ashraf S. Habib
2008	Ruth Landau	2019	Carolyn Weiniger

Acknowledgement

Dr William Camann kindly provided the curriculum vitae of Gerard W. Ostheimer.

Further reading

Lema MJ. In Memoriam Gerard W. Ostheimer, M.D. *Regional Anesthesia* 1995; **20**: 469-70.

Van Zundert A, Ostheimer GW (Eds.). *Pain Relief and Anesthesia in Obstetrics*. New York: Churchill Livingstone, 1996.

Camann W. Pioneer's Corner: Gerard Ostheimer, M.D. *SOAP Newsletter* Winter 2011-12: 11.

Neal JM, Baker J. Regional Anesthesia and Pain Medicine After 30 Years: A Historical Perspective. *Regional Anesthesia and Pain Medicine* 2006; **31**: 575-81.

GERALDINE O'SULLIVAN LECTURE

Geraldine Mary O'Sullivan (1952-2013)

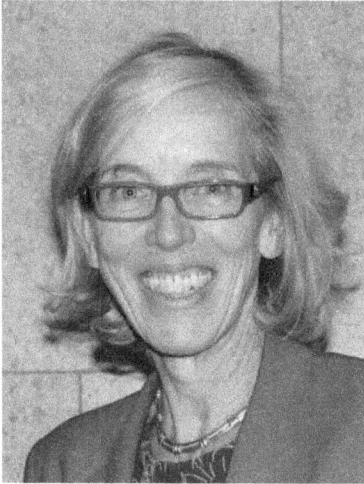

Geraldine M. O'Sullivan. Image courtesy of the Obstetric Anaesthetists' Association.

Geraldine O'Sullivan was born in September 1952 in Ireland. She completed her education at Loreto Abbey, Rathfarnham (South Dublin), Ireland in 1969 and then studied medicine, graduating MB, BCh BAO from the National University of Ireland in 1975. After junior doctor training in Dublin, she took a senior house officer post in anaesthetics at Cork Regional Hospital and at this early stage of her career contributed to a paper on attenuation of the pressor response to laryngoscopy, published in the journal *Anaesthesia* in 1980. She then moved to Oxford, England where by 1981 she had qualified with the diploma FFARCS and had a senior registrar post in the Nuffield Department of Anaesthetics at the Radcliffe Infirmary. Attracted to obstetric anaesthesia, she won (out of eight applicants) the first Research Fellowship awarded by the Association of Anaesthetists of Great Britain and Ireland – for the study of gastric function in pregnancy, using non-invasive methods. She worked with recognized experts including Roy E. S. Bullingham (who later went to Syntex Research), Henry J. McQuay and Len E.S. Carrie. Completing her appointment in March 1984, she submitted her work for an MD thesis to the National University of Ireland. Another notable aspect of her time in Oxford was that she assisted Len Carrie in introducing the combined spinal-epidural (CSE) technique into British practice.

O'Sullivan then moved to St Thomas' Hospital in London to complete her anaesthetic training. This was an ideal place to further her career in obstetric anaesthesia: it had the largest maternity unit in London and was a tertiary referral centre for high risk pregnancies; the academic unit was headed by Felicity J.M. Reynolds, then Reader in Pharmacology and Honorary Consultant in charge of obstetric anaesthesia. Soon O'Sullivan was appointed a Consultant there with sessions in obstetric, ophthalmic and vascular anaesthesia, and she continued high quality research and publications.

In 1991 O'Sullivan was on the founding editorial board of the new *International Journal of Obstetric Anesthesia*. Over the next decade she contributed chapters to textbooks and became renowned as a lecturer, particularly at the annual 3-day course on obstetric anaesthesia and analgesia organized in London by the Obstetric Anaesthetists' Association (OAA). She served two terms on the OAA Executive Committee and was elected President of the OAA in 2002 until 2005.

O'Sullivan went on to be the lead clinician for obstetric anaesthesia at St Thomas' Hospital. In November 2007, as Chair of the International Committee of the OAA, she went as one of the Faculty for a refresher course on anaesthesia and analgesia in obstetrics held in Sremska Mitrovica, Serbia. In March 2009 she went to Iasi, Romania as a member of an outreach team organized by the European Society of Anaesthesiology (ESA) to be faculty for a 2-day refresher course on obstetric anaesthesia. That year she became a member of ESA's Faculty of Euroanaesthesia Congresses and a member of the Task Force on Preoperative Guidelines (2009-2011): these guidelines on perioperative fasting were published in the *European Journal of Anaesthesiology* in 2011. In this were updates on oral intake in labour, incorporating O'Sullivan's earlier work which had dispelled much myth, by showing the relative safety of isotonic sports drinks in labour. She was elected to ESA Council in 2010. She chaired the European Regional Section of the World Federation of Societies of Anaesthesiologists (WFSA). In 2011 she was elected Chair of the National Anaesthesiology Societies Committee (NASC) and successfully organised the first ESA "Teach the Teacher" course.

Geraldine O'Sullivan had a long and courageous battle with cancer, continuing to work, lecture and write until just a few weeks before her death in December 2013. She conceived and was the principal investigator of an important study on gastric emptying, which was published in the *British Journal of Anaesthesia* in January 2014.

Socially she played tennis and was known by colleagues and visitors as an entertaining hostess. She was married to a Professor of Ophthalmology with whom she had two daughters. In all the published obituaries and tributes to her, and in correspondence to produce this article, the most striking message has been the warmth of feeling that she generated.

In 2017 the OAA Executive decided that the special lecture at its annual 3-day course, earmarked for an invited expert, should be named the Geraldine O'Sullivan Lecture.

Table 1. Geraldine O'Sullivan lecturers and lecture titles

Year	Lecturer	Title
2017	Andrew Shennan	A simple strategy to tackle global pre-eclampsia, sepsis and haemorrhage.
2018	Cynthia Wong	Maternal mortality and the role of the anaesthetist.
2019	Jose Carvalho	Dogmas in obstetric anaesthesia: the balance between evidence, common sense, habit and fear.

Acknowledgement

Dr Nuala Lucas kindly assisted with the list of Geraldine O'Sullivan lectures.

Further reading

Curran J, Crowley M, O'Sullivan G. Droperidol and endotracheal intubation. Attenuation of pressor response to laryngoscopy and intubation. *Anaesthesia* 1980; **35**: 290-4.

O'Sullivan GM, Bullingham RE. Does twice the volume of antacid have twice the effect in pregnant women at term? *Anesthesia and Analgesia* 1984; **63**: 752-6.

Carrie LE, O'Sullivan G. Subarachnoid bupivacaine 0.5% for caesarean section. *European Journal of Anaesthesiology* 1984; **1**: 275-83.

Smith I, Kranke P, Murat I, Smith A, O'Sullivan G *et al*. Perioperative fasting in adults and children:guidelines from the European Society of Anaesthesiology *European Journal of Anaesthesiology* 2011; **28**: 556-69.

Russell R. Obituary Geraldine O'Sullivan. *International Journal of Obstetric Anesthesia* 2014; **23**: 8-9.

NAGIN PARBHOO HISTORY OF ANAESTHESIA MUSEUM and MEMORIAL LECTURE

Nagin Parbhoo (1942-2009)

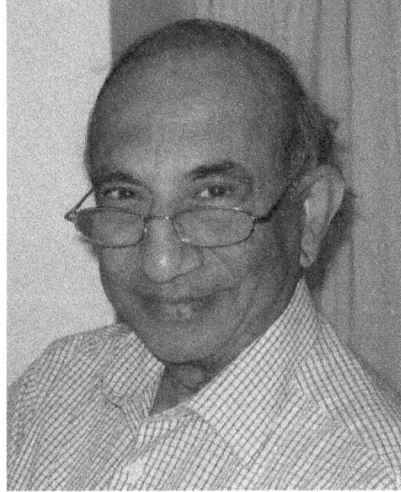

Naginlal Parag (Nagin) Parbhoo, the youngest of 8 children was born in Wynberg, Cape Town in 1942. His father Parag had travelled to South Africa (SA) from India seeking work in 1902. A cordwainer by trade, he travelled widely in SA and eventually settled in Wynberg where he opened 3 shops to take advantage of the British military presence in the area. After several trips to India, he brought the family to SA in 1936. Nagin's older brother Santilal qualified MB ChB from the University of Cape Town (UCT) and later became a surgeon in the UK. Unable to study medicine at UCT because of apartheid quotas he accepted a scholarship from the Government of India and graduated MB BS from the University of Bombay's Grant Medical College in 1969. He returned to SA and worked in Port Elizabeth as a general practitioner with an interest in anaesthesia, before specialising in anaesthesia at UCT. After qualifying FFA (SA) in 1983 he worked as a consultant at Groote Schuur Hospital until 1987 when he went into private practice whilst retaining links with the hospital as a part-time senior lecturer until 1995.

Throughout his career he devoted much time and effort to the South African Society of Anaesthesiologists (SASA) both locally in the Western Cape where he served as Chairman in 1990 and nationally as Councillor. In 1987 he accepted the position of honorary archivist of the society, a position he held until his death in 2009. He authored the history of the society in his book *Five Decades - The History of the SA Society of Anaesthetists 1943 - 1993*, released at the Society's Jubilee Congress in 1993. In the same year he took over from Tony Rocke as editor of the Societies' Newsletter, *Pipeline*, a task he relished until 2001 when he was diagnosed with leukaemia and resigned. In 2002 he was awarded the degree of Doctor of Medicine by UCT for his thesis, *The Department of Anaesthesia, UCT 1920 - 2000*. Nagin died in January 2009 and is survived by his three daughters and 5 grandchildren.

The Museum

The anaesthesia museum at Groote Schuur Hospital was started as a small collection in 1956 by the then HoD of the UCT Department of Anaesthesia Dr Cecil (Buck) Jones after the donation of equipment and papers that had belonged to SA's first specialist anaesthetist, Dr Bampfylde Daniel by his partner Dr Royden Muir. In the 1930's Muir travelled to the USA, befriended Ralph Waters and Richard von Foregger and on his return in 1933 introduced cyclopropane to Britain and South Africa. Anaesthetic equipment owned by Muir in the museum includes a rare 1917 Boyles apparatus, a Pinson ether 'bomb', a specially commissioned 2-yoke Muir Midget, and a pharyngeal airway designed by Canadian Beverly Leech in 1937. After failing to persuade the University to house the collection in the medical school library the artifacts were housed in the office of the head of the UCT anaesthetic department and became the nucleus of the museum.

In 1961 Arthur Bull was appointed to the newly created Chair of Anaesthesia at UCT. He encouraged the growing collection and contacted anaesthetic appliance companies in the UK seeking information on some of the early equipment on display. Whilst a Nuffield Clinical Assistant under Macintosh in Oxford he had worked with Raventos and Suckling in early testing of halothane in animals and later donated a rare TEC 1 vaporiser and an Oxford Miniature ventilator to the collection. The collection also possesses a rare TEC 2 type MJ halothane vaporizer (calibrated from 0 - 10) and a Gardner Oxford Ether vaporizer. The Taurus radiofrequency blood warmer in the museum was developed in a collaborative process between the UCT departments of electrical engineering and anaesthesia in the 1960s and named after Bull. On his retirement the Cape Western Branch of SASA commissioned a bronze bust of Bull that was presented to him and subsequently donated to the museum.

In 1980 Nagin approached Professor Gaisford Harrison, who had succeeded Bull as head of department and asked whether he could take charge of the collection. He was appointed Honorary Curator of the fledgling museum and spent much of his free time sourcing old equipment from various nursing homes in Cape Town. After the move to the much enlarged anaesthetic department in the New Groote Schuur Hospital in 1988, Naginlal with the approval of the new HoD, Professor Mike James, obtained sponsorship for housing the collection in 8 oak and glass cabinets (Figure 1). In March 2000 James honoured his contribution by naming the museum "The Nagin Parbhoo History of Anaesthesia Museum".

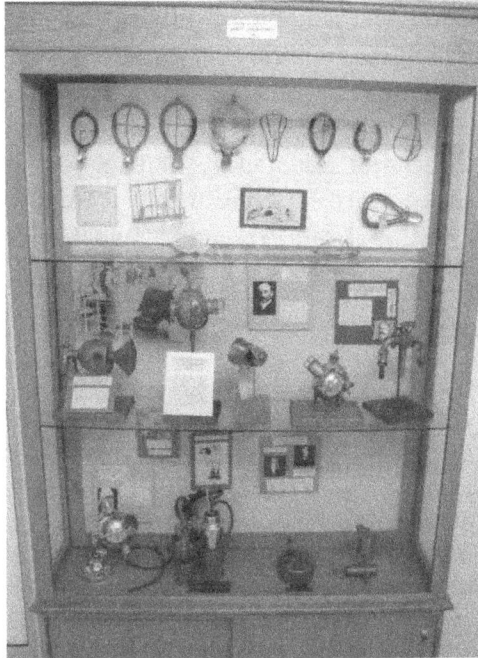

Figure 1. Display of early masks and inhalers.

Peter Gordon succeeded Parbhoo as curator of the museum and SASA archivist in 2009 and has significantly grown the collection housing new items in silver and glass display cabinets previously used in the operating theatres (Figure 2). He has also encouraged research into many of the artifacts. The displays are mainly laid out along the corridors of the Department, but also in part of two rooms – total floor space about 158 m^2.

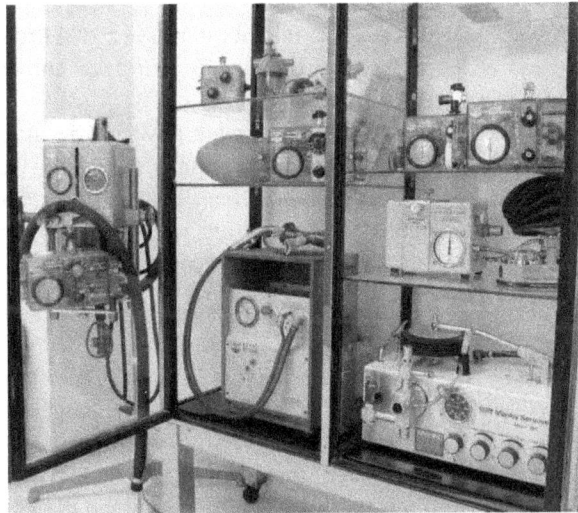

Figure 2. Ventilators in the collection.

Prof. Justiaan Swanevelder succeeded Professor James as HoD in 2012 and at his suggestion a successful History of Anaesthesia and Ethics Congress was held in Cape Town in 2013. At the meeting renowned anaesthetic historian Dr

David Wilkinson handed over a facsimile of Morton's inhaler to the museum on behalf of Dr George Bause, honorary curator of the Wood Library-Museum in Chicago. The museum has become popular with organized medical tours from abroad and in 2018 links with Australia were cemented by the donation of a Komasarrof resuscitator donated by Dr Paul Luckin on behalf of the Melbourne Ambulance Service Museum that was used in mobile intensive care ambulances in Australia from 1972, and a medallion from the Australian Society of Anaesthesia.

The Collection houses:

- Early anaesthetic and analgesia delivery systems designed by - Murphy (1847), Esmarch (1877), Schimmelbusch (1897), Hewitt (1901), Vernon Harcourt (1901), Ombrédanne (1908), Boyle (1917 - 1933), Junkers (1867) & later modifications, Shipway (1916), Pinson's 'ether bomb' (1926), McKesson (1920 & 1930), De Caux (1930), King (1936). Later vaporizers include the Copper Kettle, Rowbotham inhaler, Foregger ether drop vaporizer, Fluotecs Mark 1-6, Goldman's vinesthene and halothane vaporizers, and the Dräger Vapor Halothan vaporizer (1960).
- Ventilators displayed include: Bird mark 1, 2, 3, 4, 7, & 8; Manley; Cyclator; Dräger Iron Lung model E52, an Emerson cuirass ventilator and the hand sized Minivent designed by Johannesburg anaesthetist, Dr Anthony Cohen in 1965.
- Battlefield equipment include a USA Kreiselman resuscitator (1943), a USSR resuscitator manufactured in 1963 and an Ambubag made for use in chemical warfare.
- Anaesthetic equipment designed by SA anaesthesiologists includes the Taurus blood warmer named after the UCT's Professor Bull, Cape Town and Stellenbosch breathing circuits for paediatric anaesthesia, Samson's neonatal resuscitators, Humphrey's ADE breathing system (q.v. pages 100-104), and the Miller Maxima breathing system.

- Anaesthetic machines and monitors used at Groote Schuur Hospital between 1940 and 1984.
- Posters recording the historic human-to-human heart transplant operation performed at Groote Schuur Hospital in 1967 and Harrison's pioneering work in Malignant Hyperthermia that led to the use of dantrolene.
- A section of the museum is devoted to the history of the SA Society of Anaesthesiologists since its foundation in 1943.
- Equipment designed by South African anaesthetists on display includes the Taurus blood warmer named after Prof. Bull, and breathing circuits designed by Dr Heymie Samson, Don Miller and David Humphrey.
- Signed photographs of prominent anaesthetists from abroad who visited SA include Sir Robert Macintosh and Victor Goldman from the UK, and Prof. E Rovenstine and Ralph Tovell from the USA.

Dr Eric Hodgson from Durban succeeded Nagin as editor of *Pipeline* and at his suggestion the Society has since 2010 (except for 2015) held a Nagin Parbhoo History of Anaesthesia Memorial Lecture during its annual Congress (Table 1).

Table 1. Nagin Parbhoo Memorial lecturers and lecture titles

Year	Lecturer	Title
2010	Stephanus Potgieter	Anaesthesia in SA from Jan van Riebeek until today
2011	David Morell	The history of oxygen – from the big bang to the era of the super predator
2012	Peter C Gordon	The anaesthetic for the world's first human-to-human heart transplant
2013	Alan Weyer	The Eastern Cape's 100 years war: cattle, diamonds and ether
2014	David Wilkinson	Can we reach parity?
2015	No lecture	
2016	Louise Cilliers	Anaesthesia BC
2017	Michael James	In the beginning there was oxygen ..... or was there?
2018	David Wilkinson	Looking back to go forward: the history and future of our specialty
2019	David Morrell	Look Ma, no hands! What AI, immunotherapy and CRISPR hold for us.
2020	Arthur Rantloane	From agony to ecstasy – the gift of anaesthesia to the world

Further reading

Parbhoo NP. *Five decades The South African Society of Anaesthetists 1943-1993*. Johannesburg: South African Society of Anaesthetists, 1993.

Gordon PC, James MFM. The Nagin Parbhoo History of Anaesthesia Museum - Part 1. *South African Journal of Anaesthesia & Analgesia* 2019; **25**: 5-13.
-Part 2. *South African Journal of Anaesthesia & Analgesia* 2020; **26**: 21-25.

PATIENT CONTROLLED ANALGESIA (PCA)

Philip Haim Sechzer (1914-2004)

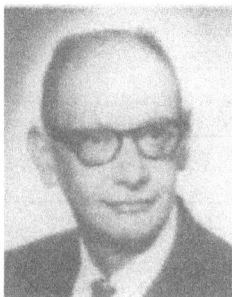

Philip Haim Sechzer was born in New York City in September 1914, the son of Jewish immigrants. He was educated at Stuyvesant High School until 1930 and then City College of New York, graduating BS in 1934. He then studied medicine at New York University, where he graduated in 1938.

After being a house physician at Harlem Hospital (1938-1940) Sechzer chose to be a resident in anaesthesiology at Fordham Hospital in New York City. Then he served in the Second World War as a Major in the US Army Air Forces Medical Corps, stationed in Texas from 1942 to 1946. After the war, he was Director of Anesthesiology at Fordham Hospital from 1947 to 1955. He moved to the post of Assistant Professor of Anesthesiology at the University of Pennsylvania School of Medicine in 1956. Next, through 1963-65 he taught at the Baylor University College of Medicine in Houston, Texas and worked in Michael De Bakey's cardiac surgery team. He published a book on how to operate and maintain the Bird Respirator in 1965.

Philip H. Sechzer. Credit: Maimonides Medical Center.

At Baylor in February 1965, while attending the Nathan B. Eddy (National Institute of Health) Conference on Drug Addiction and Narcotics, a new concept occurred to him: the idea of 'patients controlling their own analgesia' electronically. His hypothesis was that if a patient could register pain by pressing a button which activated delivery of a dose of analgesic, this could be used to measure pain, analgesic efficacy and placebo effect. A simple apparatus was constructed, and initial data was collected in the Cardiovascular Intensive Area of the Methodist Hospital, Houston. Sechzer first reported on this at the Argentinian Angiology Congress held in Buenos Aires in 1966. In the same year he moved to the Maimonides Medical Center in Brooklyn, New York where he was appointed Director of Anesthesiology. He was also appointed Professor of Anesthesiology at the State University of New York (SUNY) – Health Science Center at Brooklyn.

In January 1968 Sechzer published a study on the use of his analgesic-demand system on 20 postoperative patients: when a patient pressed the button, a nurse-observer administered 1 ml of analgesic solution (morphine or pethidine) intravenously (i.v.) and also recorded its effect. The results indicated that the system provided improved analgesia with relatively low total drug dosage. However, it clearly placed impractical demands on the nursing staff.

At the SUNY, Sechzer developed an apparatus which included an electronic recorder and timer, and a roller pump (Holter Co.) which delivered an i.v. dose of opioid or placebo, on demand, but restricted to a fixed interval. The results of its use on treating postoperative pain in 118 patients were presented at the 1970 Congress of the International Anesthesia Research Society and published in January the following year in *Anesthesia and Analgesia*. The first sentence of this paper began "A patient-controlled analgesic ....": **hence the acronym PCA**.

Sechzer was mainly interested in the study of pain and pain relief *per se* rather than developing PCA as a clinical treatment modality. The latter aim was taken forward by others, initially most effectively by Michael Keeri-Szanto, who was the Professor of Anaesthetics in London, Ontario, Canada. He collaborated with Sechzer and over the next ten years developed a commercial PCA pump – US patent 4, 275, 727 (1981). His team reported that use of the device decreased postoperative pain and shortened hospital stay.

In the UK, Professor Michael Rosen at Cardiff developed a PCA apparatus for delivering incremental doses of pethidine in labour: the 'Cardiff palliator' which came to market in 1976. Rosen organized an international symposium on PCA at Leeds Castle in Kent, England in 1984. There it was agreed that the title for the new modality should indeed be 'Patient Controlled Analgesia' (PCA). The Cardiff Palliator became obsolete because it did not have a means to lock up the drug syringe.

The development of microprocessors accelerated the advance of programmable PCA pumps. It became accepted that PCA gives the patients self-control of their own pain, exact titration of dose, rapid pain relief without having to bother the nurses; good analgesia is usually achieved with less total opioid. The method has been adopted widely in the developed world, with pre-setting but possible adjustment of two main variables: the dose and the 'lockout' time; in addition, it is possible to provide a background infusion. Alarms with indicators for various problems have been devised.

A low incidence of complications including death have been reported. Throughout the world most healthcare authorities have produced their own guidelines for safe use of the PCA system. Most important is adequate explanation to the patient. A one-way Y-connector enables use with i.v. infusions; anti-reflux valves are recommended to prevent reflux delivery of drug into gravity fed infusion tubing in the event of an occlusion. The patients must be monitored by use of a chart which includes pain score, respiration, sedation and nausea.

At Maimonides Medical Center, Sechzer directed the Pain Therapy Center, which included nerve blocks, acupuncture, biofeedback, hypnosis, physical therapy, TENS, psychiatric and psychological help. In 1985 he was awarded Honorary FFARCS by the Royal College of Surgeons in Ireland. He retired in 1986, but published a summary of his pioneering work on the PCA system in 1990.

The term PCA has come to be universally applied to the system whereby a patient can get analgesics *injected* on-demand. As described, this was pioneered by Sechzer from 1965. Some historians have pointed out that the concept of self-administration of *inhalational* analgesia was noted as far back as 1847 by William Hooper and introduced in the form of nitrous oxide with air for labour by Robert Minnitt in 1933.

Further reading

Pearce J. Philip H. Sechzer, 90, Expert On Pain and How to Ease It. *The New York Times* 4 October 2004.

Sechzer PH. *The Bird respirator*. Houston: D.H. White & Co., 1965.

Sechzer PH. Objective Measurement of Pain. *Anesthesiology* 1968; **29**: 209-10.

Sechzer PH. Studies in Pain With the Analgesic-Demand System. *Anesthesia and Analgesia* 1971; **50**: 1-10.

White PF. Use of Patient-Controlled Analgesia for Management of Acute Pain. *Journal of the American Medical Association* 1988; **259**: 243-7.

Sechzer PH. Patient-Controlled Analgesia (PCA): A Retrospective. *Anesthesiology* 1990; **72**: 735-6.

PAYNE STAFFORD TAN AWARD

James Patrick Payne (1922-2015)

James Payne was brought up in Larkhall, South Lanarkshire, Scotland until he was fourteen, when his father died and the family moved to Leith, the port of Edinburgh. After secondary education he began medical studies at the University of Edinburgh, funding himself by working on the Edinburgh to London railway. During Army Training Corps exercises he sustained a partially detached retina, so that he was unable to read for some weeks – this prompted him to volunteer for work in the casualty department of Leith Hospital. There he was introduced to the administration of anaesthetics and he accumulated over 5000 administrations by the time he qualified MB, ChB in 1946.

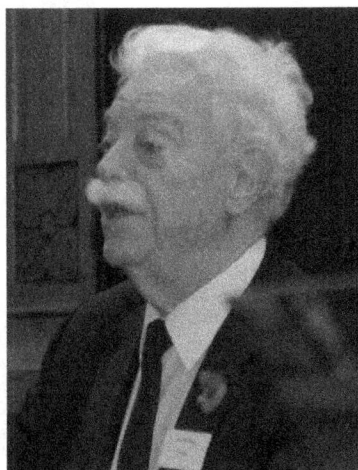

James P. Payne. Image courtesy of the History of Anaesthesia Society.

In 1950 he joined the Department of Anaesthetics under Dr John Gillies at the Royal Infirmary of Edinburgh. Next, he moved to the University of Manchester and then in 1954 he was appointed a Lecturer at the Department of Anaesthetics of the Postgraduate Medical School, Hammersmith, London. Qualified FFARCS at this time, he worked there with another lecturer, J.F. Nunn and the pair jointly published a landmark paper on postoperative hypoxaemia in 1962. Payne assisted J.F. Nunn and R.P. Harbord in setting up the Anaesthetic Research Society in 1958.

Payne was appointed to the British Oxygen Company (BOC) endowed Professorial Chair at the Royal College of Surgeons of England in 1963 (succeeding Ronald Woolmer). Three years later he published (with Hill and King) a notable paper in the *British Medical Journal* on the distribution of alcohol in blood, breath and urine. Based on this research, the breathalyser was introduced in Britain in 1967 – leading to a great reduction in deaths caused by car crashes from drink driving. In 1970 Payne delivered the Joseph Clover Lecture of the Faculty of Anaesthetists – on the quality of measurement.

Becoming well known as "Jimmy Payne" he published extensively on monitoring of neuromuscular blockade (1970s) and the new muscle relaxants atracurium and vecuronium (1980s). Other topics on which he published much were technology as well as ethics (1970s) and in 1980 he and J.A. Bushman co-edited a book *Artificial Ventilation: Technical, Biological and Clinical Aspects*. In 1981 he produced a review of chloroform in clinical anaesthesia. Through 1980-83 he was Chairman of the Manpower Advisory Standing Committee, Department of Health and Social Security (DHSS). He was a member of the Council of the Association of Anaesthetists of Great Britain and Ireland (AAGBI) for 1984-86 and served as Vice President. In 1986 he co-edited a book *Pulse Oximetry* with Professor John W. Severinghaus of San Francisco.

Payne retired from his Chair at the Royal College of Surgeons in 1987, having been Professor there for 24 years. The University of London named him Emeritus Professor of Anaesthesia. He was elected an Honorary Member of the AAGBI in 1989. In retirement he was active in the history of anaesthesia, publishing many articles through the 1990s and up to 2005. A plain-speaking, but colourful character, Jimmy Payne was proud of his Scottish roots and unstintingly praised his mentor, John Gillies (q.v. page 76).

The Royal College of Anaesthetists began in 2009 an annual Payne Stafford Tan Award. This came about through the generosity of the Norman Knight Charitable Foundation of Boston, Massachusetts, USA. It was created in honour of the medical careers of Professor James P. Payne and two researchers he mentored at the Royal College of Surgeons, London – Dr Timothy J. Stafford and Dr Oon T. Tan. In 1982 they jointly published a paper on the suppression of alcohol-induced flushing by a combination of H1 and H2 histamine antagonists. Later in 1982 Timothy J. Stafford went to work for Kontron Inc. in Boston and while there he published on instrumentation for computerized monitoring. Oon T. Tan also subsequently went to Boston where she became a Lecturer on Otolaryngology at Harvard Medical School and Director of the Carolyn and Peter Lynch Center for Laser and Reconstructive Surgery.

The Payne Stafford Tan award has provided funding for travel and research, the aim being to mark excellence in clinical practice, teaching or research in anaesthesia, critical care or pain management.

Table 1. Payne Stafford Tan award winners

Year	Recipient
2009	Dom Hurford
2010	Isabelle Reed and Eleanor Walker
2011	No award
2012	Zahid Khan
2013	No award
2014	Danielle Huckle
2015	Rebecca Szekely
2016	No award
2017	Vasileios Zochios
2018	Yohinee Karuna Rajendran
2019	No award

Further reading

Obituary: JP Payne. *The Guardian* 28 May 2015.

J.P. Payne MB Edin FFARCS DA. In: Harrison MJ. *British Academic Anaesthetists 1950 – 2000 Volume 1*. Wellington NZ: Michael J Harrison, 2011; 77-96.

Nunn JF, Payne JP. Hypoxaemia after general anaesthesia. *Lancet* 1962; **2**: 631-2.

Payne JP. Chloroform in clinical anaesthesia. *British Journal of Anaesthesia* 1981; **53**: 11S-15S.

Tan OT, Stafford TJ, Sarkany I, Gaylarde PM, Tilsey C, Payne JP. Suppression of alcohol-induced flushing by a combination of H1 and H2 histamine antagonists. *British Journal of Dermatology* 1982; **107**: 647-52.

PENDER COLLECTION OF LIVING HISTORY OF ANESTHESIOLOGY

John William Pender (1912-2001)

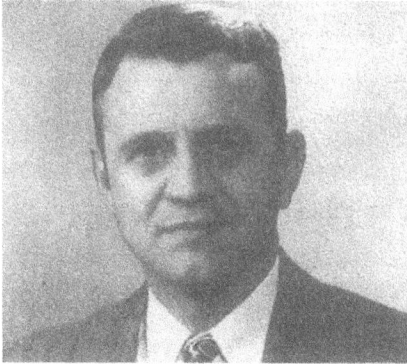

John William "Bill" Pender was born in Hesterville, Mississippi, USA in 1912. After schooling, he went to the University of Mississippi where he received his BS degree in 1933. This being during the Great Depression, his further education at Tulane Medical School in New Orleans was funded by a grant from the Commonwealth Fund of New York. Obtaining his MD in 1935, he proceeded to internship at the US Public Health Hospital in San Francisco.

John W. Pender. Image reproduced with permission from *Bulletin of Anesthesia History*.

Pender entered general practice (GP) in rural Mississippi in 1937 and after a while took over the GP of his ill father in Hesterville. However, he missed the specialist work he had seen at Tulane, and in 1940 he moved to anaesthesia training at the Mayo Clinic in Rochester, Minnesota. In 1942, after the USA entered the Second World War, he was called up for active duty in the Navy. Soon he was stationed at the Bethesda Naval Hospital, Maryland near Washington, DC.

At Bethesda in February 1944, President Franklin D. Roosevelt presented for excision of a sebaceous cyst on the back of his head. Pender was the anaesthesiologist who infiltrated the local anaesthetic for this and of course he checked the President's blood pressure – he found severe hypertension, but he did not declare this at the time. The operation was uneventful; however, the following month the President was investigated for heart failure.

Later in 1945 Lt. Pender invented an endotracheal vaporizer for convenient administration of open drop ether without having to hold a mask. The device consisted of wire basket about the size of a lemon, which fitted into an endotracheal adapter; cotton gauze was wrapped over the basket and the liquid anaesthetic agent was dripped onto this. He also experimented with electrical anaesthesia, but this project ceased when he was sent to a US Naval Hospital ship in the Pacific Theatre of Operations.

After the War in 1946, Pender returned to the Mayo Clinic for a consultant post and became involved in the development of the open-heart surgery programme. He was also involved in the teaching of regional anaesthesia. He contributed to John S. Lundy's Travel Club and later began interviewing senior staff to document the history of the Department of Anesthesiology at Mayo. In 1954 (after Lundy retired) Pender moved to Palo Alto in California. This was initially for private practice only, but later he took academic sabbaticals at the University of Pennsylvania and the University of Wales, working with Professor William Mushin (q.v. page 151).

Pender was associate editor of the journal *Anesthesiology* for 1956-1965 and President of the Academy of Anesthesiology in 1965. The following year he got the idea of being trained in oral interviewing by David Seegal, MD of Columbia University and joined Dr John Leahy of Philadelphia in the "Men of Anesthesia" recordings, interviewing many famous anaesthesiologists himself – see Table 1. The initial efforts were recorded on 16 mm cine film. The problem of self-funding caused a lack of interviews in the years 1968-75. Then, under the Presidency of K. Garth Huston, the Wood Library-Museum (WLM) supported it under the name "Living History Series" as an ongoing project. From the late 1970s videotape became available and this improved the quality. From then on, interviews were consistently added to the collection every year. Pender himself was interviewed by Alan D. Sessler in 1996. The collection has grown to over 150 and are available in various formats for loan or purchase from the WLM.

On retiring in 1977, Pender was made Emeritus Director of Anesthesiology, Palo Alto Clinic. He was also honoured by Stanford University as the first Clinical Professor Emeritus of Anesthesia. He delivered the Lewis H. Wright Memorial Lecture in 1980. His last enjoyable years were spent with his family in the Los Altos Hills, California.

Pender made a substantial donation to the WLM for the creation in its building of a Curator's Room dedicated to the Mayo Clinic. In 2000, just a few months before his death, he contributed to an editorial in the journal *Anesthesiology*. The Living History Collection of the WLM was endowed by Pender posthumously. The full list of interviews is available in alphabetical order on the website of the WLM.

Table 1. Oral interviews conducted by JW Pender

Year	Interviewee
1961	Ralph T. Knight, University of Minnesota
1966	Donald E. Hale, Cleveland Clinic
1960s	John W. Dundee, Queens University, Belfast
1966	John S. Lundy, Mayo Clinic
1966	Stevens J. Martin, Hartford, Connecticut
1981	William B. Neff, Stanford University
1990	Charles F. McCuskey, University of S. California

Acknowledgement

The Anesthesia History Association kindly gave permission to reproduce the portrait photograph from the *Bulletin of Anesthesia History*.

Further reading

Pender JW, Lane JN. An endotracheal vaporizer. *Anesthesiology* 1945; **6**: 418-20.

Calmes SH. John William "Bill" Pender, M.D., 1912-2001. *Bulletin of Anesthesia History* 2001; **19** (2): 2-3.

Leahy JJ. Twenty-five years of living history. In: Fink BR, Morris LE, Stephen CR (Eds.) *The History of Anesthesia Third International Symposium Proceedings*. Park Ridge, Illinois: Wood Library-Museum of Anesthesiology, 1992; 277-8.

Bacon DR, Albin M, Pender JW. Editorial: Anesthesiology's Greatest Generation? *Anesthesiology* 2001; **94**: 725-6.

Bause GS. The Nine Lives of Paul Wood's Collection: The Wood Library-Museum of Anesthesiology. In: Bacon DR, McGoldrick KE, Lema MJ (Eds.). *The American Society of Anesthesiologists – A Centenary of Challenges and Progress*. Park Ridge, Illinois: Wood Library-Museum of Anesthesiology, 2005; 55-73.

PINKERTON MEMORIAL LECTURE

Herbert Harvey Pinkerton (1901-1982)

Herbert Pinkerton was born in Belfast, Northern Ireland in 1901 and educated at the High School of Glasgow. He enrolled at the University of Glasgow initially in the Faculty of Engineering before transferring to Medicine, and he graduated MB, ChB in 1926 with honours and as Brunton Medallist. Then he had resident posts at the Western Infirmary, Glasgow before entering general practice. While in practice in Busby, near Glasgow he turned more to the administration of anaesthesia and focused on the problems of pulmonary tuberculosis. Deciding to be a full-time anaesthetist, he undertook postgraduate training under Dr John Challis at the London Hospital in 1936. He passed the examinations for the Diploma in Anaesthetics (RCP&S) in 1938. On return to Glasgow, he was appointed as a visiting

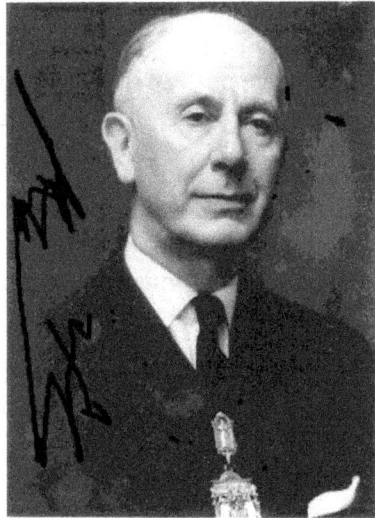

Herbert H. Pinkerton. Image courtesy of The Anaesthesia Heritage Centre, AAGBI.

anaesthetist at the Western Infirmary and the Royal Samaritan Hospital for Women in Glasgow, and Hairmyres Hospital, Lanarkshire. In 1948, at the start of the National Health Service, he was appointed a Consultant Anaesthetist at the Western Infirmary, Glasgow.

Known to most as 'Tony', Pinkerton was President of the Glasgow and West of Scotland Society of Anaesthetists for 1948-49. Two years later he was elected President of the Scottish Society of Anaesthetists for 1951-52 – his Presidential address was "General anaesthesia in collapse treatment for pulmonary tuberculosis".

Being particularly interested in the training of doctors recruited to anaesthesia, Pinkerton established in 1954 the Glasgow academic Department of Anaesthesia, becoming the first consultant-in charge. Clinically, he published on cyclopropane and thiopentone and in 1957 he devised a cuirass belt for negative pressure ventilation in general anaesthesia for bronchoscopy.

Pinkerton was a member of the Board of the Faculty of Anaesthetists of the Royal College of Surgeons of England and of the Council of the Association of Anaesthetists of Great Britain and Ireland (AAGBI). He was elected President of the AAGBI in 1964 and in the final year of his Presidency, 1967 he established the Junior Anaesthetists' Group (JAG). This group went from strength to strength – at its Annual Scientific Meeting in 1973 an annual guest lecture was inaugurated by J. Alfred Lee.

Pinkerton was also a member of the Board of Management and the Editorial Executive of the *British Journal of Anaesthesia* (BJA) for more than 20 years. He retired from the Glasgow Western Infirmary in 1966, but he continued his BJA duties until 1969.

In 1971 Pinkerton was elected an Honorary Member of the AAGBI. He was awarded the Gold Medal of the Faculty of Anaesthetists in 1980 and was appointed an Honorary Member of the Section of Anaesthetics, Royal Society of Medicine in 1981.

In the year of Pinkerton's death, 1982, the guest lecture at the Annual Scientific Meeting of the JAG became the eponymous "Pinkerton Lecture" and the first to deliver it was Chris J. Hull, the Professor of Anaesthesia at Newcastle upon Tyne. Since then the lecture has been delivered by many more illustrious men and women! In 1991 the JAG was renamed the Group of Anaesthetists in Training (GAT) and in 2019 it was again renamed: Trainee Committee. For many years, each Pinkerton Lecturer was awarded a bronze medal by the AAGBI (similar to the John Snow medal) as well as an honorarium, but this was discontinued after 2015.

Table 1. Pinkerton lecturers and lecture titles

Year	Lecturer	Title
1982	Chris J. Hull	Dangerous ground
1983	D. J. Gee	Criminal view of life and death
1984	D. C. Flenley	Sleep, breathing and oxygen
1985	A. Maynard	Rationing care and efficiency
1986	K. Rawnsley	The sick doctor
1987	J. W. Dundee	A travelling professor
1988	M. J. Halsey	Basic science and anaesthesia
1989	R. Dyson	Clinical and resource management. What are the options for anaesthetists?
1990	W. C. Bowman	What's new at the neuromuscular junction?
1991	T. B. Boulton	From black gas to propofol
1992	J. S. M. Zorab	Twenty-five years of development in European and World Anaesthesia
1993	Brian Edwards	Have we seen the high point of the development of the health service?
1994	A. Taylor	A professional agenda for anaesthetists
1995	S. Brandon	The cost of caring

1996	J. S. Milledge	High altitude medicine
1997	I. Calder	Lead kindly light
1998	G. Hume	Medicine in the media
1999	Mike Stroud	Survival of the Fittest
2000	D. K. Whittaker	Forensic dental science in investigation of serious crime
2001	John Clark	Genetic Modification, Home of Dolly the Sheep
2002	Philip Routledge	Drug Safety – a titanic struggle
2003	D. Boxall	Over, around and out of this world – taking balloons to the limit
2004	Frank Golden	Immersion related deaths
2005	Kevin Fong	Medicine for Mars – the next small step
2006	John Burn	Running in the blood
2007	James Reason	Error Management
2008	Michael Grocott	Caudwell Xtreme Everest
2009	Nick Wilson	In the Beginning was the Word – an etymological history of everyday anaesthetic terminology
2010	Patricia Oakley	Planning for the future Anaesthetic workforce – a research agenda
2011	Neil McGuire	Lessons from the battlefield
2012	Linda Ruxton	Fatal accident inquiries and their role in improving patient safety
2013	Daniele Bryden	Who are your competitors?
2014	H. A. McLure	Charge of the Night Brigade
2015	Vicky Osgood	The future of training
2016	Alan Aitkenhead	Healthcare professionals and criminal law
2017	Peter Maguire	Training: past, present and future
2018	*Cancelled*	
2019	Peter Homa	Leadership within the NHS

Acknowledgement

Felicia El Kholi, Heritage Assistant at the AAGBI, kindly provided the list of Pinkerton lectures.

Further reading

Wishart HV, Holloway KB, Spence AA. Obituary Henry Harvey Pinkerton. *Anaesthesia* 1982; **37**: 1143-5.

Spence AA. Herbert Harvey Pinkerton. *The History of Anaesthesia Society Proceedings* 1995; **17**: 17-21.

Boulton TB. *The Association of Anaesthetists of Great Britain and Ireland 1932-1992 and the Development of the Specialty of Anaesthesia*. London: AAGBI, 1999; 348, 720, 750-2.

PULSE OXIMETRY

Takuo Aoyagi (1936-2020)

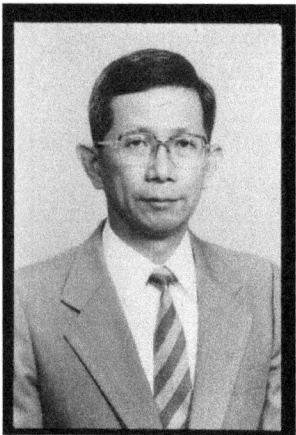

Takuo Aoyagi is widely regarded as the inventor of pulse oximetry. Before Aoyagi, non-invasive oximetry was available in the form of Earl Wood's (rather unreliable) method of expelling blood from the ear to obtain 'zero', then readmitting it and measuring the transmission of two wavelengths of light to compute the arterial blood oxygen saturation (SaO_2). However, it was Aoyagi who first combined *pulsation* with oximetry to enable reliable, continuous, long-term monitoring of SaO_2 with the probe not restricted to the ear.

The first ear oximeter was invented by Glen Millikan in 1941, in response to the need to measure blood oxygen saturation of fighter pilots, who could black-out at high altitude in the Battle of Britain. After the war in 1948, Earl Wood at the Mayo Clinic improved Millikan's device by adding an inflatable cuff to the earpiece to obtain a bloodless 'zero', before measuring the light transmitted through the blood. In 1950 Wood and colleagues further improved the accuracy of the oximeter by dividing the red signal by the infrared signal to display SaO_2 continuously. They also described the isobestic points (wavelengths where the absorbance by oxyhaemoglobin and deoxy-haemoglobin are identical) and plotted the calibration curves.

Takuo Aoyagi. Image courtesy of Prof. Hirosato Kikuchi.

Takuo Aoyagi was born in Niigata Prefecture, Japan in 1936. He graduated in electrical engineering at Niigata University in 1958 and went to work at Shimadzu Corporation in Kyoto, where he became attracted to patient-monitoring. In 1971 he moved to the Research and Development Division of Nihon Kohden Corporation in Tokyo. There in the following year he conceived the idea of using Wood's oximeter earpiece to measure cardiac output by the dye dilution method: after calibration with a blood sample, the ear oximeter could be used to record a dye dilution curve. But, using two wavelengths, arterial pulsation "noise" prevented accurate extrapolation of the indo-cyanine green dye downstroke. Then he realised that he could eliminate this "noise" by calculating the *ratio* of optical densities of the two wavelengths. Testing this with an ear dye densitometer on himself, he noticed that holding his breath (i.e. decreasing oxygen saturation) caused pulsatile waves to be reintroduced by changing the ratio of densities at the two wavelengths. This was a "eureka" moment – he realised that the pulsating portion might be used to measure arterial oxygen saturation!

Early in 1973 Dr S. Nakajima, a surgeon at the Sapporo Minami National Sanatorium, was involved in the idea and encouraged the production of a prototype *pulse oximeter*. By September this was ready and was evaluated clinically by Nakajima. In October 1973 Aoyagi submitted a preliminary abstract to the Japan Society of Medical Electronics and Biological Engineering (MEBE) and in March 1974 a patent application was sent to the Japanese Patent Office by Nihon Kohden Corporation. Aoyagi delivered an oral presentation at the MEBE meeting in Osaka the next month.

In September 1975 personnel transfers at Nihon Kohden resulted in Aoyagi moving from research to be manager in the division of patient monitoring, and the company did not pursue improving its pulse oximeter, the performance of which was not yet satisfactory. However, another Japanese company, Minoruta Camera (known as Minolta in the USA), developed a device with a fingertip probe and two fibreoptic cables: the Oximet-1471, marketed in 1977.

The first commercial pulse oximeter in the USA was introduced by Biox Technology, Inc. (led by Mr Scott A. Wilber) in 1981: the focus of its use was in respiratory care. In the same year anaesthesiologist William New and engineer Jack Lloyd plus Jim Corenman and Bob Smith in Hayward, California started a company called 'Nellcor' to develop and market pulse oximetry systems. Their N-100, released in 1983, utilised light-emitting diodes (LEDs), a sensitive photodiode and a microcomputer. It was accurate, relatively portable and led to widespread adoption of pulse oximetry for monitoring during anaesthesia in operating theatres. New worked at Stanford University School of Medicine with Assistant Professor Mark Yelderman, and they published the evaluation of the device in 1983.

In 1984 Biox became part of the Ohmeda division of the British Oxygen Company (BOC). Then the Ohmeda Biox 3700 pulse oximeter was developed: its liquid crystal display provided both plethysmographic waveform and numeric SaO2 and pulse rate – see Figure 1.

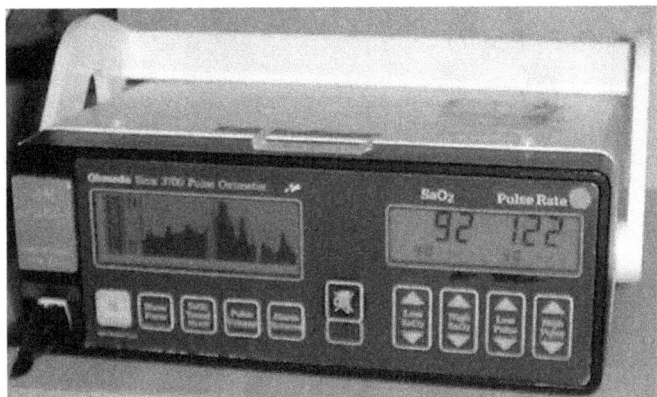

Figure 1. Ohmeda Biox 3700 pulse oximeter, c. 1986. Photograph by Dr Alistair McKenzie.

Takuo Aoyagi further contributed to the theory of pulse oximetry from 1985, when he was able to resume research. He collaborated with Professor M. Saito of Tokyo University, Dr K. Miyasaka of the National Children's Hospital, Dr John Severinghaus of the University of California in San Francisco, and Mr A. Yamanishi of Minolta. Using a blood pulsator, he noted that the pulse oximetry oxygen saturation S_pO_2 was not consistent with the oxygen saturation of the blood in the pulsator SO_2. Thus, he came to understand that blood in the body is surrounded by light scattering tissue and that the effect of pulsation of tissue other than blood is included in the measured pulse. Hence the blood optical density should be measured with scattering light. He used this information in developing pulse spectrophotometry which yielded useful theory for improving the performance of pulse oximeters.

Aoyagi was awarded his PhD in Engineering at Tokyo University in 1993. Honours came his way in 2002: the "Social" award by the Japanese Society of Anaesthesiologists and the Purple Ribbon Medal from the Emperor of Japan. Aoyagi's legacy is that the adoption of pulse oximetry as a standard for intraoperative monitoring has greatly reduced anaesthesia-associated deaths.

Acknowledgement

Professor Hirosato Kikuchi kindly provided information about Takuo Aoyagi.

Further reading

Aoyagi T, Kishi M, Yamaguchi K, Watanabe S. Improvement of an earpiece oximeter. Abstracts, 13th Annual Meeting of the Japan Society of Medical Electronics and Biological Engineering, Osaka, Japan, 26-27 April 1974; pp. 90-91.

Yelderman M, New W, Jr. Evaluation of Pulse Oximetry. *Anesthesiology* 1983; **59**: 349-52.

Aoyagi T. Pulse oximetry: its invention, theory, and future. *Journal of Anesthesia* 2003; **17**: 259-66.

Severinghaus JW. Takuo Aoyagi: Discovery of Pulse Oximetry. *Anesthesia & Analgesia* 2007; **105**: S1-S4.

RAVUSSIN TRANSTRACHEAL CATHETER

Patrick Ravussin (1950-)

Patrick Ravussin was born in Winterthur, Switzerland in 1950. After schooling, he studied medicine at the University of Lausanne, graduating in 1975. Then he began training in surgery at the Centre Hospitalier Universitaire Vaudois (CHUV) and became attracted to anaesthesia; he obtained his MD in 1977.

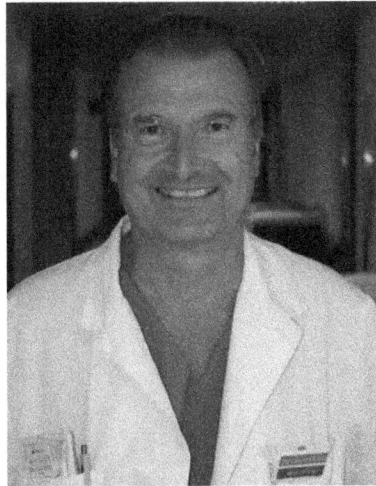

He took a Fellowship at the Department of Anaesthesia at McGill University in Montreal, Canada, returning to register as a Specialist in Anaesthesiology with the Swiss Medical Association (FMH) in 1982. While practising anaesthesia especially for ENT and neurosurgery, he was dissatisfied with the available needles and catheters for transtracheal ventilation. In 1984 he designed his own device, tested it at CHUV and patented it – soon it was manufactured by the VBM Laboratories of Medizintechnick in Sulz/Neckar, Germany. It facilitated smooth insertion of the catheter through the cricothyroid membrane or between the first and second tracheal rings. Moreover, it had a dual attachment system: either conventional ventilation equipment (e.g. Ambu bag) could be connected to the 15 mm male end, or jet ventilation (e.g. Sanders injector) could be delivered by its Luer-lok fitting. He published on this in the *Canadian Anaesthetists' Society Journal* in 1985 – he was Assistant Professor of Anaesthesia at McGill University for 1984-85. Returning to CHUV in 1986, he used the paediatric size of the transtracheal catheter and published on this in 1987. In time the device became known worldwide as the 'Ravussin cannula' – see Figure 1. Further features include:

- available in both adult size (13 G) and paediatric sizes (14 G, 18G);
- Teflon catheter (kink-resistant) has a stainless steel cannula within it, curved with an angled flange on the connector so that it points down the trachea when fully inserted;
- the cannula, with a Luer-Lok (q.v. page 126) syringe attached, is inserted through the cricothyroid membrane, with aspiration of air to confirm intratracheal placement;
- the syringe assembly is held steady while the catheter is advanced forward off the cannula;

- there are three small lateral holes at the distal tip of the catheter, which centre the device in the trachea during jetting and prevent 'whipping'.

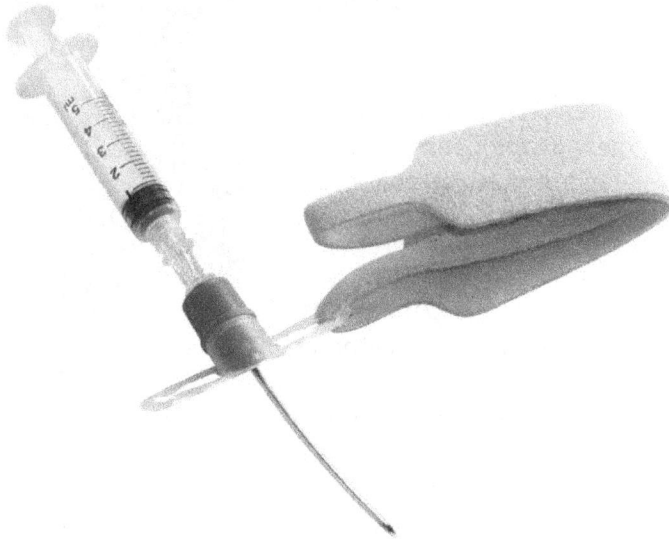

Figure 1. Ravussin cannula with Luer-Lok syringe attached. Image courtesy of VBM Medizintechnik GmbH.

By 1992 Ravussin was registered with the FMH as a Specialist in Intensive Care. In 1996 he became Chief of the Department of Anaesthesiology and Resuscitation of central Valais, while maintaining a part-time activity at CHUV. He was appointed (extraordinary) Associate Professor ad personam, University of Lausanne. In addition, he chaired the Commission of the Swiss Society of Anaesthesia and Resuscitation for postgraduate training. He went on to be President of the Association of Anaesthesia and Resuscitation for ENT (CARORL). For the Latin portion of Switzerland, he became President of the Association of Neuroanaesthesia-Resuscitation in the French language (ANARLF), and he was a founding member of the Commission for Training and Engagement in Anaesthesia of Latin Switzerland (COMASUL). Internationally, he was a founding member of the European Society of Anaesthesiology (ESA), representing Switzerland for many years.

In 2001 Ravussin contributed to a tri-centre study (France and Switzerland) on complications recorded in 643 patients receiving high frequency jet ventilation (HFJV) for endoscopic airway surgery. Two brands of transtracheal catheter were used: either Ravussin or Seldicath; the HFJVs had an automatic cut-off device which disallowed inflation if a pre-set pressure (usually 4 cm of water) was exceeded. The authors found a low incidence of complications: subcutaneous emphysema 8.4%, pneumothorax 1%, failure to insert the transtracheal catheter 0.3% – the rate did not depend on either the type of catheter or the experience of the anaesthetist. They concluded that HFJV is a reliable technique in the hands of trained personnel and that control of airway pressure did not prevent a low incidence of pneumothorax.

In 2004 concern over the risk of barotrauma from raised intratracheal pressures during transtracheal jet ventilation (TTJV) led to a study by Patel and Diba at the Queen Victoria Hospital in East Grinstead, England. Consecutively in ten adult patients, who required TTJV and fibreoptic tracheal intubation as part of their routine anaesthetic management, a 13-G Ravussin catheter was inserted through the cricothyroid membrane under local anaesthetic. Then the catheter was connected to a Manujet variable pressure injector which delivered oxygen at 4 bar. After induction of general anaesthesia, the tracheal airway pressures were measured at three anatomical levels during fibreoptic intubation. The peak airway pressures generated at the carina during TTJV were found to be small (5 – 13 mm Hg), indicating a low risk of barotrauma.

Ravussin was President of the Swiss Society of Anaesthesiology and Resuscitation for 2006-8. He received the annual award of the Faculty of Biology and Medicine (FBM) of the University of Lausanne in 2015. This was the year in which he retired to enjoy mountaineering and golf.

Further reading

Ravussin P, Freeman J. A new transtracheal catheter for ventilation and resuscitation. *Canadian Anaesthetists' Society Journal* 1985; **32**: 60-64.

Ravussin P, Bayer-Berger M, Monnier P, Savary M, Freeman J. Percutaneous transtracheal ventilation for laser endoscopic procedures in infants and small children with laryngeal obstruction: report of two cases. *Canadian Journal of Anaesthesia* 1987; **34**: 83-6.

Bourgain JL, Desruennes E, Fischler M, Ravussin P. Transtracheal high frequency jet ventilation for endoscopic airway surgery: a multicentre study. *British Journal of Anaesthesia* 2001; **87**: 870-5.

Patel C, Diba A. Measuring tracheal airway pressures during transtracheal jet ventilation: an observational study. *Anaesthesia* 2004; **59**: 248-51.

RENTON PRIZE

Douglas George Renton (1899-1955)

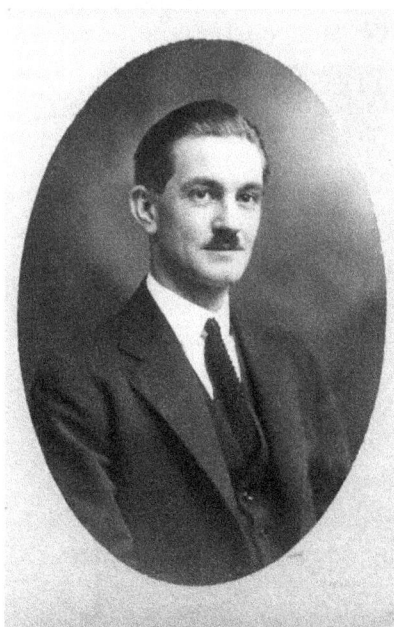

Douglas G. Renton. Image courtesy of the Geoffrey Kaye Museum of Anaesthetic History, ANZCA.

Douglas Renton was born in Parkville, Victoria, Australia in 1899 and educated at Scotch College, Melbourne. He then studied medicine at the University of Melbourne, graduating MB BS in 1922, and proceeded to two years of local hospital appointments. In 1924 he set up in general practice in rural Rochester, Victoria. Unfortunately, that year he developed adhesions from appendicitis, which impacted permanently on his health and caused him to be invalided for much of 1929.

Renton moved to Melbourne in 1929 to specialize in anaesthesia. Initially appointed honorary assistant anaesthetist at the Alfred Hospital and Melbourne Hospital, by one year he had honorary anaesthetist appointments at the Alfred and Austin hospitals – at a time of having to be self-taught. An adept fitter and turner, in 1931 he built in his own machine shop a compact circle system with valves and a canister for soda lime. With this he pioneered carbon dioxide absorption anaesthesia in Australia. He became an examiner for the Diploma in Anaesthetics, D.A. (Melbourne).

In 1934 Renton was one of the co-authors of the first Australian textbook on anaesthetics *Practical Anaesthesia*. Two years later he was a founder member of the Australian Society of Anaesthetists. The D.A. (RCP&S) was conferred on him in 1939. During the Second World War he was in the reserve of the Australian Army Medical Corps, advising on the manufacture and design of anaesthetic equipment.

After the War Renton was co-author with Kaye and Orton in the publication of a second textbook *Anaesthetic Methods*, produced in 1946. That year he became part-time salaried anaesthetist to the neurosurgical unit at the Alfred Hospital. The FFARCS was conferred on him by election in 1949. In 1952 he played a prominent role in the formation of the Faculty of Anaesthetists of the Royal Australasian College of Surgeons, becoming its interim Dean in

1953. Naturally the FFARACS was conferred on him the following year when he was the first constitutional Dean. Sadly, his term of office was cut short by his untimely death in May 1955 as his ill health reached a crisis.

From 1958 the Australasian Faculty (later the ANZCA) awarded the Renton Prize to the trainee achieving the highest marks in the primary examination for the Fellowship (provided the examiners consider the standard sufficiently high). The Prize has taken the form of a medal.

Table 1. Renton Prize winners

Year	Recipient	Year	Recipient
1958	Vera Gallagher	1991	Anton E. Loewenthal
1959	Bryan E. Sharkey	1991	Rex A. Smith
1959	James Loughman	1992	Andrew J. Patrick
1960	Ian R. Philpott	1992	Brian T. Spain
1962	Michael F. O'Rourke	1993	Shane C.T. Townsend
1963	Warren H. Millist	1994	Ai Yu Cheng
1965	David Komesaroff	1994	Peter A. Watt
1965	Robert McKay Hare	1995	Catherine S. Downs
1966	Richard Gun	1995	Kwok Wing Hong
1967	Michael H. Harpur	1996	Angela G. Playoust
1967	Peter G. Thomson	1996	Anthony N. Coorey
1968	Colin R. Brown	1997	David R.R. Lardner
1968	Dennis L. Fitzsimmons	1997	Stephen B. Gibson
1968	Eric J. Micklethwaite	1998	Brian S. Cowie
1969	Barbara G. Burrows	1998	Craig Hargreaves
1969	William J. Herlihy	1999	Nicole A. Healy
1970	Aleksander Joost	1999	Tyron R. Crofts
1970	Isobel A. Perry-Keene	2000	Ben Jon Di Luca
1971	George R.J. McEwin	2000	Gary L. Hopgood
1971	Terence F. Little	2001	Andrew H. Jackson
1972	Richard W. Davis	2001	Michael P. Clifford
1972	Victor I. Callanan	2002	James N. King
1973	Harry Kay	2002	Michael S. Paleologos
1973	Roderick J.B. Tiernan	2003	Markus H. Schmidt
1974	Ivan P. Sergejev	2003	Tamara J. Culnane
1975	John L. Moran	2004	Jamie P. Stevens
1975	Raymond T.C. Soon	2005	Daniel J. Faulke
1976	Bin Bin Lee	2005	Luke E. Torre
1976	David Kault	2005	Pedro Diaz
1977	Geoffrey R. Cutfield	2006	Damien Wallman
1977	Helen J. Bridgman	2006	Raymond Tiong Chin Hu

1978	Jacob Boon	2007	Amanda Kruys
1979	Christopher D. Clay	2007	Siu Wah Sylvia Au
1979	Robert H. Woog	2008	Ann-Lynn Kuok
1980	Keith A. Streatfeild	2008	Stanley Tay
1980	Rusli Arshad	2009	Alexander Smirk
1981	Jeremy A. Foate	2009	Tung Hoi Ying Queenie
1982	David A. Scott	2010	Lachlan F. Miles
1982	Roger E. Traill	2010	Vivian N. Nguyen
1983	Anne M. Cunningham	2011	Katrina P. Pirie
1983	Tan Lee Choo	2011	Wong Ong Yat
1983	Keith J. Kelly	2012	Ing-Kye Sim
1984	Ian M. McKenzie	2012	Mark P. Plummer
1984	Jeremy O. Cooper	2013	Duncan J.M. Brown
1984	Simon C. Body	2013	Adam I. Mossenson
1985	Alexandra D. Moore	2014	Adam J. Mahoney
1985	Terence Buckman	2014	Steven M. De Luca
1986	John H. Reeves	2015	Kaylee A. Jordan
1986	Roger M.O. Hall	2015	Frank B. Marroquin-Harris
1987	Elizabeth M. Ashwood	2015	Daniel R. Frei
1987	Ian R. Jenkins	2016	John A. Newland
1988	Bruce G. Marks	2016	Andrew P. Melville
1988	Linda J. Cass	2017	Blagoja Alampieski
1988	Philip G. Ragg	2017	Jana L. Vitesnikova
1989	Neale N. Mushet	2018	Brian Nee Hou Chee
1990	Keith B. Laubscher	2018	Grace B. Hollands
1990	Lam Kwok Key	2019	Andrew W.T. Burch; Stuart N. Watson
		2019	Nathaniel J. Hiscock

Further reading

Obituary Douglas George Renton. *The Medical Journal of Australia* 1955; **2**: 145-6.

Renton DG. Gas Anaesthesia: The Closed-Circle Absorption Technique. *Anesthesia and Analgesia* 1937; **16**: 9-15.

RITCHIE WHISTLE AND JOHN RITCHIE PRIZE

John Russell Ritchie (1909-1976)

John Ritchie was born in Dunedin, New Zealand in 1909, the son of an obstetrician/anaesthetist. Following schooling at Christ's College in Christchurch he entered the University of Otago at Dunedin and completed the medical degree course in 1933. He did house jobs at Auckland Hospital in 1934, then proceeding to overseas experience in anaesthetics. Through 1935 to 1937 he worked in London, England as an assistant to Dr Ronald Jarman (a future President of the AAGBI) and as locum at St George's and Queen Charlotte's Hospitals. Further, he worked at the Rotunda in Dublin, Ireland and was Ship's Surgeon on the journeys between New Zealand and UK.

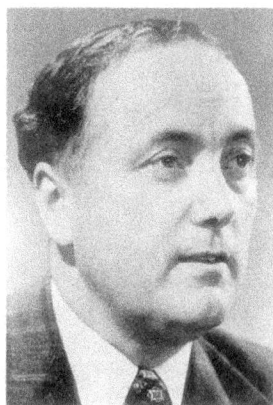

John R. Ritchie. Image courtesy of the NZSA.

Ritchie passed the examination for the Diploma in Anaesthetics held in London in May 1937 (the first New Zealander to do so) and he returned to Dunedin at the end of the year. From 1938 to 1949 he established himself in general practice with anaesthetics, being appointed Lecturer in Anaesthetics to the Otago Dental School in 1940. He used his home as a venue in 1948 to meet anaesthetists from Auckland, Wellington and Christchurch, resulting in the founding of the New Zealand Society of Anaesthetists (NZSA) the following year.

Ritchie was appointed Director of Anaesthetics at Dunedin Hospital in 1949 and this became a fulltime post the following year, when he also became Senior Lecturer. Mechanically minded, he focused on the improvement in performance and safety of anaesthetic equipment rather than publishing. In 1951 he was elected to the British Fellowship of the Faculty of Anaesthetists of the Royal College of Surgeons (FFARCS). From that year he maintained the collection of anaesthetic data and set up a New Zealand-wide system of reporting on deaths associated with anaesthesia. In 1952 he became a Foundation Fellow of the Australasian Faculty of Anaesthetists and he was a member of the Board from 1956 to 1960.

In the mid-1960s he designed an oxygen failure warning device, which was successfully used at Dunedin Hospital. He published this by way of a letter to the *British Journal of Anaesthesia* in 1974. It was the first device to rely just on the failing oxygen supply for its power. The device was manufactured by

Penlon Ltd. of Abingdon, England. The principle of the device is illustrated in Figure 1.

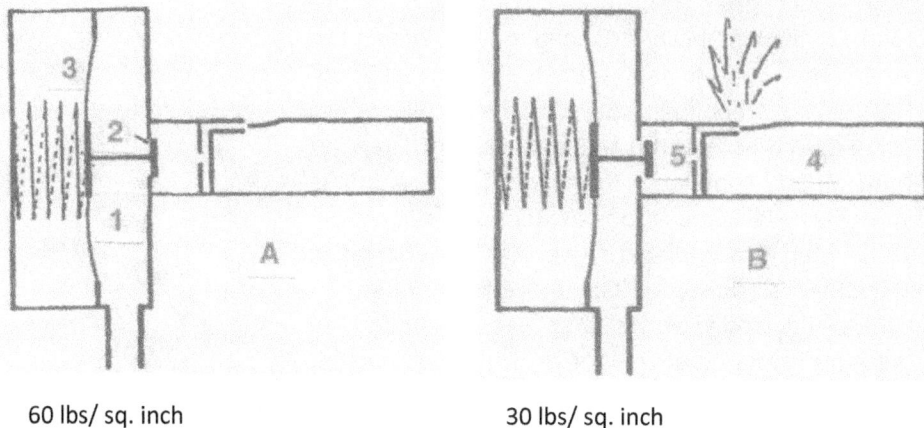

60 lbs/ sq. inch   30 lbs/ sq. inch

Figure 1. Principle of Ritchie's oxygen failure warning device. 1- chamber connecting to oxygen line; 2- valve; 3- diaphragm attached to spring; 4- whistle; 5- orifice. (A): oxygen pressure of 60 PSI pushes the diaphragm so that the valve is sealed. (B): at lower oxygen pressure of 30 PSI, the diaphragm can no longer oppose the spring so that the valve opens, allowing oxygen to escape and sound the whistle; the orifice-5 restricts the flow of oxygen at 30 PSI to about 2 L/min.

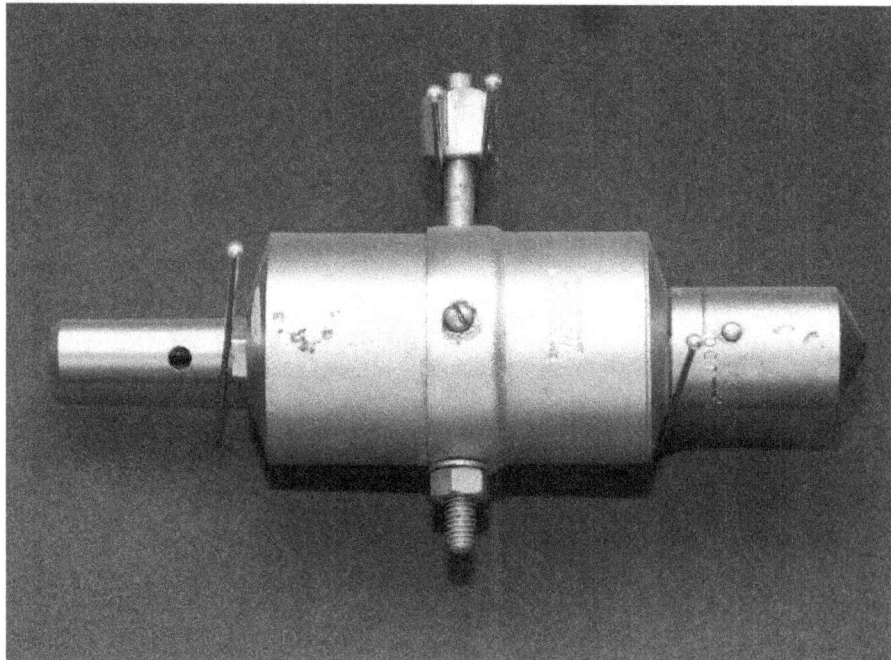

Figure 2. Ritchie whistle. Image Credit: Mushin Museum.

The manufactured product is shown in Figure 2. After some time, the device became known as the 'Ritchie whistle'; a magnet keeper was added to the spring mechanism. Although the original Ritchie whistle now only remains on older anaesthetic machines still in use, its principle forms the basis of most oxygen failure warning devices.

Ritchie was awarded the Orton Medal (q.v. page 158) of the Faculty of Anaesthetists, Royal Australasian College of Surgeons (later ANZCA) for distinguished service to anaesthesia in 1974. He retired at the end of that year. In 1975 he was appointed an OBE in the New Zealand Honours List. He suffered from fibrosing alveolitis, to which he succumbed the following year.

In his honour, the Ritchie Memorial Lecture was inaugurated by Professor Barry Baker in 1981 at the Department of Anaesthesia and Intensive Care, Dunedin Hospital. Although this was initially held annually, it was discontinued after 2013. However, named after him in the Dunedin Anaesthesia Department is the John Ritchie seminar room, in which his portrait and Robert Orton Medal are displayed. The eponym has further survived as the 'John Ritchie Prize' for the best paper by a member of the New Zealand Society of Anaesthetists (NZSA), which was worth $500 when it began in 1984. The prize was presented annually at the NZSA meeting from 1984 until 1995 when there was a lull as the rules for the contest were reviewed. The award was recommenced in 2003 – see Table 1.

The standard checklist for anaesthetic machines used to include, for gas supplies, disconnection of pipelines via Schrader valves – so that the deliberate interruption of oxygen supply would be marked by the sound of the Ritchie whistle. This section of the AAGBI guideline on checking anaesthetic equipment was changed in 2004 to a simple 'tug test' which was upheld in the next revision of 2012. So, a whole generation of trainees have not routinely heard the Ritchie whistle.

Table 1. John Ritchie Prize winners

Year	Recipient	Paper
1984	Leona F. Wilson	Venous tolerance to a mixed micelle preparation of diazepam.
1985	Duncan C. Galletly	Comparative cutaneous histamine release by neuromuscular blocking drugs.
1986	Record lost	
1987	J.W. Stokes	The patient with unexpected intraoperative hypoxaemia – update on monitoring and management.

1988	Vaughan G. Laurenson	Comparison of Mapleson A and ADE circuits.
1989	Ross R. Kennedy	A simple exponential infusion device.
1990	No award	
1991	Record lost	
1992	Duncan C. Galletly	The effect of anaesthesia on the phase space attractor and correlation dimension of the human ECG.
1993	Record lost	
1994	Record lost	
1995	P.R. Hicks and Alan J. McKenzie	The crash of Ansett Flight 703.
2003	A. Neil Pollock	Genotype-phenotype comparison of five New Zealand MHS families.
2004	Ross R. Kennedy	The relationship between end-tidal sevoflurane and bispectral index or burst suppression during routine anaesthesia and surgery.
2005	Philip B. Cornish	The axillary tunnel – redefining the limits and dynamics of brachial plexus blockade.
2006	Alexander L. Garden	Altered patterns of speech in fatigued anaesthetic registrars.
2007	Brian J. Anderson	Investigating the pharmacodynamics of ketamine in children.
2008	Philip B. Cornish	The 100k mouth and the laryngoscope – friends or foes?
2009	Sheila Barnett	Preoperative oral paracetamol versus intra-operative intravenous paracetamol; plasma levels in the recovery room.
2010	No award	
2011	Era Soukhin	A single centre study of outcomes from fractured neck of femur; a 5-year audit.
2012	Paul Baker	Visual acuity at different illuminance levels during direct laryngoscopy.
2013	Colin Marsland	Emergency percutaneous transtracheal ventilation in an obstructed airway model in sheep: oxygenation, airway pressure and carbon dioxide clearance using the Ventrain and Manujet.
2014-17	No ASM	
2018	Brian J. Anderson	Acetaminophen, ibuprofen and tramadol analgesic interactions after adenotonsillectomy.
2019	David Choi	Characterisation of aluminium release by the EndFlow Fluid-Warming System in crystalloids and blood products.

Acknowledgement

The New Zealand Society of Anaesthetists kindly provided the list of John Ritchie Prize winners.

Further reading

Baker AB. Ritchie of the Whistle a New Zealand pioneer anaesthetist. In: Diz JC, Franco A, Bacon DR, Rupreht J, Alvarez J (Eds.) *The History of Anaesthesia: Proceedings of the Fifth International Symposium on the History of Anesthesia*. Amsterdam: Elsevier, 2002; 299-307.

Ritchie JR. A simple and reliable warning device for failing oxygen pressure. *British Journal of Anaesthesia* 1974; **46**: 323.

Loader J. Would you recognize the Ritchie whistle? *Anaesthesia* 2009; **64**: 574.

ROBERTSHAW DOUBLE-LUMEN TUBE

Frank Leonard Robertshaw (1918-1991)

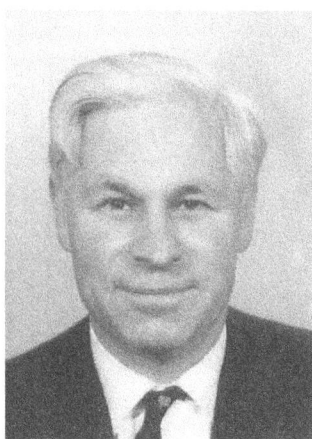

Frank Robertshaw was born in London, England in 1918. After education at St Christopher's School in Letchworth, he proceeded to St Andrew's University and graduated MB, ChB in 1944. Then he worked in obstetrics at St Mary's Hospital in Manchester, followed by several jobs in obstetrics and anaesthetics in the London area and Essex.

After the end of the Second World War in 1945 he was called up for national service in the RAF, initially in Oxfordshire. He came under the spell of Air Commodore (Professor) Robert Macintosh, who arranged an anaesthetic post for him in Cheshire. On completing his national service in 1947, he worked at various civilian hospitals in England and passed both the DOBSTRCOG and the DA. Finally, he opted for a career in anaesthetics and took a Consultant post covering hospitals in Hartlepool and Sedgefield in 1950.

Frank L. Robertshaw. Image courtesy of Dr K. George Lee.

In 1954, when he was elected FFARCS, Robertshaw moved to another Consultant post at Park Hospital, Davyhulme, Greater Manchester to do anaesthesia for thoracic surgery. He soon became an expert at one-lung anaesthesia and noted the shortcomings of the Carlens' double-lumen endobronchial tube, which was the only one available at that time. From the late 1950s until 1961 he designed prototypes of his own double-lumen tube, which he got made by the Leyland and Birmingham Rubber Company of Preston, Lancashire. He tested these on patients undergoing major thoracic surgery and guided by the performance of the tubes, made improvements until his final design, which he published in 1962. Differences from the Carlens' tube (manufactured by Rusch in Germany) included: absence of carinal hook, no latex outer coating (which disallowed repeated sterilization), larger lumens (D-shaped) which permitted passage of suction catheters and ensured lower resistance to gas-flows. The material was a rubber compound (firmer than ever before, yet elastic) and the cuff-inflating tubes were colour-coded: red for tracheal cuff and blue for bronchus. The tip of the left-sided version was angled at 45° to enter the left main bronchus, while the right-sided tube had a tip angled at 20° and a slotted endobronchial cuff to allow inflation of the right upper lobe – see Figures 1 and 2. There were three sizes: large, medium and small. His tubes were marketed by Medical & Industrial Equipment Ltd., London.

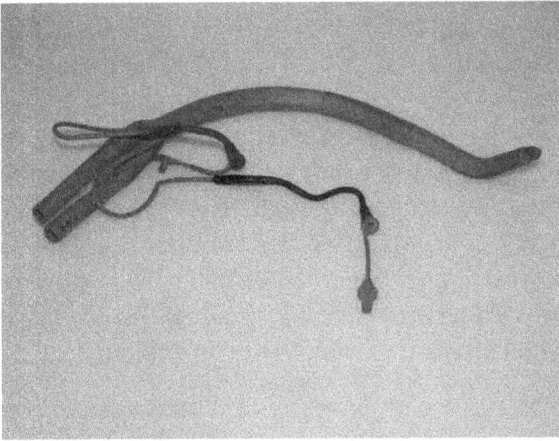

Figure 1. Robertshaw left-sided double-lumen tube. Image courtesy of The Anaesthesia Heritage Centre, AAGBI.

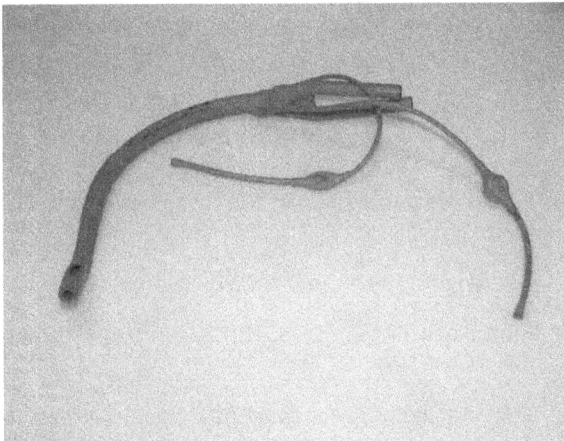

Figure 2. Robertshaw right-sided double-lumen tube. Image courtesy of The Anaesthesia Heritage Centre, AAGBI.

Robertshaw was one of the first to use halothane in cardiothoracic anaesthesia, as the company ICI had arranged to have Fluothane evaluated clinically in Manchester. He maintained his links with Oxford and in September 1962 he accompanied Neville Ripley of the Longworth Scientific Instrument Co. Ltd., Abingdon to demonstrate the company's laryngoscopes and other equipment at the first European Congress of Anaesthesiologists in Vienna. At that time Robertshaw liaised with Macintosh and developed a new paediatric laryngoscope blade, which he went on to publish two months later. This laryngoscope blade was made by Longworth, which later became Penlon, Ltd.

His double-lumen endobronchial tubes soon became widely known as "Robertshaw's" and were listed as such in the sixth edition of Lee's Synopsis of Anaesthesia. They became very popular in cardiothoracic anaesthesia. In 1968 Robertshaw was a founder member of the Riverside Club, an informal group of anaesthetists and senior staff of the Longworth Scientific Instrument Co. Ltd., which met three or four times a year at the Riverside Restaurant, Burcot – a few miles from Abingdon. He attended their meetings into the 1970s. In 1978 he sustained a minor stroke and therefore retired, moving to his dream area for fell and rock climbing, the Lake District. Sadly, he suffered a further stroke soon afterwards, which left him with nominal dysphasia.

From 1992 to 1994 there was some concern that the Robertshaw double-lumen tubes of the original design and red rubber material would no longer be available, because the Leyland Company had ceased trading. The merits of the original device were extolled by Conacher in 1994 and then a new manufacturer came forward to produce the original design for single use only: Phoenix Medical Ltd., Preston. This is now a company of P3 Medical Ltd.

Further reading

Robertshaw FL. Low resistance double-lumen endobronchial tubes. *British Journal of Anaesthesia* 1962; **34**: 576-9.

Robertshaw FL. A new laryngoscope for infants and children. *Lancet* 1962; **280**: 1034.

Dark J. Obituary F L Robertshaw FFARCS DOBSTRCOG. *British Medical Journal* 1991; **303**: 1329.

Conacher ID, Herrema IH, Batchelor AM. Robertshaw Double Lumen Tubes: A Reappraisal Thirty Years On. *Anaesthesia and Intensive Care* 1994; **22**: 179-83.

Lee KG. FL Robertshaw and the double-lumen tube. In: Drury PME, Armitage EN, Bacon DR et al (Eds.) *The History of Anaesthesia – Proceedings of the 6th International Symposium on the History of Anaesthesia*. Reading: Conservatree, 2007; 551-7.

SAMUEL THOMPSON ROWLING ORATION

Herbert Samuel Thompson Rowling (1874-1950)

Samuel Thompson Rowling was born in Leeds, England and educated at Leeds Grammar School. He studied medicine at Leeds Medical School and graduated MB, ChB with honours in 1896 at the Victoria University in Manchester as this was before the royal charter for Leeds University.

After qualifying, Rowling was house surgeon at the Leeds General Infirmary, where his interest was captured by anaesthesia. He then became an assistant in general practice for a short period, before setting up his own family practice. In 1910 he was appointed as Honorary Anaesthetist to Leeds General Infirmary and later he obtained further appointments to the Ministry of Pensions Hospital, Leeds and the West Riding County Council Hospital at Otley.

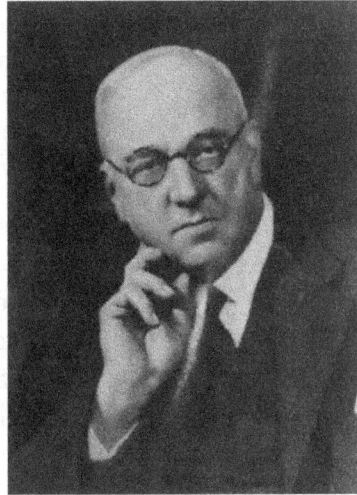

S. Thompson Rowling. Image by kind permission of the Royal College of Anaesthetists.

In 1911, at a meeting of the Yorkshire Branch of the British Medical Association held in York, Rowling described the calibration of his modified Clover's inhaler. He served in the Royal Army Medical Corps for about three years during the First World War at Becketts Park Army Hospital, Leeds. During this time, he was one of the few early exponents of intubation in anaesthesia using Kuhn's tube.

Rowling successfully defended his MD thesis in 1920. This was based on his previous work and expounded on the measurement of the concentrations of the components of anaesthetic gas mixtures. Highly respected at Leeds University, he was elected Chairman of Convocation for 1924-26.

In 1932 when he was Lecturer in Anaesthetics at Leeds University, Rowling published on his chloroform-paraffin bottle, which he devised as a simple means to deliver accurate concentrations of the anaesthetic. Into the bottle 6 drachms of chloroform (SG 1.497) was added to 12 oz. liquid paraffin (SG 0.88) as an inert diluent, resulting in 3.5% chloroform with SG 0.914. The glass bottle (see Figure 1) had a rubber stopper through which passed one inlet and one outlet tube and a small funnel for replenishing chloroform. There were four different coloured specific gravity beads within the bottle: red 0.914, blue 0.908, yellow 0.903 and green 0.897. All the beads would float at the start (3.5% chloroform). As the chloroform got used up, the red bead would sink, indicating 3 – 3.5%. Below 3% the blue bead would sink, below 2.5% the yellow bead would sink, and below 2% the green bead would sink – so nil beads floating represented < 2%. The nitrous oxide/oxygen was passed through the liquid and the vapour from the outlet tube delivered to the facepiece of an inhaler. A short-circuiting tap enabled the chloroform to be reduced in strength or even cut out if desired.

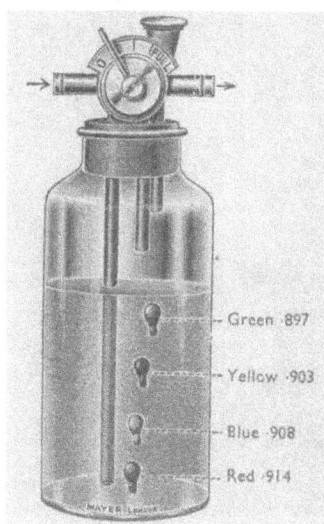

At a time when most anaesthetists had abandoned inhalers such as Vernon Harcourt's (q.v. page 27) because of its delicacy and protracted induction, Rowling's bottle (Figure 1) was welcomed in the early editions of C.L. Hewer's *Recent Advances in Anaesthesia and Analgesia*. It was also fully described in Minnitt and Gillies' *Textbook of Anaesthetics*.

Figure 1. Rowling's chloroform-paraffin bottle. From Mayer & Phelps Ltd. Catalogue, 1939.

Rowling was a member of Council of the Association of Anaesthetists of Great Britain and Ireland for 1933-36. He was awarded the Diploma in Anaesthetics (DA) without examination in 1935. On the formation of the Faculty of Anaesthetists of the Royal College of Surgeons in 1948, he was elected a Foundation Fellow. Regionally, in 1948 he became the first President of the Yorkshire Society of Anaesthetists.

He was a corps surgeon in the St John Ambulance Brigade and an officer of the Order of St John of Jerusalem. As he loved ships, he took many of his 'holidays' as Ship's Surgeon, often to Norway. He served as a lay preacher in the Church of England until doctors advised him to stop because of the angina from which he suffered in the last decade of his life. At the age of 75 in 1950 (the year of his death) he was co-author of a paper on an indicator method for measurement of carbon dioxide concentrations in anaesthetic gas mixtures.

Samuel Thompson Rowling had two daughters (one of whom became an orthopaedic surgeon) and a son, John Thompson Rowling who became a general surgeon. The son endowed a fund to the Royal College of

Anaesthetists, which facilitated an annual Samuel Thompson Rowling Oration from 2011.

Table 1. S T Rowling lecturers and lecture titles

Year	Lecturer	Title
2011	Robert Sneyd	Taking the lead.
2012	Charles Hinds	Generic influences on sepsis, susceptibility and outcome. Where next?
2013	Charles Hogue	Monitoring cerebral blood flow.
2014	Michael James	Magnesium – the once and future ion.
2015	Julian Bion	7 day services – policies and evidence.
2016	Jeremy Lambert	The role of GABA receptors in mediating the behavioural effects of general anaesthetics.
2017	No award	
2018	No award	
2019	Duminda Wijeysundera	Cardiopulmonary fitness and perioperative risk: insights from the METS study.
2019	Paul Wischmeyer	What patients need their doctors to know: keeping the care in healthcare.

Further reading

Harbord RP. Obituary Samuel Thompson Rowling. *British Journal of Anaesthesia* 1950; **23**: 134-7.

Rowling ST. An original clinical method of giving chloroform in definite percentage dosage. *British Journal of Anaesthesia* 1932; **9**: 59-66.

Ringrose HT, Rowling ST, Harbord RP. A practical means of determining CO_2 concentrations in samples of anaesthetic and other gases. *British Journal of Anaesthesia* 1950; **22**: 25-33.

Davison MHA, Essex L, Pask EA. Older methods of vaporisation of liquid anaesthetics. *Anaesthesia* 1963; **18**: 302-10.

FRANCIS RYND LECTURE

Francis Rynd (1801-1861)

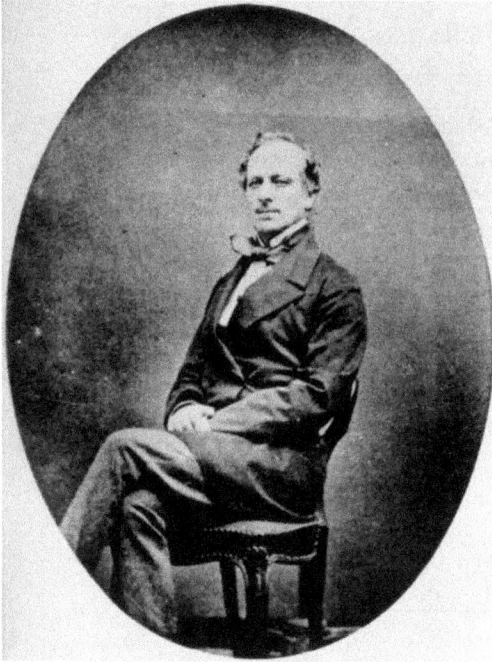

Francis Rynd. Credit: Wellcome Collection. Reproduced under Creative Commons Attribution (CC BY 4.0).

Francis Rynd was born into landed gentry in Dublin, Ireland. He was the second of five sons of James Rynd of Ryndville House, County Meath (20 miles west of the city) and his third wife, Hester Fleetwood. In 1817 he went to medical school at Trinity College, Dublin and in 1818 was apprenticed under the surgeon, Sir Philip Crampton at the Meath Hospital. He graduated BA in 1821 and in 1830 he obtained the MRCS (Ireland), followed by MA from Dublin University in 1832. Four years later he was appointed to a surgical post at Meath Hospital, where he worked with Robert James Graves (eponym 'Graves disease') and William Stokes (eponyms 'Cheyne-Stokes breathing' and Stokes-Adams syndrome').

Tall and dapper, Francis Rynd was very much a part of 'high society' – a dedicated follower of fashion and popular with the ladies. He enjoyed fox hunting and was a member of the Medico-Philosophical Society. He even attained membership of the exclusive Kildare Street Club in Dublin, which did not readily admit doctors. Known as an able surgeon with empathy for his patients, he had a lucrative private practice, which included much of the nobility of Ireland.

While surgeon to the Meath Hospital in June 1844, Rynd treated a lady with tic douloureux (trigeminal neuralgia) by injecting a solution of morphine acetate in creosote subcutaneously into branches of the trigeminal nerve. Relief of pain occurred within a minute; recurrence of some pain was ended by a repeat treatment about a week later. Soon after he successfully treated a man with sciatica by injecting morphine acetate along the course of the sciatic nerve, repeated after 3 days. He reported these two cases in the 12

March 1845 issue of the *Dublin Medical Press*. However, he failed to include a description of the instrument used.

It was not until 1861 that Rynd published an account of his apparatus, having performed his method on a larger number of patients. His illustration and description are shown in Figure 1. Clearly it was an ingenious trocar and cannula, by means of which fluid could be introduced subcutaneously through the cannula by gravity. By this time Alexander Wood in Edinburgh, Scotland had published two papers on the relief of pain by subcutaneous injection of opiates to painful points. However, as Rynd's 1845 paper was the first publication, arguably he was the inventor of the hollow needle – although this is not accepted by some historians. Wood is credited as the first to combine the syringe and hollow needle together. The term "hypodermic" needle was not used until 1863, when it was coined by Charles Hunter of London, England.

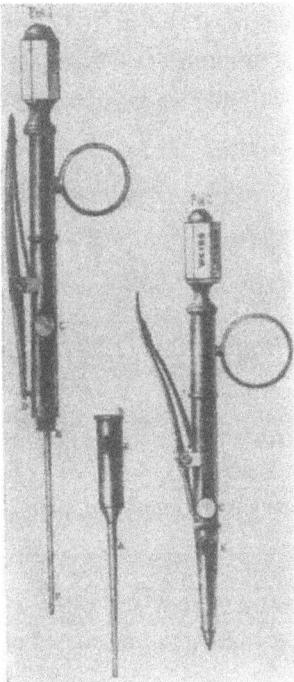

The canula (A) screws on the instrument at (B); and when the button (C), which is connected to the needle (F), and acted on by a spring, is pushed up (as in Fig. 2), the small catch (D) retains it in its place. The point of the needle then projects a little beyond the canula. The fluid to be applied is now to be introduced through the hole (E), either from a common writing-pen or the spoon-shaped extremity of a silver director; a small puncture through the skin is to be made with a lancet, or the point of the instrument itself is to be pressed through the skin, and on to the depth required; light pressure now made on the handle raises the catch (D), the needle is released, and springs backwards, leaving the canula empty, and allowing the fluid to descend.

Figure 1. Rynd's retractible trocar and his description of its use. From Rynd F., 1861: *Dublin Quarterly Journal of Medical Science*; 32: 13.

An interesting reference was made by Florence Nightingale in a letter she wrote on 12 July 1866 to Julius von Mohl, the Professor of Persian at the Collège de France in Paris. She wrote "Nothing did me any good but a new-fangled operation of putting opium under the skin, which relieved one for 24 hours".

Rynd was appointed honorary medical secretary to the Meath Hospital, medical superintendent of the Mountjoy Prison (1847-57) and consulting surgeon to the Coombe Hospital. As Surgeon to the Meath Hospital and County of Dublin Infirmary, Rynd's medical practice included urology, on which he published a book of 196 pages in 1849: *Pathological and Practical Observations on Strictures: And Some Other Diseases of the Urinary Organs.*

Rynd married Elizabeth Alley, the daughter of Alderman John Alley, who was elected Lord Mayor of Dublin. They had four sons and three daughters. At the age of sixty he was involved in a minor accident while driving a phaeton. In the stress of the ensuing altercation, he suffered a heart attack and died.

The Faculty of Pain Medicine of the College of Anaesthesiologists in Ireland was formally inaugurated in 2008. The coat of arms of the Faculty features a cross like structure, reminiscent of a surgical instrument, in the lower half of the shield; this has been taken from the Rynd family crest. From 2012 the Faculty has held the Francis Rynd Lecture as a central component of its Annual Scientific Meeting (Table 1). A Medal has been struck and this Francis Rynd Medal is awarded to the lecturer.

Table 1. Francis Rynd lecturers and lecture titles.

Year	Lecturer	Title
2012	Robert Levy	Use of medical devices in the management of pain.
2013	Michael Cousins	The Future of Pain Medicine.
2014	Michael Stanton-Hicks	Pain Medicine – A perspective from the Cleveland Clinic and career spanning three continents.
2015	Clifford J. Woolf	From the Gate theory to molecular mechanisms of pain.
2016	Frank Huygen	New Insights into the Pathology of CRPS.
2017	Andrew Rice	Heterogeneity in neuropathic pain.
2018	Ralf Baron	Phenotyping the pain patient: preparing for the advent of precision medicine.
2019	Daniel Rawluk	Integrated approach to cranial pain.
2020	Henrik Kehlet	Enhanced recovery after surgery focus: on the role of pain medicine.

Acknowledgement

Dr Declan Warde kindly assisted with information.

Further reading

Andrews H. Rynd, Francis. In: Dictionary of Irish biography. http://dib.cambridge.org (accessed 13 October 2020).

Rynd F. Neuralgia – introduction of fluid to the nerve. *Dublin Medical Press* 1845; **13**: 167-8.

Rynd F. Description of an instrument for the subcutaneous introduction of fluids in affections of the nerves. *Dublin Quarterly Journal of Medical Science* 1861; **32**: 13.

Howard-Jones N. A critical study of the origins and early development of hypodermic medication. *Journal of the History of Medicine and Allied Sciences* 1947 (Spring); **2**: 201-49.

Editorial. Francis Rynd (1801-1861). *Journal of the American Medical Association* 1970; **212**: 1208.

Boulton TB. Classical File. Alexander Wood, M.D. (1817-1884) and the use of the syringe and hollow needle for parenteral medication. *Survey of Anesthesiology* 1984; **28**:346-54.

BRUCE SCOTT LECTURES

Donald Bruce Scott (1926-1998)

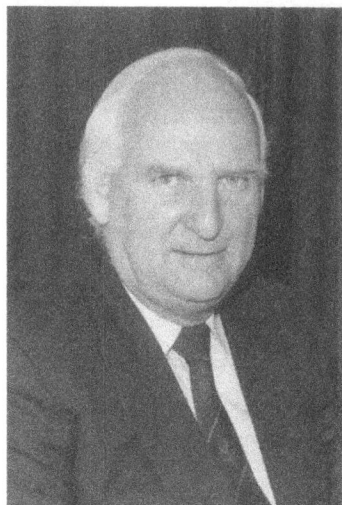

D. Bruce Scott. Photograph in the possession of Dr Alistair McKenzie.

D. Bruce Scott was born in Sydney, Australia in December 1925. He was moved to Britain at the age of three as his family settled in Sussex and he was educated at Hove Grammar School. Then he went to the Medical School of the University of Edinburgh, graduating in 1948. Next, he did a year in house jobs at hospitals in Sussex and then joined the Colonial Medical Service – serving for four years in Gold Coast (now Ghana).

On return to the UK, Scott pursued training in the Department of Anaesthetics at the Royal Infirmary of Edinburgh (RIE), where his interest in regional anaesthesia was encouraged by the head, John Gillies (q.v. page 76). He obtained the FFARCS and by 1957 was a Senior Registrar. He produced his MD thesis on epidural blockade in 1959, in which year he was appointed a Consultant at the RIE and Senior Lecturer in the University of Edinburgh. In 1960 he took a year's sojourn in Ibadan University, Nigeria where he accomplished a safe technique of anaesthesia to facilitate surgery for the facial deformity caused by cancrum oris.

Back at the RIE, Scott next focused his attention on researching cardiovascular dynamics. Working in the 1960s at the Simpson Memorial Maternity Pavilion, he was the anaesthetist in the multi-disciplinary team which elucidated the supine hypotensive syndrome of pregnancy – demonstrating the occlusion of the inferior vena cava by the gravid uterus. He also promoted epidural anaesthesia and introduced a modification to the hub of the Tuohy needle. Continuing into the 1970s and 1980s he published much on systemic toxicity and pharmacokinetics of local anaesthetics, but always promoting the safe use of regional anaesthesia. At the RIE he inspired a large cohort of trainees to get involved in research, and he was a natural choice for Acting Head of Department on the retirement of Professor J.D. Robertson in November 1982 – until 1984.

Scott served for many years on the Editorial Board of the *British Journal of Anaesthesia* and on the Board of the Faculty of Anaesthetists, fostering high standards of regional anaesthesia in both. He was a member of Council of the Association of Anaesthetists of Great Britain and Ireland (AAGBI) for 1976-79. The Obstetric Anaesthetists' Association (OAA) elected him its second President for 1976-79, and he was the first President of the European Society of Regional Anaesthesia (ESRA, founded in 1980).

For many years Scott served in Scotland on the Confidential Enquiries into Maternal Deaths. In an editorial in the February 1977 issue of the *British Journal of Anaesthesia*, he suggested that instead of the unique requirement in Britain for deaths associated with anaesthesia to be subject to legal processes, there should be a confidential and peer reviewed enquiry modelled on the Department of Health's triennial enquiry into maternal deaths in England and Wales. This led to the setting up by the AAGBI of a working party, followed by a Central Committee with Scott as Secretary – which went on to conduct a large survey of deaths within 6 days of anaesthesia/surgery in 5 regions of over 12 months; a report was published by J.N. Lunn and W.W. Mushin (q.v. page 151) in 1982.

Scott was elected President of the Scottish Society of Anaesthetists for 1983-84. He was co-author with B.G. Covino of *Handbook of Epidural Anaesthesia and Analgesia* in 1985. Although he retired from clinical work in 1986, his collaboration with Astra Pharmaceuticals led to the endowment of an annual Clinical Research Fellowship for an anaesthetic trainee, and establishment of its Clinical Research Centre in Edinburgh of which he was Deputy Director for six years. His numerous honours included election as a Fellow of the Royal College of Physicians of Edinburgh in 1980, the Frederick Hewitt Lectureship of the Faculty of Anaesthetists in 1987, the Gaston Labat Award of the American Society of Regional Anesthesia in 1988 and the Carl Koller Gold Medal from ESRA in 1990.

In 1999 the Great Britain & Ireland (GB&I) zone of ESRA named the guest lecture at its annual meeting the 'Bruce Scott Lecture'. This lecture was continued at the annual Regional Anaesthesia-UK (RA-UK) meeting after 2010 when ESRA (GB&I) split to form RA-UK and the Irish Society of Regional Anaesthesia (ISRA).

Table 1. ESRA (GB&I zone)/Regional Anaesthesia-UK's Bruce Scott lecturers and lecture titles

Year	Lecturer	Title
1999	Dag Selander	Transient neurological symptoms – neurotoxicity or 'potato picker's back'?
2000	Nick Scott	It gets better.
2001	Henrik Kehlet	The future role of regional anaesthesia in fast-track surgery.
2002	Anthony P. Rubin	Following on the inspiring work of Bruce Scott.
2003	Edmond Charlton	On the shoulders of giants.
2004	J. Anthony W. Wildsmith	Is this Cockfosters?
2005	Barrie Fischer	A road less well travelled.
2006	William Harrop-Griffiths	The history of regional anaesthesia.
2007	Jonathan Richardson	Paravertebral blocks.
2008	Vincent Chan	Ultrasound guided regional anaesthesia – is it here to stay?
2009	Alain Delbos	Interactive anatomy DVD.
2010	Peter Marhofer	Ultrasound guided regional anaesthesia – what we have learnt during the last 15 years.
2011	Guy Weinberg	Lipid resuscitation.
2012	Franco Carli	How to merge regional anaesthesia with modern surgical protocols.
2013	No meeting	
2014	Jeff Gadsden	Does regional analgesia improve outcome in trauma?
2015	Rob Raw	Is intraneural injection so bad and are we just missing the point?
2016	Paul Bigeleisen	Lessons from the past, challenges of the present and the future is intraneural injections.
2017	Admir Hadzic	From humble beginnings to the road ahead.
2018	Michael Barrington	From anatomy to patient-centred outcomes – meaningful participation from all is required.
2019	Ki Jin Chin	Opportunities and challenges in the renaissance of regional anaesthesia.

From 2003 the Obstetric Anaesthetists' Association started holding a Bruce Scott Lecture at its annual meeting.

Table 2. OAA's Bruce Scott lecturers and lecture topics/titles

Year	Lecturer	Title
2003	Sanjay Datta	Spinal anaesthesia "sweet or sour"
2004	No lecture	
2005	Philip Steer	Evolution of pain in childbirth
2006	No lecture	
2007	David Birnbach	Patient safety and communication on the labour suite. Where have we been, where are we now, and where should we be going?
2008	Cynthia Wong	Above all do no harm
2009	Gordon Lyons	How to approach postnatal neurologic pathology
2010	Lawrence Tsen	Epidural equinox: 10 tips to optimize your epidural technique
2011	Andrew Calder	Simpson and Scott: innovators in obstetrics and anaesthesia
2012	David Gabbott	"Dangerous airways" – nightmares in obstetric anaesthesia
2013	Mike Paech	A fortunate life – reflections on the (recent) evolution of obstetric anaesthesia
2014	Brendan Carvalho	The customer is always right: understanding our role in the obstetric pain experience
2015	David Bogod	Mothers in law
2016	Judith Hall	Sustainable anaesthesia: the Millenium Mums of Africa
2017	Roshan Fernando	Forever running but never quite catching up ..... tales from obstetric anaesthesia
2018	S Mike Kinsella	Lateral thinking by obstetric anaesthetists
2019	Lesley Regan	Global maternal mortality

Acknowledgement

Professor Tony Wildsmith kindly assisted with the list of ESRA Bruce Scott lectures, and Dr Nuala Lucas with the OAA Bruce Scott lectures.

Further reading

Wildsmith JAW. Obituary Donald Bruce Scott, MD FRCA FRCPEd 1925-1998. *The Annals of the Scottish Society of Anaesthetists* 1999; **39**: 6-7.

McClure JH, Loudon JDO. Obituary Donald Bruce Scott. *British Medical Journal* 1999; **318**: 469.

Kerr MG, Scott DB, Samuel E. Studies of the inferior vena cava in late pregnancy. *British Medical Journal* 1964; **I**: 532-3.

Scott DB. Death associated with anaesthesia. *British Journal of Anaesthesia* 1977; **49**: 95-96.

OLE SECHER LECTURE

Ole Secher (1918-1996)

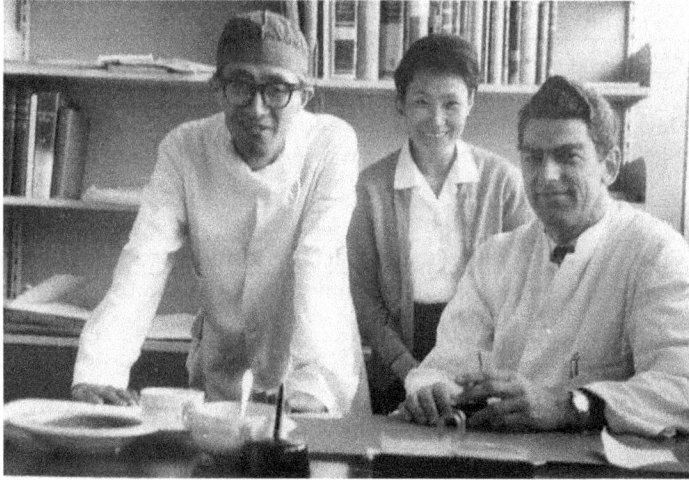

Ole Secher (R) in 1958 with Dr Kim Young Wo (L) and Dr JS Shin (middle) at the National Medical Centre in Seoul. Image provided by Dr Preben Berthelsen.

Ole Secher was born in Denmark in 1918, the son of a professor of internal medicine. As a youth he was outstanding at rowing, but after the occupation of Denmark by Germany in April 1940, he enrolled in medical school of Copenhagen University. While a medical student, he joined the Danish resistance and from October 1943 was involved in the rescue of Danish Jews to Sweden. Before long (December) the Gestapo raided the Bispebjerg Hospital and arrested Secher, who then had to endure six weeks in prison.

After the liberation, Secher graduated in medicine in 1945. He then did his internship and junior doctor jobs in the Copenhagen area, and worked as an anaesthesiologist. Indeed, he was a founder member of the Danish Anaesthesiologists Association (DAA) and its Chair from 1949 to 1951. The WHO-sponsored Anaesthesiology Training Centre in Copenhagen began in May 1950 and Secher was in the founding group of instructors. He was a research fellow at the Institute of Pharmacology, and he completed his MD thesis on the peripheral effects of ether in 1952. That year he travelled to the USA to do a residency in anaesthesiology at the Children's Hospital of Philadelphia (University of Pennsylvania). Later in 1952 and extending into 1953 he was in the Danish Military Medical Mission sent to the Korean War. He worked in the Danish Red Cross on the hospital ship *Jutlandia*, which was moored at Busan (Pusan).

Having returned Copenhagen, in 1953 Secher was appointed head of the Department of Anaesthesiology at the Rigshospitalet. He was Chair of the Danish Society of Anaesthesiologists (DSA, reorganized from the DAA) for 1955-57. During this period, he was involved in further medical missions: WHO mission to Egypt (1955) and Red Cross mission to Hungary (1956).

Besides the Danish hospital ship, during the Korean War (1950-53) two other Scandinavian countries gave medical aid. Sweden provided a hospital at Busan; Norway provided a Mobile Army Surgical Hospital (MASH) in the UN Army serving north of Seoul and this did not close until November 1954. The Koreans realised that they needed a medical training facility and by 1956 it was formally agreed that the three Scandinavian countries would establish this. So, in October 1958 the extended old city hospital in Seoul was opened as the National Medical Centre (NMC). There Ole Secher was head of anaesthesia for the first year 1958-59, after which a Norwegian, Bjorn Hegar, took over as head for the next two years. In 1968, the running of the NMC was transferred to the Koreans.

In 1964 Secher became the first full Professor of Anaesthesiology in Denmark. For 1965-67 he served again as Chair of the DSA and during this period he was President of the Second European Congress of Anaesthesiology, held in August 1966 in Copenhagen. He continued to serve as an instructor on courses at the Anaesthesiology Training Centre in Copenhagen until 1973.

Secher published about 100 articles on various aspects of anaesthesia mainly in Scandinavian journals. He was called upon to be visiting professor in Europe, the Middle East and the Americas. From the 1970s he took increasing interest in the history of anaesthesia and he presented at the First International Symposium on the History of Modern Anaesthesia held in Rotterdam in 1982. Notably he produced a short Bibliography of books, journals and articles on the history of anaesthesia in 1987, which stimulated others to expand on this work. He again presented at the Second International Symposium on the History of Anaesthesia held in 1987 in London. Again in 1992 he delivered a paper at the Third International Symposium on the History of Anaesthesia held in Atlanta. He passed away in 1996. His son, Niels H. Secher, also became Professor of Anaesthesiology at the Rigshospitalet and his elder grandson became an anaesthesiologist in the thoracic department of the Rigshospitalet – so there have been three generations of Secher anaesthesiologists.

Honours bestowed on Secher from Denmark included a Knighthood, the Jutlandia Medal and the Danish Red Cross Order of Merit. His international awards included Honorary Fellowship of the Faculty of Anaesthetists, Royal

College of Surgeons (England), the United States Service Medal (Korea), the Korean Presidential Citation and the Korean War Service Medal.

From 1989 the Danish Society of Anaesthesiology and Intensive Care Medicine arranged the Ole Secher Lecture to be held in Denmark. Initially it alternated with the Bjorn Ibsen Lecture (q.v. page 107), but since 2005 it has occurred triennially due to the addition of the Henning Ruben lecture to the series.

Table 1. Ole Secher lecturers and lecture titles

Year	Lecturer	Title
1989	Ole Secher	The first blood transfusion in Denmark
1991	Tapani Tammisto	Neuromuscular block versus muscle relaxation – clinical applications of the difference
1993	Torstein Stefanson	Anaesthesia and surgical risk in the elderly patient
1995	Niels H. Secher	Can normovolaemia be defined and, if so, maintained through surgery?
1997	Henning Ruben	Taken from a life as an anaesthesiologist
1999	Mads Gilbert	Boundless anesthesia: Challenges to a new art!
2001	Petter Andreas Steen	Guidelines 2000 for Cardiopulmonary Resuscitation and Emergency Cardiovascular Care
2003	Peter Baskett	Resuscitation
2005	James E. Caldwell	How to become an anaesthesiologist in USA/UK – differences and similarities
2008	Herwig Gerlach	"And not a word about sepsis". Barriers for improvement
2012	Lars S. Rasmussen	Is it something acute?
2015	Kirsten Moller	Anaesthesia for the heart and brain
2018	Doris Ostergaard	What promotes good clinical learning – and have you downloaded the latest update?

Acknowledgements

Dr Preben Berthelsen kindly provided the list of Ole Secher lectures. Professor Niels Secher provided information about Ole Secher's time in Korea and his family life.

Further reading

Lewis MC. Ole Secher: A True Hero of Anesthesiology. *Israel Medical Association Journal* 2007; **9**: 215-16.

Secher O. Anaesthesiology Centre Copenhagen. In: Rupreht J, van Lieburg MJ, Lee JA, Erdmann W (Eds) Anaesthesia Essays on Its History. Berlin: Springer-Verlag, 1985; 321-34.

Lockertsen J-T, Fause Å. The nursing legacy of the Korea Sisters. *Nursing Open* 2018; 5: 94-100. https://doi.org/10.1002/nop2.117 (accessed 8 July 2020).

Secher O. *Bibliography of the History of Anaesthesia* (2nd Ed.). Albertslund: S&W Medico Teknik A/S, 1988.

Secher O. Forty-six "first anaesthetics in the world". *Acta Anaesthesiologica Scandinavica* 1990; **34**: 552-6.

SELDINGER WIRE TECHNIQUE

Sven-Ivar Seldinger (1921-1998)

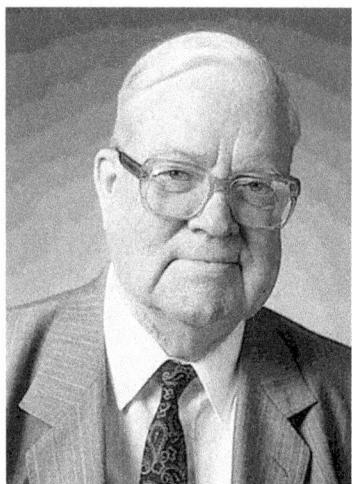

Sven-Ivar Seldinger was born in Mora, a village in central Sweden in 1921 and educated at local schools. As a child he spent much time with his grandfather, who was a mechanical toolmaker, and he developed a liking for precision manufacturing. In 1940 he began medical school at the Karolinska Institute, Stockholm and graduated in 1948.

Seldinger opted to specialize in diagnostic radiology, in which he began training at the Karolinska Sjukhuset in 1950. He soon faced the problem attendant on angiography at that time: inserting catheter-through-needle into blood vessels was often traumatic with much haemorrhage. His *first attempt* at solving the problem was to provide a catheter with a side-hole (a short distance from the tip) through which the needle passed to puncture the blood vessel – the needle was then removed and the catheter advanced: this method failed because the floppy polyethylene catheter kinked. *Secondly* he tried introducing a piano wire inside the catheter to make it more rigid: considering the risk of the wire tip breaking off, he collaborated with A.B. Stille-Werner, who manufactured a metal-spiral armed wire with a central core: prototype of the modern guidewire. However, this also failed and there remained still the risk of rupture of the catheter at the side-hole. *Thirdly*, in a 'eureka moment' he realised the means of using needle, guidewire (which he called "leader") and catheter appropriately – introduce the needle into the vessel, thread the guidewire through the needle, remove the needle, insert the proximal tip of the guidewire into the catheter which is then advanced over the wire, and finally remove the guidewire.

Sven-Ivar Seldinger. Image provided by his family and in the public domain.

This technique was tried successfully the next day and within a week in June 1952 on Seldinger's behalf, his supervisor Professor Knut Lindblom, presented the new method at the Congress of the Northern Association of Medical Radiology in Helsinki, Finland. Seldinger duly published the technique in the journal *Acta Radiologica* the following year.

Seldinger published his application of the new technique for the first localization of parathyroid adenomata by arteriography in 1954 and for the first selective renal arteriography in 1955. He was one of the pioneers of percutaneous transhepatic cholangiography in 1962 and this was the subject of his thesis which he defended in 1966. A further examination in teaching earned him the title of Docent in Radiology in 1967, when he moved back to Mora to become the Chief of Radiology in Mora Lasarett.

Within a few years of Seldinger's 1953 paper, the new technique was adopted by radiologists in Europe, but it took longer to be accepted in the USA and the UK. Certainly, it accelerated the rise of interventional radiology. However, Seldinger could not have foreseen the huge impact it would come to have in emergency medicine, anaesthesia and critical care. A letter in the *Journal of the American Medical Association* by Thomas J. Conahan (Professor of Anesthesiology in Philadelphia) in 1977 drew attention to the advantages of the technique in facilitating central venous cannulation and use of the Swan-Ganz catheter. In the 1980s in the USA and the UK, Seldinger kits began to gradually replace the cannula-over needle devices marketed for central venous catheterisation. The technique was soon also applied to arterial cannulation for monitoring.

In the 1990s Melker applied the Seldinger technique to insertion of a cricothyrotomy catheter and produced a commercial kit. This could be used for laryngeal surgery or for emergency front of neck access (FONA) in airway management.

The Seldinger technique has been accepted all over the world and is employed by anaesthetists every day. However, complications began to be reported soon after it became adopted in anaesthetic practice. These included kinking, knotting and loss of the guidewire; cardiac tamponade due to perforation of the heart (sometimes fatal) has rarely been reported. Recently the importance of operators being adequately trained became clear and guidelines for safe insertion were published.

Seldinger was invited to give lectures in several continents. Honours bestowed on him included honorary membership of the Swedish Association of Medical Radiology and of the German Roentgen Association, and the Valentine award from the New York Academy of Medicine. He retired in 1986.

Further reading

Varon J, Nyman U. Sven-Ivar Seldinger: The revolution of radiology and acute intravascular access. In: Baskett JF, Baskett TF (Eds.) *Resuscitation Greats*. Bristol: Clinical Press Ltd., 2007; 267-71.

Seldinger SI. Catheter replacement of the needle in percutaneous angiography: a new technique. *Acta Radiologica* 1953; **39**: 368-76.

Doby T. A tribute to Sven-Ivar Seldinger. *American Journal of Roentgenology* 1984; **142**: 1-11.

Conahan TJ, Schwartz AJ, Geer RT. Percutaneous Catheter Introduction: The Seldinger Technique. *Journal of the American Medical Association* 1977; **237**: 446-7.

SPROTTE SPINAL NEEDLE

Günter Sprotte (1945 –)

Günter Sprotte was born in Heigenbruecken, Bavaria in 1945. From 1965 to 1970 he studied medicine at the Julius Maximilian University of Würzburg. For the next two years he did medical assistantships in hospitals.

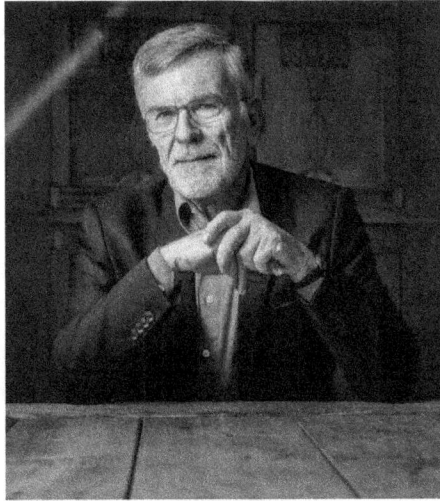

Sprotte obtained his PhD in 1971 at the Institute of Anaesthesiology of the University of Würzburg, where he then proceeded to four years of specialist training. As a newly qualified specialist anaesthetist, he was responsible for the anaesthetic department at the Orthopaedic University Clinic in Würzburg. To improve the peri-operative care of the patients he tried to shift the emphasis to regional anaesthesia. In this regard he had to face up to the fact that inherent in spinal anaesthesia was the problem of post-dural puncture headache (PDPH). He ordered Whitacre pencil-point spinal needles from the USA and tried these (instead of cutting tip needles) to reduce PDPH, but was disappointed: due to the very small orifice near the tip, which was not occluded by the stylet, blockage by tissue could occur, impeding the flow of cerebrospinal fluid (CSF).

Sprotte had the idea to modify the pencil-point needle, but he was rebuffed by the major German medical products manufacturer. In 1979 he visited the Pajunk company in Geisingen and explained to the two Pajunk brothers the changes that he envisaged making to the Whitacre needle. A prototype was produced the same day and a week later Sprotte received 100 sterilized needles of the new design. In the first 100 spinal procedures with the new needle there were zero headaches. Encouraged, Sprotte applied for a German patent in 1980 and after one year of development, the Pajunk company began mass production of the needles. The new design incorporated a more elongated, ogive-

Pencil-point   Ogive
Figure 1.

shaped point. In comparison with the rotationally symmetrical circular cone of the pencil-point, here was shoulder-edge curved in two radii (Figure 1).

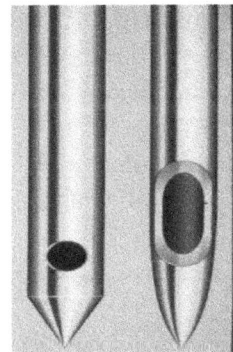

Whereas with a circular cone, the tissue-pressure is maximum on the shoulder edge – in advancement of the ogive, pressures are evenly distributed over all parts of the tip. This new needle facilitated more gradual parting of the dural fibres with less CSF leakage; the side orifice was much larger – allowing a faster flow of CSF and easier injection of local anaesthetic solution.

Sprotte was granted a patent for an "atraumatic universal cannula for spinal anaesthesia and diagnostic lumbar puncture" in 1983. Within 6 years of introduction, 30000 procedures with the new spinal needle had been performed at the University Clinic where he worked. In 1987 he published the results of the 6-year trial of the "atraumatic universal needle"; soon it became known as the Sprotte needle.

In 1990 a paper from France compared use of a 24G Sprotte needle with a 25G cutting tip (diamond) needle in a randomised trial of 110 women undergoing caesarean section under spinal anaesthesia. The incidence of PDPH was 14.5% in the cutting tip group (62% requiring an epidural blood patch) compared with zero in the Sprotte group. The authors noted that lumbar puncture was easy to perform with the Sprotte needle, but there was one failure despite free flow of CSF: it was presumed that the needle's distal orifice straddled the dura, so that the local anaesthetic was injected into the epidural space. The news of removal of PDPH ushered in a huge rise in the use of spinal anaesthesia for operative obstetrics.

Aglan and Stansby proposed (based on an experimental flow study) in 1992 that the lateral orifice of the 24G Sprotte spinal needle could be reduced to the size of the internal cross-sectional area – to avoid some of the local anaesthetic being injected outside the subarachnoid space. Their measurements of the dimensions of the lateral orifice were length 1.7 mm and width 0.32 mm. Günter Sprotte responded with counter argument in a letter to the same journal (*Anaesthesia*). Later the Pajunk company manufactured the 24G Sprotte needle with the dimensions of its lateral orifice being length 0.9 mm and width 0.25 mm (see Figure 2).

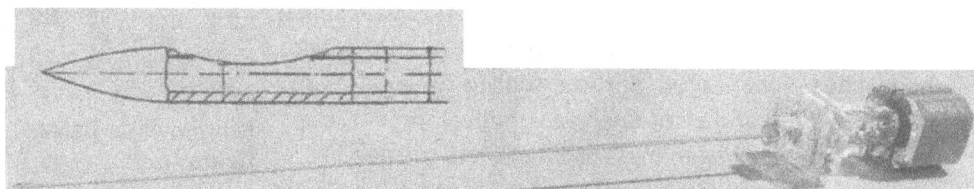

Figure 2. Sprotte spinal needle and diagram of ogive point and large side orifice. From Pajunk Magazine, September 2019.

The Sprotte spinal needles were marketed by the Pajunk company worldwide and became standard equipment for a great number of anaesthetists practising regional anaesthesia. Unfortunately, use of 'conventional' cutting tip spinal needles for diagnostic lumbar puncture was continued for decades by physicians and neurologists, who eschewed atraumatic needles – with consequent distress from PDPH in their patients.

Sprotte advanced his career in the field of pain medicine. He and colleagues investigated the use of immunoglobulin to treat chronic pain conditions. In 2000 he received a European Patent grant for oral administration of immunoglobulin preparations for treatment of chronic pain syndromes. From 2003 to 2008 he was Lecturer at the Academy for Palliative Medicine, Palliative Care and Hospice Work at the Juliusspital Foundation in Würzburg, and a member of the Scientific Advisory Board of the Academy. Honours he has received include the Karl Ludwig Schleich award from the German Society of Anaesthesiology in 1982, and the German Pain Award in 2009. He retired in 2010.

Further reading

An interview with Prof. Dr. Sprotte. The Pajunk Magazine September 2019; issue **01**: 1-4.
Sprotte G, Schedel R, Pajunk H. Eine atraumatische Universalkanule für einzeitige Regionalanaesthesien. *Regional Anaesthesie* 1987; **10**: 104-8.

Cesarini M, Torrielli R, Lahaye F, Mene JM, Cabiro C. Sprotte needle for Caesarean section: incidence of postdural puncture headache. *Anaesthesia* 1990; **45**: 656-8.

Aglan MY, Stansby PK. Modification to the Sprotte spinal needle. *Anaesthesia* 1992; **47**: 506-7.
Sprotte G. No need to modify the Sprotte needle. *Anaesthesia* 1992; **48**: 1103-4.

Nath S, KoziarzA, Badhiwala JH, Alhazzani W *et al*. Atraumatic versus conventional lumbar puncture needles: a systematic review and meta-analysis. *Lancet* 2018; **391** (10126): 1197-1204.

C. RONALD STEPHEN LECTURE AND RESIDENT ESSAY AWARD

Charles Ronald Stephen (1916-2006)

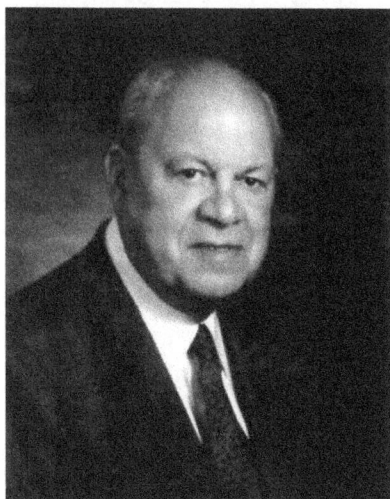

C. Ronald Stephen was born in Montreal, Canada in 1916. After schooling locally, he entered McGill University in 1934 for a science-based curriculum. While a student he was editor of the *McGill Daily* newspaper. By 1936 he decided to study medicine and was admitted to the first year of the McGill medical school. He graduated B.Sc. and M.D.C.M. in 1940 and he then did a one-year internship at Montreal General Hospital.

C. Ronald Stephen. Image courtesy of Department of Anesthesiology, Washington University School of Medicine, St. Louis MO.

For a year 1941-42 Stephen was a resident at the Jeffery Hale Hospital in Quebec City. Then in July 1942 he joined the Royal Canadian Army Medical Corps with the ambition of becoming a specialist physician. However, from December 1943 he was assigned to a three-month intensive course in anaesthesiology with teaching from doctors Wesley Bourne, Harold R. Griffith and Digby Leigh. He was sent to Great Britain in May 1944, arriving about two weeks before D-Day. Stationed at a 1200 bed hospital in Bramshott, Sussex he gained much experience in the care of war casualties. He felt that the Canadian Army was privileged to have the use of cyclopropane. When the casualty rate declined in 1945, he was granted leave to spend three months at the Nuffield Department of Anaesthetics in Oxford where he received instruction from Robert Macintosh and William Mushin (q.v. page 151). Following this period of training he passed the examinations for the Diploma in Anaesthetics (RCP&S) in London.

Stephen returned to Canada in 1946 and was discharged from the Army with the rank of Lt. Colonel. He was persuaded to forsake his aspirations to specialise in internal medicine work and with help from Dr Bourne he was appointed Chief of Anaesthesia at the Montreal Neurological Institute, where he anaesthetized for the neurosurgeon Wilder Penfield. Then from 1947 to 1950 he was Director of Anaesthesia at the Children's Memorial Hospital, where in 1948 he published with H.M. Slater a landmark paper 'A nonresisting, nonrebreathing valve', which was key to the advancement of inhalation anaesthesia for paediatrics. He passed the examinations of the American

Board of Anesthesiology and was duly certified as a Diplomate in 1950. That year he was head hunted to move to an academic appointment in the USA: Professor of Anesthesiology at Duke University School of Medicine in Durham, NC. There he established a training programme for resident physicians in anaesthesiology. In 1952 he published the textbook *Elements of Pediatric Anesthesia* (Charles C. Thomas, Publisher). At Duke in 1956 he introduced halothane into clinical practice in the USA and in 1961 he published with David M. Little (q.v. page 121) another textbook *Halothane (Fluothane)*. Notably in 1957 he was the founding editor of *Survey of Anesthesiology*; in 1964 he was awarded an Honorary FFARCS at a ceremony in London, England.

After sixteen years at Duke Hospital, Stephen moved in 1966 to take up the Chair of Anesthesiology at the Southwestern Medical School, University of Texas and head of anaesthesia at the Children's Medical Center in Dallas. From there he was recruited in 1971 to become the Henry E. Mallinckrodt Professor of Anesthesiology at Washington University School of Medicine in St. Louis, Missouri. He was also Chief of Anesthesiology at Barnes and St. Louis Children's Hospitals. On retirement from his academic role in 1980, he served as head of a private practice anesthesia group at St. Luke's Hospital in St. Louis for five years. In 1986 he co-edited with Richard Assaf of Dublin, Ireland another textbook *Geriatric Anesthesia Principles and Practice*. He seems to have been unique in producing textbooks on anaesthesia for the two extremes of age!

Stephen was also a National Consultant in Anesthesia to the United States Air Force and the United States Navy for over twenty years. He was awarded in 1981 the highest honour of the American Society of Anesthesiologists, the Distinguished Service Award. However, in the main, he was renowned for his teaching and lecturing. After his full retirement, the Washington University School of Medicine in St. Louis (WUSM-SL) set up the Annual C.R. Stephen Lecture – see Table 1.

Table 1. WUSM-SL's Annual C.R. Stephen lecturers and lecture titles

Year	Lecturer	Title
1988	Leroy D. Vandam, MD	Schools of Anesthesia
1989	M.T. Jenkins, MD	Archeology of Fluid Balance in Infants, Birds, Sharks, and Other Strange Milieus
1990	James E. Eckenhoff, MD DSc	Random Thoughts About The Practice of Anesthesiology: A Half Century Perspective
1991	Robert K. Stoelting, MD	Pharmacology of Anesthetic Drugs – Past Problems and Future Promises
1992	Nicholas M. Greene, MD	The ASA's East African Anesthesia Program
1994	Warren M. Zapol, MD	Inhaled Nitric Oxide: A Selective Pulmonary Vasodilator

1995	Howard L. Fields, MD PhD	Neural Circuits Underlying Opioid Analgesia
1996	Marcus E. Raichle, MD	An Expanded View of Human Memory Systems
1997	Steven E. Hyman, MD	How Dopamine and Psychostimulant Drugs Regulate Gene Expression in the Striatum: Implications for Behaviour
1998	Clifford J. Woolf, PhD	Pain and Plasticity
1999	David A. McCormick, PhD	General Activating Systems and Their Role in Sleep, Arousal, and Anesthesia
2000	Allan I. Basbaum, PhD	The Neurochemistry of Acute and Persistent Pain
2001	Nicholas P. Franks, PhD	How Do General Anesthetics Work? – Light at the End of the Tunnel
2002	Eric R. Kandel, MD	Genes, Synapses and Long-Term Memory
2003	Erwin Neher, PhD	Ca++ signals controlling neurotransmitter release and short term synaptic plasticity
2004	Mervyn Maze, MB,ChB FRCP	Molecular Mechanisms and Neural Substrates for the Behavioural Effects of General Anesthetics: Clinical Implications
2005	David Julius, PhD	From Peppers to Peppermints: Molecular Insights into Thermosensation and Pain
2006	Kevin J. Tracey, MD	HMGB1 and the Inflammatory Reflex
2007	Clifford B. Saper, MD PhD	Relationship of Sleep and Anesthesia
2008	Jeffrey R. Balser, MD PhD	Personalized Healthcare – the Next Manhattan Project
2009	Gregg L. Semenza, MD PhD	Regulation of Oxygen Homeostasis by Hypoxia-Inducible Factor 1
2010	Irene Tracey, PhD	Imaging Pain and Its Relief in Controls and Chronic Pain Patients
2011	James C. Eisenach, MD	Can We Prevent Chronic Pain After Injury?
2012	Guilio Tononi, MD PhD	Consciousness, Sleep and Anesthesia
2013	Beverley Orser, MD PhD FRCPC	Memory Loss and Anesthesia: The Good, The Bad, and The Ugly
2014	Albert Dahan, MD PhD	Ketamine's Second and ..... Third Life
2015	Emory N. Brown, MD PhD	Unlocking the Mysteries of the Brain Under General Anesthesia
2016	Paul Myles, MBBS MPH MD	The Special Value and Importance of Large Trials in Perioperative Medicine
2017	E. Wesley Ely, MD MPH	A New Frontier in Critical Care: Saving the Injured Brain
2018	Vamsi Mootha, MD	Mitochondrial Systems Biology: Understanding the Whole from the Parts
2019	John P. Ioannidis, MD DSc	Reproducible, Transparent, True, Useful Research

In 1986 Stephen became the second editor of the *Bulletin of Anesthesia History* published jointly by the Anesthesia History Association (AHA) and the Wood Library-Museum. Retirement enabled him to renew his interest in philately: he compiled an exhibit of about 200 stamps on 'blood transfusions and blood donors' and a larger exhibit (some 500 stamps) on 'famous people in medicine' which was donated to the Wood Library-Museum of Anesthesiology. After his death in 2006, the AHA resolved to name the prize for its annual contest for best resident's essay on the history of anaesthesia, pain medicine or intensive care the 'C. Ronald Stephen Resident Essay Award' – see Table 2.

Table 2. AHA's C. Ronald Stephen Resident Essay Award winners

Year	Recipient	Essay
2008	Edward Kosik	Four Decades of Suspending Disbelief: Milestones in Anesthesia
2009	Anup Pamnani	Dr Joseph Artusio and the early days of the Physician Anesthetist
2010	NIL	
2011	Pervez Sultan	Developments in Maxillofacial Orthognathic Anesthesia over the Past Four Decades
2012	Sarah Smith	A History of Ethics in Anesthesiology
2013	Casey B. Wiley	Anesthesia and the Lone Star State
2014	Julia M. Rosenbloom	Toward an Understanding of the Equality of Pain: Crawford Long and the Development of Anesthesia in Antebellum Georgia
2015	Peter Featherstone	The Tenacious Terrier and His Tubes
2016	Yan Cui	The Dolorimeter, Randomized Controlled Trials, and Patient Controlled Analgesia – A Journey through Pain Management History at The New York Hospital
2017	Jane Moon	William Jones, Nitrous Oxide, and the "Anesthetic Revelation"
2018	Daniel A. Hansen	"Without the Slightest Hitch" A Brief History of the First Successful Orotracheal Intubations
2019	Thomas Hamilton	Leo Fabian: A Life of Shocking Accomplishment
2020	Rohan Jotwani	From Electric Fish to the Spinal Cord Stimulator: The Historical Journey of Neuromodulation and Analgesia

Further reading

Stephen CR. A Chronology of Events. In: Fink BR (Ed). *Careers in Anesthesiology Autobiographical Memoirs*. Volume II. Park Ridge, Illinois: Wood Library-Museum of Anesthesiology, 1998; 60-88.

Stephen CR, Slater HM. A nonresisting, nonrebreathing valve. *Anesthesiology* 1948; **9**: 550-2.

Stephen CR, Fabian LW. Introduction of halothane to the USA. In: Atkinson RS, Boulton TB (Eds.) *The History of Anaesthesia*. London: Royal Society of Medicine Services, 1989; 221-2.

Stephen CR, Assaf RAE (Eds). *Geriatric Anesthesia Principles and Practice*. Stoneham (MA): Butterworth Publishers, 1986.

TARGET CONTROLLED INFUSION (TCI)

John Baird Glen (1940 –)

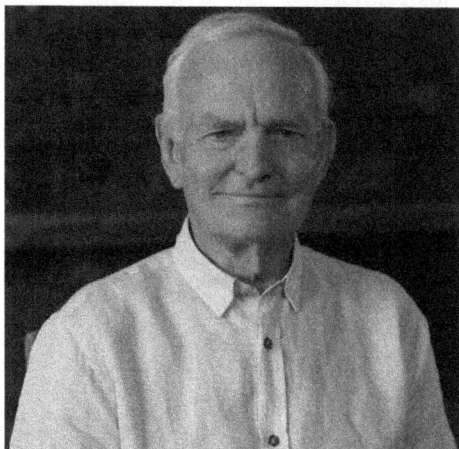

John (Iain) Glen was born in Glasgow, UK in October 1940. In 1948 the family moved to a small 50 acre farm in Corriecravie on the Island of Arran, in the Firth of Clyde, when his father, till then an Agricultural Adviser, decided to practice what he had been preaching. Glen completed his education at Keil School in Dumbarton and decided to study veterinary medicine at Glasgow University, graduating in 1963. After a year in Kenya dealing with tropical veterinary medicine, Glen returned to Glasgow University Veterinary School as a house surgeon in the small animal surgery department. His Professor, Sir William Weipers, in his role as President of the Royal College of Veterinary Surgeons, had encouraged the recent introduction of speciality diplomas, and Glen was the first to study for and gain a Diploma in Veterinary Anaesthesia in 1968. He became responsible for teaching the subject and clinical work extended to both large and small animals.

Around this time, a number of new drugs had been introduced for use in medical practice. These included, ketamine, propanidid, the steroid combination of alphaxalone and alphadolone and drugs used in the technique of neuroleptanalgesia. Glen took the opportunity to evaluate these agents and to assess their potential role in veterinary anaesthesia. This interest in research prompted him in 1972 to join the Anaesthesia Project Team in the research department at ICI Pharmaceuticals Division in Cheshire. He was able to combine research work done at Glasgow with later studies done at ICI to obtain his PhD on 'Studies on the pharmacology of injectable anaesthetic agents'.

Glen headed the team that evaluated the anaesthetic properties of compounds synthesised by project team chemists or selected from the company compound collection. The project was looking for a compound which would reproduce the desirable properties of thiopentone, but would be rapidly metabolised such that anaesthesia or sedation could be maintained by infusion or repeated injection without delaying recovery time. He first observed the anaesthetic properties of propofol in 1973, but difficulties in obtaining a satisfactory formulation delayed its introduction until 1986 in Europe and 1989 in the USA.

Propofol was introduced to anaesthetic practice as an agent for induction of anaesthesia and maintenance for short procedures by incremental injection, while studies with maintenance of anaesthesia or sedation for longer procedures continued. It became clear to Glen that improved equipment to facilitate the latter was required. Syringe pumps available at the time generally had a maximum delivery rate of 99 ml/hr and volumetric pumps were not considered suitable. Glen contacted a number of syringe pump manufacturers and alerted them to the potential for improved devices. A promising response was received from Ohmeda, who produced a prototype for clinical evaluation. This led to the Ohmeda 9000, the first of a new generation of syringe pumps with the ability to deliver rapid infusions of 300, 600 or 1200 ml/hr for induction of anaesthesia, continuous infusions up to 200 ml/hr for maintenance, and a facility to allow computer controlled operation. Thereafter similar devices were produced by Graseby Medical, Cardinal Health and Fresenius Kabi in Europe, Terumo in Japan and Bard, Medex and Baxter in the USA.

Schwilden, a mathematician and anaesthesiologist in Bonn, in 1981 was the first to demonstrate the use of a computer controlled infusion pump to deliver exponentially declining drug infusion rates, based on the concept proposed earlier by Kruger-Theimer. While Glen had heard of this work and a similar approach being adopted by other international research groups, studies with propofol for maintenance of anaesthesia were progressing satisfactorily with conventional syringe pumps and he remained to be convinced that the added complexity of computer control would be of benefit. However in 1990, he persuaded ICI to allow him to organise a workshop on computer simulation and control of i.v. infusions in anaesthesia. This workshop was attended by representatives from all the key groups advocating this approach. At the end of this meeting Glen was convinced that this approach would facilitate maintenance of anaesthesia or sedation with propofol. However, only after another two years and after Glen had organized a second workshop (Figure 1) held in 1992, was the Company (now Zeneca and later AstraZeneca) persuaded to begin the development of a commercial system.

Glen had first suggested the term, 'Target Controlled Titration' as an alternative to the various acronyms that had been proposed by the different groups working in this area (Figure 2) when speaking at a Swedish Postgraduate Anaesthesia meeting in Lejondals Castle in October 1991. Gavin Kenny, another speaker, was in the audience and he acknowledged the

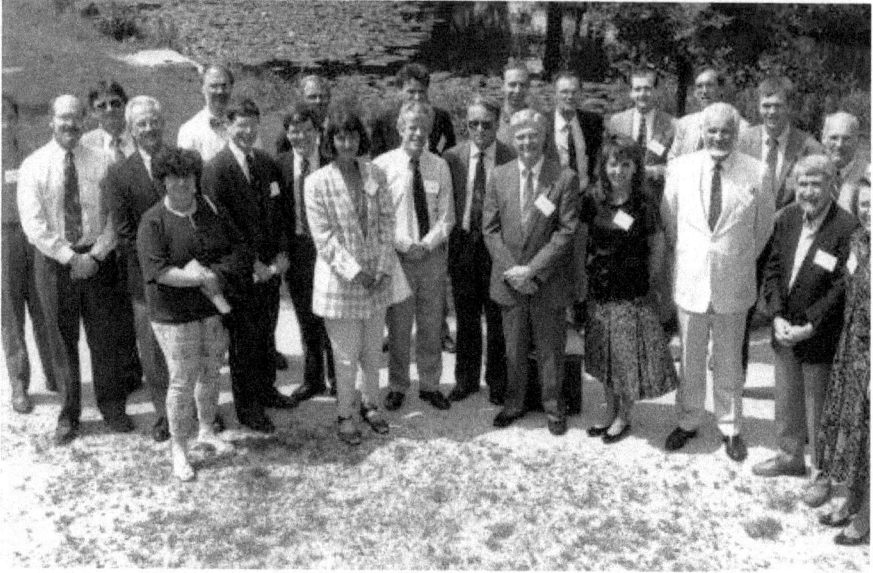

Figure 1. Academic delegates at a workshop on 'Target Controlled Titration' of anaesthetic drugs held in The Hague in 1992.

desirability of avoiding the implication that a computer rather than an anaesthesiologist was controlling the depth of anaesthesia. Thereafter, he began to use the slightly modified term, 'Target Controlled Infusion' in his subsequent publications. In 1997, Glen drafted a document on nomenclature in relation to TCI, which was endorsed by representatives of research groups working in this area.

Glen was closely involved in the clinical evaluation of the first commercial TCI system. For this project, it was considered desirable to delineate the responsibility of the pharmaceuticals company in selecting the pharmaco-kinetic model and providing guidance on appropriate target concentration settings from those of the infusion pump manufacturer. The strategy used required the development by the Company of an electronics 'Diprifusor' module which contained the pharmacokinetic model published by Marsh and colleagues and the infusion rate control algorithms and software developed at Glasgow University. This module could be installed within an infusion pump

Research Systems

CATIA Computer Assisted Total Intravenous Anaesthesia (Schuttler & Schwilden)

TIAC Titration of Intravenous Anaesthesia by Computer (Ausems, Stanski & Hug)

CACI Computer Assisted Continuous Infusion (Glass, Jacobs & Reves)

CCIP Computer Controlled Infusion Pump (Shafer, Varvel, Aziz & Scott)

Computerised Infusion System (White and Kenny)

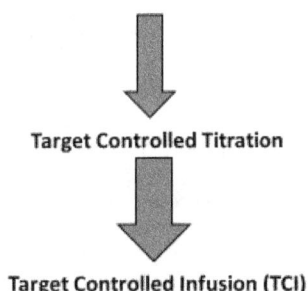

Target Controlled Titration

Target Controlled Infusion (TCI)

Figure 2. Acronyms describing early research TCI systems.

such as the Ohmeda 9000 or equivalent, with no need for an external computer. Zeneca conducted a series of clinical studies with prototype systems to determine appropriate blood target concentration settings for induction and maintenance of anaesthesia or sedation to allow appropriate guidance to be provided in 'Diprivan' propofol drug labelling. A number of drug delivery profiles were provided to device manufacturing companies to ensure that drug delivery from devices incorporating the 'Diprifusor' module was accurate.

An added complication in this development was the commercial decision to present propofol for use in syringe pumps containing the Diprifusor module in a glass prefilled syringe with an electronic tag in the finger grip and software in the module to confirm the presence and concentration of Diprivan in the syringe. While recognised as a useful safety feature, this was a more expensive preparation and, when propofol became available as a generic product, created a demand for 'Open' TCI pumps with the addition of alternative pharmacokinetic models for propofol and the addition of other drugs such as remifentanil. While the latter is to be welcomed, particularly if there is a consensus on the most appropriate pharmacokinetic model to select, having alternative models for propofol has led to a degree of confusion as such systems, which deliver a somewhat different infusion profile, have been approved without reference to drug regulatory authorities. An early example of a syringe pump containing the Diprifusor TCI module is shown in Figure 3.

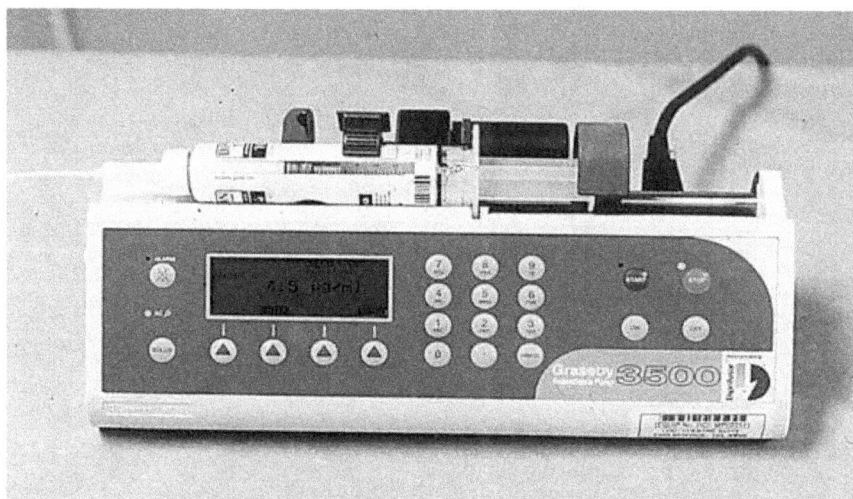

Figure 3. Graseby syringe pump containing Diprifusor TCI module as indicated by the logo at the bottom right hand corner of the face plate.

In the development of the Diprifusor TCI system there was close collaboration between Device and Drug authorities and Glen believes it would be beneficial if, in the process of adding new drugs and new pharmacokinetic models, such contact could be maintained to ensure that the presence of appropriate advice on target concentrations is included in drug labelling.

Further reading

Struys MMRF, De Smet T, Glen JB, Vereecke HEM, Absalom AR, Schnider W. The history of Target-Controlled Infusion. *Anesthesia and Analgesia* 2016; **122**: 56-69.

Glass PSA, Glen JB, Kenny GNC, Schuttler J, Shafer SL. Nomenclature for computer-assisted infusion devices. *Anesthesiology* 1997; **86**: 1430-1.

Glen JB. The development of 'Diprifusor': a TCI system for propofol. *Anaesthesia* 1998; **53**: Supplement 1: 13-21.

TRAIN OF FOUR (TOF) MONITORING NEUROMUSCULAR BLOCK

David Grob (1919-2008)

David Grob was born in New York City in February 1919. He finished high school at the age of 14 and graduated from the City College of New York at the age of 18. He then read medicine at Johns Hopkins University in Baltimore, graduating MD in 1942. He served as a physician in the US Army in the Second World War and was among the first liberators of the concentration camps in Germany. He was awarded a Bronze Star.

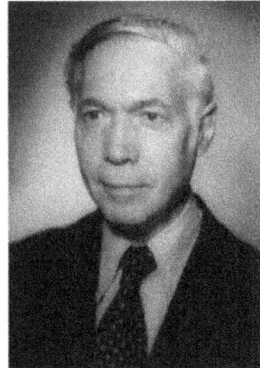

After the war, Grob joined the Department of Medicine and the Division of Clinical Pharmacology at Johns Hopkins University School of Medicine. From 1947 he was involved in clinical research on the effects of neuromuscular blocking drugs (NMBD) and anticholinesterase drugs. His main interest in these

David Grob. Credit: Dr Murali Pagala.

activities was the study and treatment of myasthenia gravis. In 1948 he used a nerve stimulator to assess neuromuscular transmission in man: percutaneously with supra-maximal pulses. The muscle action potentials were recorded. In 1956 he adopted the 'train of four' (TOF) as the standard pattern of intermittent nerve stimulation.

Grob moved to the Maimonides Research Foundation where he chaired the department of medicine from 1958 to 1989. He became an expert on the disease myasthenia gravis and its treatment. From 1989 to 2006 he was medical director at Maimonides.

In 1958 Harry C. Churchill-Davidson with T.H. Christie at St Thomas's Hospital, London introduced a nerve stimulator for use in the operating theatre. However, it was capable only of either a slow rate of twitch (3 Hz) or a fast rate (tetanus, 50 Hz) – with no facility for train of four. It did not become very popular.

The train of four twitch technique was adopted for assessment of residual curarization in human anaesthetic practice at the University of Liverpool in 1970. Hassan H. Ali working with John E. Utting under the supervision of Professor T. Cecil Gray experimented with various frequencies of ulnar nerve stimulation and settled on the following pattern: train of four at 2 Hz which was delivered every 10 seconds. The response of adductor pollicis activated a compressor transducer. This work was presented at the June 1970 meeting of the Anaesthetic Research Society held in Aberdeen, followed by three definitive papers in the *British Journal of Anaesthesia*: one in November that year and two in 1971. After administration of a non-depolarizing NMBD, the fourth twitch (T4) decreased first followed by the third (T3), then the second (T2) and lastly the first twitch (T1). Recovery of twitches when the NMBD wore off and on reversal by neostigmine, occurred in the reverse order – see Figure 1. The train of four technique caused less discomfort to the conscious patient recovering from anaesthesia than tetanic rates of stimulation (50 Hz or more). The ratio of T4/T1 was suggested for quantitative assessment as it correlated with the ability of a patient to lift the head off the pillow and sustain it in space unsupported. A TOF ratio of < 0.6 was associated with clinically obvious muscle weakness.

NON-DEPOLARIZING NMBD　　　　　　　　**NEOSTIGMINE**

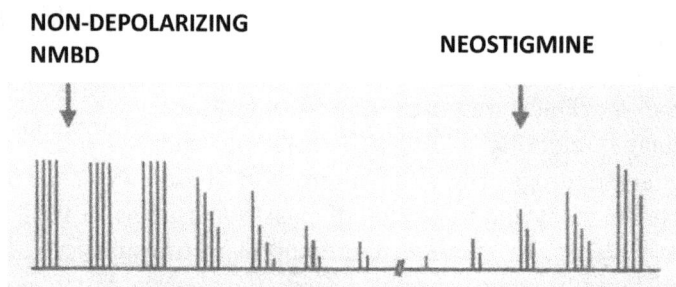

Figure 1. TOF monitoring of onset of neuromuscular block produced by a non-depolarizing NMBD, followed by antagonism with neostigmine, given when 3 twitches of the TOF are detectable.

Monitoring of neuromuscular block had some advocates, but it certainly did not become routine in anaesthetic practice until decades later. In 1988 the Association of Anaesthetists of Great Britain and Ireland (AAGBI) published a glossy guideline *Recommendations for Standards of Monitoring during Anaesthesia and Recovery*. In this the section on monitoring neuromuscular function was somewhat lacking in commitment: it stated simply that when NMBDs are used, a nerve stimulator should be readily available. A study conducted in France in 1995 (but not published until 2000) found residual curarization (TOF ratio < 0.7) in 42% of patients in the postoperative recovery room after vecuronium. The anaesthetists neither administered reversal nor used a nerve stimulator. This prompted an editorial by J. Viby- Mogensen, who remarked that ideally, at a minimum, the TOF ratio should be measured during recovery whenever a non-depolarizing NMBD is not antagonized. However, he noted that in many anaesthetic departments, clinicians did not have access to equipment for measuring the degree of neuromuscular block.

Furthermore, he noted that recent research indicated that normal vital muscle function, including normal pharyngeal function, required the TOF ratio at the adductor pollicis to be 0.9 rather than 0.7.

It was not until 2015 that the AAGBI upgraded the requirement of a peripheral nerve stimulator to be a minimum monitoring standard when NMBDs are administered – in the fifth edition of *Recommendations for Standards of Monitoring during Anaesthesia and Recovery*.

Further reading

Ricks D. David Grob; Medical Research Pioneer. *The Washington Post* 8 April 2008.

Grob D, Johns RJ, Harvey AM. Studies in neuromuscular function I: Introduction and Methods. *Bulletin Johns Hopkins Hospital* 1956; **99**: 115-124.

Christie TH, Churchill-Davidson HC. The St. Thomas's Hospital nerve stimulator in the diagnosis of prolonged apnoea. *Lancet* 1958; **i**: 776.

Ali HH, Utting JE, Nightingale DA, Gray TC. Quantitative assessment of residual curarization in humans. *British Journal of Anaesthesia* 1970; 42: 802-3.

Ali HH, Utting JE, Gray TC. Stimulus frequency in the detection of neuromuscular block in humans. *British Journal of Anaesthesia* 1970; **42**: 967-77.

Viby-Mogensen J. Postoperative residual curarization and evidence-based anaesthesia. *British Journal of Anaesthesia* 2000; **84**: 301-3.

VIENNA SCORE FOR ULTRASONOGRAPHIC-GUIDED NERVE BLOCKS

Peter Marhofer (1964-)

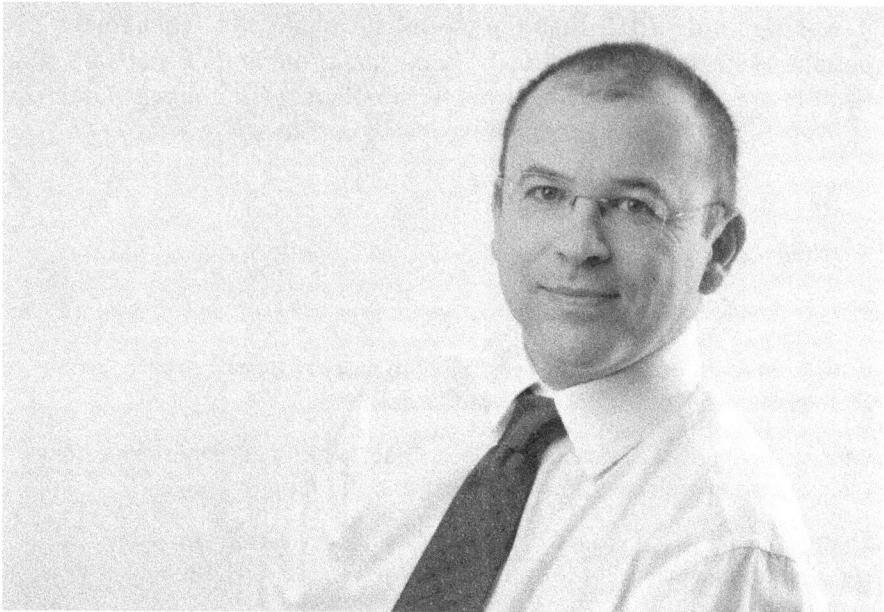

Peter Marhofer was born in Vienna in 1964. He attended schools in Vienna and Lower Austria until 1984, then proceeding to the School of Medicine at the University of Vienna. After graduating in medicine in 1991, he undertook specialist training in anaesthesia and critical care.

Together with his colleagues, Professor Stephan Kapral and Dr Manfred Greher, Marhofer participated in the development of ultrasound guidance in regional anaesthesia. The first studies and publications in that field were performed in 1993-1994, and from that time this technique was spread all over the world and contributed significantly to the efficacy and safety in regional anaesthesia.

From 1995 Marhofer and colleagues developed the Vienna score: a 4-point observational scoring tool which describes the echogenicity of nerve structures. They observed that every (for regional anaesthesia purposes) peripheral nerve shows a particular ultrasound behaviour. The sciatic nerve, to mention just one example, shows (despite its large size) an isoechoic behaviour and careful ultrasound probe adjustment is required to identify this nerve via ultrasound guidance (Vienna score for proximal approaches 3-4 and for distal approaches 2-3). The median nerve serves as an example of a smaller nerve (relative to the sciatic nerve) with a Vienna score of 1.

The visibility of peripheral nerves is dependent on their internal structure and depth. Due to physical limitations of ultrasound technology, deeper structures are less visible as compared to more superficial structures. The visibility of nerve structures in ultrasound is the main factor in the performance of regional anaesthetic block using ultrasound guidance.

In 1999 Marhofer was appointed attending anaesthesiologist and critical care physician; the following year he became Associate Professor at the Department of Anaesthesia, General Intensive Care and Pain Control at the Medical University of Vienna. At the same institution he became Professor and Head of Paediatric Anaesthesia and Paediatric Intensive Care Medicine in 2000. This was followed by his appointment in 2003 as Director of Paediatric Anaesthesia and Paediatric Intensive Care Medicine.

Having attracted worldwide participants to his practical workshops in the field of ultrasound guided regional anaesthesia for many years, Marhofer published his book *Ultrasound Guidance for Nerve Blocks* in 2008. He was appointed a Board Member of the *British Journal of Anaesthesia* in 2009, by which time he had published over 70 scientific papers on regional and paediatric (regional) anaesthesia. The second edition of his book came in 2010 with a new title *Ultrasound Guidance in Regional Anaesthesia*. In this book the expected Vienna scores of all relevant nerves were described. Importantly the author highlighted that these scores are variable and also dependent on individual patients' factors, such as artefacts and body mass index. The ultrasound visibility of nerves is also influenced by the hand skills of the operator.

Marhofer delivered the prestigious Bruce Scott Lecture (q.v. page 208) at the 2010 Annual Scientific Meeting of the European Society of Regional Anaesthesia (ESRA), held in Belfast, NI. A further appointment in 2016 was as Emergency Physician in Vienna. For the past decade he has travelled internationally to give invitation lectures at international meetings of various societies of anaesthesiologists – speaking on regional anaesthesia in both adults and paediatrics. Recognized as an authority, he cautioned in 2018 that there was not enough evidence of benefit to recommend dexamethasone as a perineural additive to local anaesthetics. In 2020 he is Executive Managing Physician at the Department of Anaesthesia, General Intensive Care and Pain Control at the Medical University of Vienna.

Table 1. The Vienna score for ultrasonographic-guided nerve blocks

Score	Description
1	The internal structure of the nerve visualized
2	The nerve is visualized as a circular or oval bright halo (epineurium)
3	The nerve is visualized as reflections determined by the anatomy of the surrounding tissue
4	The anatomical position of the nerve shows no response to the ultrasound beam (isoechoic behaviour)

Further reading

Marhofer P. *Ultrasound Guidance in Regional Anaesthesia* (2nd edition). Oxford: Oxford University Press, 2010.

Marhofer P, Ivani G, Santhanam S, Melman E, Zaragoza G, Bosenberg A. Everyday regional anesthesia in children. *Pediatric Anesthesia* 2012; **22**: 995-1001.

Marhofer P, Columb M, Hopkins PM. Perineural dexamethasone: the dilemma of systematic reviews and meta-analyses. *British Journal of Anaesthesia* 2018; **120**: 201-3.

BENJAMIN WEINBREN MEMORIAL LECTURE

Benjamin Weinbren (1889-1965)

Benjamin Weinbren was born in Lithuania on 7 January 1889 and like many Jewish families at that time emigrated to South Africa with his parents at a very young age. After schooling at Marist Brothers College and Jeppe High School in Johannesburg he travelled to the United Kingdom to study medicine. After graduating MB, ChB from Edinburgh in 1912 he worked in England for two years before returning to Johannesburg to set up practice as a general practitioner. He developed an interest in anaesthesia and in 1916 was appointed to the Johannesburg General Hospital as a part-time honorary anaesthetist, a position he held until 1944.

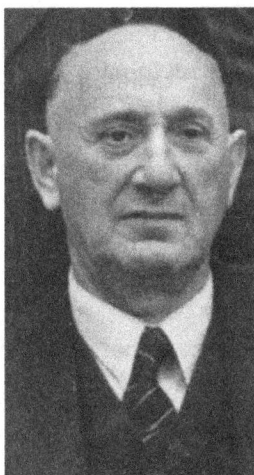

In 1916 the Witwatersrand Branch of the British Medical Association recognised the need to establish a medical school and a Witwatersrand University Committee was formed. Three years later Parliament passed the Anatomy Act that provided for the creation of a medical school at the South African School of Mines and Technology (SASTM) in Johannesburg and teaching of anatomy and physiology to students began. In 1922 the SASTM became the University of the Witwatersrand (Wits) and admitted the first students to the clinical years of training at the Johannesburg General Hospital and its associated hospitals.

In 1920 Weinbren decided to confine his practice to anaesthesia and was appointed Lecturer in Anaesthetics by the University when anaesthesia began to be taught as a subject. In 1933 he like several other SA medical practitioners in that era journeyed to the UK and USA to study new developments in anaesthesia. (They included Royden Muir, Eric van Hoogstraten, and Harry Grant Whyte who all played major roles in the development of the specialty in South Africa). Whilst in the US, Weinbren worked under Dr E.I. McKesson and on his return introduced cyclopropane and McKesson's method of administering anaesthesia with nitrous oxide and oxygen to Johannesburg practitioners.

Following the introduction of the world's first formal qualification in anaesthetics, the Diploma in Anaesthetics of the Conjoint Board of the Royal College of Surgeons and Physicians of London in 1935, Weinbren was awarded the DA (RCS RCP London) without examination the following year.

Highly respected he was elected President of the Southern Transvaal Branch of the Medical Association of South Africa (MASA) in 1935 and two years later was elected a member of the MASA Ethical Committee. His growing stature in the field led to him being appointed to a Government's commission appointed to investigate the death rate from anaesthesia in South Africa.

With the outbreak of war in 1939 Weinbren volunteered for military duty but after being rejected on medical grounds took control of the administration of anaesthetics at Johannesburg's Cottesloe Military Hospital. At that time, the status of anaesthesia in SA was poor. Anaesthetists in State Hospitals were employed in the Department of Surgery, and anaesthetists in private practice were remunerated by the surgeon they worked with in private practice and worked as honorary anaesthetists in state hospitals.

The South African Society of Anaesthetists was formed during the WW2 at a meeting held at the Johannesburg General Hospital on 1st August 1943. At the meeting attended by 13 of the 26 registered specialist anaesthetists in SA at that time Weinbren was elected as the Society's first president – see Figure 1. In his opening address as President he stated that the chief aims of the society would be to safeguard the economic status of anaesthetists, to educate so that the specialty might be recognized, and to encourage self-criticism, lest local anaesthetists fell behind in the scientific advances in anaesthesia.

In 1954 the SASA Council honoured Weinbren by electing him as the Society's first Honorary Life Vice-President in recognition of his special services to anaesthesia in SA, and in 1960 he was elected an Emeritus Member of MASA.

Dr Weinbren passed away in October 1965. Two years later at the 1967 AGM of the Society, SASA archivist Dr Jack Abelsohn's proposal that a Weinbren Memorial Lecture be held at the Society's 25th Anniversary Congress the following year was accepted. The inaugural lecture was delivered by the Society's official guest, Professor John W. Dundee from Belfast. The Weinbren Memorial Lecture has been held annually since then and by tradition is the opening lecture at the Congress. See Table 1.

In the obituary to Dr Weinbren published in the *South African Medical Journal*, J. Schwartz wrote- "Dr Weinbren had a grand sense of humour and enlivened the lives of surgeons in operating theatres by keeping them in good humour even under the most difficult conditions."

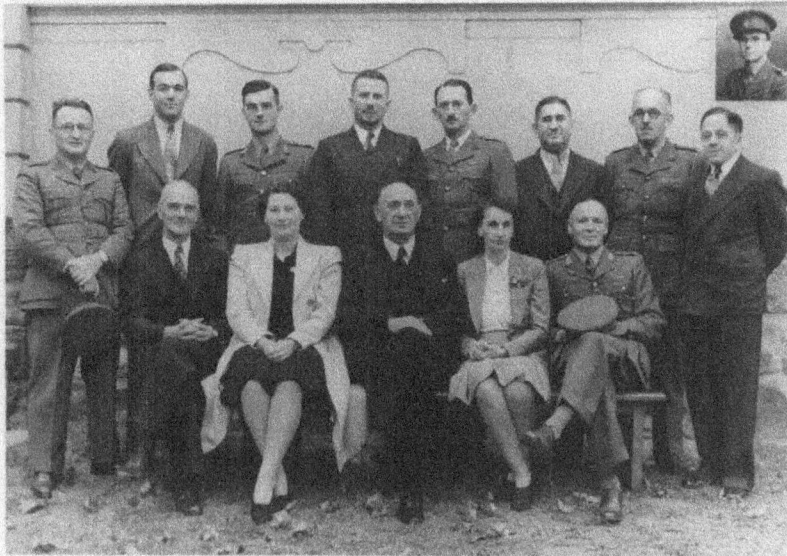

SOUTH AFRICAN SOCIETY OF ANAESTHETISTS
INAUGURAL MEETING

Johannesburg

1st August 1943

PRESENTED BY DR. J. ABELSOHN TO THE
DEPARTMENT OF ANAESTHETICS, SEPT, 1968

Standing left to right:
Capt. C. Arkles, Dr. D. Feldman, Capt. J. R. Dulfield, Dr. H. Grant-Whyte, Capt. H. H. Samson, Dr. S. Lipron,
Major R. A. Moore Dyke (Secretary-Treasurer), Dr. S. Hoffmann.

Sitting left to right:
Dr. D. Crawford, Dr. Blumy Segal, Dr. B. Weinbren (President), Dr. M. B. Barlow, Major C. C. Becker.

Inset: Maj. J. Abelson.

Figure 1. South African Society of Anaesthetists inaugural meeting, 1st August 1943.

Note

Benjamin's brother Maurice became a leading radiologist in South Africa, was a founder of the Radiological Society of SA and has since 1959 been honoured by the Colleges of Medicine of South Africa through the annual awarding of the Maurice Weinbren Award in Radiology for a publication of sufficient merit. His son Ian worked as a physician in England.

Table 1. Benjamin Weinbren Memorial lecturers and lecture titles

Year	Lecturer	Title
1968	John W. Dundee	Iatrogenic diseases
1970	James E. Eckenhoff	Shock

1972	E. Cooper	The place of the anaesthetist in modern anaesthetic practice.
1974	John F. Nunn	Mechanisms of action of inhalational anaesthetic agents
1976	M. Keith Sykes	Machines in medicine
1978	John J. Bonica	History and current activities of the WFSA
1981	Arthur B. Bull	History of anaesthesia in the Cape
1983	E.S. Siker	What we learn from each other
1985	John F. Nunn	Oxygen – friend or foe
1987	Burnell Brown	Where are we going with new drugs in anaesthesiology?
1989	S.A. Strauss	Doctor, patient and the law in the late 1980s
1990	Clive Walker	The fate of the black rhino in Africa
1991	A. Cunningham	Heart of the matter: what Graham Greene forgot to say
1992	Ophelia Jutta	How to prosper financially & succeed in new SA
1993	Soloman Benatar	Scientific & social influences on the future of medicine and healthcare in SA
1994	Pierre Oliver	South Africa's Bill of Rights
1995	Michael Todd	Cerebral metabolic depression and brain protection
1996	Jerrold Lerman	Current thoughts on fasting and general premedication in children
1997	NIL	
1998	Mike Ellis	Healthcare in SA – can any government achieve its aims?
1999	Stephen Slogoff	*Record of title lost*
2000	J.C. de Villiers	Medicine during Anglo-Boer War
2001	Desmond Tutu	*Record of title lost*
2002	Ronald Miller	The future of anaesthesia
2003	Barry Baker	Macintosh – before anaesthesia
2004	George Bizos	South Africa – 10 years post the fall of apartheid
2005	Clive Torr	Wines of the Cape
2006	Piet Naude	Ethics
2007	David Wilkinson	Why are we here today? The history of mistakes.
2008	NIL	
2009	Barbara Hogan	Health in South Africa
2010	Charles Cote	The history of paediatric anaesthesia
2011	Alex Harris	Journey on foot to the South Pole
2012	Tim Noakes	Character, teamwork and the search for perfection.
2013	Justice Malala	South Africa after Mangaung
2014	David Block	The power of vision
2015	D. Moodley	Artificial intelligence – threat or hype?
2016	Matie Hoffman	Cosmic change
2017	Imtiaz Sooliman	"Gift of the Givers"
2018	Glenda Gray	H.I.V.
2019	Lungile Pepeta	Training fit for purpose medical practitioners.
2020	Michael Pepper	Cell and gene therapy

Further reading

Schwartz J. Benjamin Weinbren Obituary. *South African Medical Journal* 1965; **39**: 1128.

Obituary. *South African Jewish Times* 5 November 1956.

Keene R. *Our Graduates 1924-2012*. Adler Museum of Medicine, Faculty of Health Sciences, University of the Witwatersrand.

Orenstein AJ, Robertson IS. Report of the Committee on Deaths under Anaesthesia. *South African Medical Journal* 1936; **10**: 729-34.

Parbhoo NP. *Five decades The South African Society of Anaesthetists 1943-1993*. Johannesburg: South African Society of Anaesthetists, 1993.

Horace Wells (1815-1848)

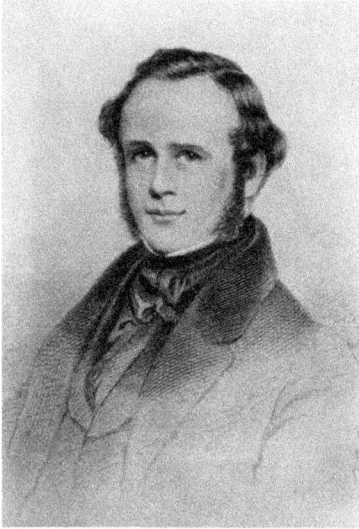

Horace Wells. Photograph of reproduction of stipple engraving by H.B. Hall. Credit: Wellcome Collection. Reproduced under Creative Commons Attribution (CC BY 4.0).

Horace Wells was born in Hartford, Vermont, USA on 21 January 1815. He was educated from 1821 to 1834 at select academies in that area and then became a teacher at a district school for a short while. From 1834 he studied dentistry in Boston for about two years and in 1836 he set up practice in Hartford, Connecticut.

Wells was quite successful in his Hartford practice where he offered improved methods of filling teeth and he published articles in dental journals. In 1838 he married Elizabeth Wales, who bore him a son, Charles Thomas, the following year. In 1842 he took on a student dentist, William Thomas Green Morton, who had previously studied in Baltimore, Maryland. Morton moved to Boston in 1843 and Wells assisted him in establishing a practice there. However Wells formed a poor opinion of Morton, describing him in a letter to his mother and sister as being "without any principle", possessing "no self denial" and "the most deceitful man I ever knew". So, after a matter of weeks Wells returned to Hartford, CT.

According to his own record of events with supporting testimony by two doctors and a dentist (1847), Wells in the autumn of 1844 had the idea of relieving the pain of surgical operations by the inhalation of exhilarating gas. He therefore procured some nitrous oxide gas and under its influence he had one of his own teeth extracted by the dentist John M. Riggs – feeling no pain. According to Riggs, this was about the 1st of November. Wells then extracted teeth from 12-15 patients under nitrous oxide (assisted by Riggs) with similar results.

By January 1845 Wells had proceeded to Boston to present his discovery to the medical faculty. He contacted William Morton, who introduced him to John Collins Warren, the Professor of Anatomy and Surgery at Harvard University and Drs George Hayward and Charles T. Jackson. He told them of his discovery, and it was arranged to have a demonstration at a hall in Boston before the medical class of Warren. A volunteer for tooth extraction was duly administered nitrous oxide by Wells, but he cried out during the extraction and several spectators declared the affair was "humbug". A disheartened Wells returned to Hartford.

Wells then became depressed and relinquished his professional business. His mental state was not helped by the news of Morton's successful public demonstration of ether as an anaesthetic in October 1846 followed by the dispute between Morton and Jackson claiming to being the discoverers of anaesthesia. However, on 24 December 1846 Wells sailed for Liverpool, England and proceeded to sight-seeing in London. Then he proceeded to Paris, France where he was befriended by an American dentist, C. Starr Brewster, who helped him to present his case to the Académie des Science and the Académie de Médecine and the Paris Medical Society. Wells was well received and through his last ten days in Paris was invited to celebrity balls and parties given in his honour.

Arriving back in Hartford in March 1847, Wells began collecting sworn statements and on 30 March he published his 'A History of the Discovery'. However, it did not reverse what he saw as injustice. Seemingly becoming psychotic, he moved at the end of 1847 to New York City with intent to experiment further with nitrous oxide, ether and chloroform. He opened a dental office, but it did not prosper. On 21 January 1848 (his birthday) under the influence of chloroform to which he had become addicted, he spattered a prostitute with sulphuric acid. He was arrested and placed in the Tombs prison. On the following day he inhaled smuggled chloroform and cut his left femoral artery with a razor; he wrote a suicide note before dying that night. He was buried at Cedar Hill Cemetery in Hartford, Connecticut.

Ironically, twelve days after his death, a letter arrived from C. Starr Brewster in Paris conveying the news that the Paris Medical Society had voted Horace Wells to be "due all the honours of having first discovered and successfully applied the uses of vapours or gases, whereby surgical operations could be performed without pain". They had also elected him an honorary member of their Society. This tragic story must surely strike a chord of sympathy in even the most hardened of practitioners.

Later a statue of Wells was erected in Paris. Wells' widow, Elizabeth strove to vindicate his memory. The son, Charles Thomas Wells, acquired considerable influence and financial resources, which he used to honour his father's contributions. A statue of Horace Wells was sculptured and placed in Bushnell Park, Hartford in 1875.

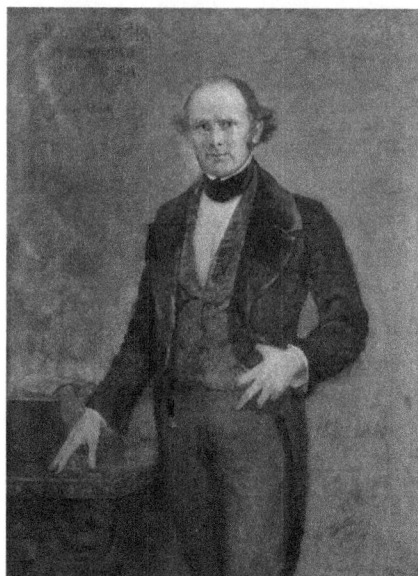

Horace Wells. Oil painting 1899 by Chas Noel Flagg. Credit in full: page iv.

In Hartford, CT in 1894, on the 50th anniversary of Wells' discovery, the Horace Wells Club was founded by a group of Connecticut dentists. The first task they completed that year was to place a bronze plaque of Horace Wells at the location of his old office, the original structure no longer existing. The Horace Wells Club has since met annually on the first Saturday of December to honour the great man. In 1899 the American artist, Charles Nöel Flagg, produced an oil painting of Horace Wells; this was later gifted to the Wadsworth Atheneum Museum of Art, Hartford CT (Figure 1).

In 1944 the Horace Wells Club together with the American Dental Association coordinated a worldwide celebration for the centenary of Horace Wells' discovery. The Club took on responsibility for maintaining the statue of Horace Wells. From 1956 the Horace Wells Club Award has been presented annually to a dentist or physician who has made a meritorious contribution to the art and science of anaesthesia (Table 1).

Note

Many articles, chapters and books state that Wells first got the idea of using nitrous oxide at a public exhibition of exhilarating or laughing gas (nitrous oxide) by the itinerant lecturer, Gardner Quincy Colton, in Hartford on 10th December 1844, followed by a private exhibition on the morning of 11th December. However, these dates did not appear in the literature on Wells until 1853.

Acknowledgement

Dr William MacDonnell, President of the Connecticut Society of Dentist Anesthesiologists, kindly provided the list of Horace Wells Club Award winners.

Table 1. Horace Wells Club Award winners

1956	Ralph Moore Tovell, MD	Hartford Hospital
1957	John Silas Lundy, MD	Mayo Clinic
1958	Jay A. Heidbrink, DDS	Minneapolis General Hospital
1959	Stevens J. Martin, MD	St. Francis Hospital
1960	Nicholas M. Greene, MD	Yale University School of Medicine
1961	Leonard M. Monheim, DDS	University of Pittsburgh
1962	Curtis B. Hickcox, MD	Hartford Hospital
1963	NIL	
1964	E. Clayton Gengras	Hartford (Benefactor)
1965	Leroy D. Vandam, MD	Peter Bent Brigham Hospital
1966	Robert D. Dripps, MD	University of Pennsylvania
1967	Edward J. Driscoll, DDS	National Institute of Health, Bethesda
1968	John Keet, MD	Waterbury Hospital
1969	John Adriani, MD	Charity Hospital, New Orleans
1970	NIL	
1971	Robert B. Sweet, MD	University of Michigan
1972	David M. Little, MD	Hartford Hospital
1973	Joseph F. Artusio, MD	Cornell Medical Center
1974	Donald W. Benson, MD	Johns Hopkins University Medical Center
1975	John Abajian, Jr., MD	Medical Center Hospital of Vermont
1976	General Robert Shira, DDS	Tufts University (ADA President)
1977	Maynard K. Hine, DDS	University of Michigan
1977	Howard R. Raper, DDS	Retired author of "Dental Radiography & Diagnosis" and "Man against Pain"
1978	Joseph P. Cappuccio, DDS	University of Maryland (ADA President)
1979	Thomas W. Quinn, DMD	Tufts University (ADSA President)
1980	Edwin M. McCluskey, MD	St. Francis Hospital
1981	Edmund T. Welch, MD	Hartford Hospital
1982	Egidio Fulchiero, MD	Lawrence Memorial Hospital
1983	Paul G. Barash, MD	Yale School of Medicine
1984	William J. Gacso, MD	St. Vincent's Hospital
1985	Anthony J. Dougherty, MD	St. Francis Hospital
1986	Clark A. Sammartino, DMD	Rhode Island Hospital
1987	Ronald J.M. Steven, MBBS	Hartford Hospital
1988	Katherine A. Shaw, MD	Greenwich Hospital
1989	Augustine M. McNamee, MD	Rhode Island Hospital
1990	James S. Harrop, MD	St. Francis Hospital
1991	Peter H. Jacobsohn, DDS	Marquette University
1992	James J. Richter, MD PhD	Hartford Hospital
1993	William D. Conrad, MD	Hartford Hospital
1994	C. Richard Bennett, DDS PhD	University of Pittsburgh
1994	Stanley Malamed, DDS	University of Southern California

1994	Neil L. Schecter, MD	St. Francis Hospital
1995	Gwendolyn H. Moraski, MD	St. Francis Hospital
1996	Hanumanthaiah Balakrishna MD	New Britain General Hospital
1997	Connecticut Society of Oral and Maxillofacial Surgeons	
1998	Norma V.B. Maderazo, MD	Rockville Hospital
1999	William A. MacDonnell, DDS	University of Connecticut
2000	James P. Phero, DMD	University of Cinninnati
2001	Morton B. Rosenberg, DMD	Tufts University
2002	Stuart E. Lieblich, DMD	University of Connecticut
2003	NIL	
2004	Peter J. Deckers, MD	Dean, University of Connecticut
2005	Robert Galvin, MD	Health Commissioner Connecticut
2006	Kurt Koral, DDS	Yale University
2007	Jeffrey Gross, MD	University of Connecticut
2008	Andrew Herlich, DMD MD	University of Pittsburgh
2009	Christian Stoller, DMD	Dean, University of Maryland
2010	Robert Faiella, DMD	ADA President
2011	Bruce Koeppen, MD	Dean Quinnipiac University
2012	NIL	
2013	Karen Crowley, DDS	ADSA President
2014	NIL	
2015	Joel M. Weaver, DDS PhD	Ohio University, ASDA/ADSA President
2016	Peter Tan, DDS	ADSA
2017	NIL	
2018	Robert C. Bosack, DDS	University of Illinois at Chicago
2019	NIL	
2020	American Society of Dentist Anesthesiologists	

Further reading

Nuland SB. *The Origins of Anesthesia*. Birmingham (Alabama): The Classics of Medicine Library, 1983; Chapter VII: Nitrous Oxide: A Discovery in Vain.

Bunker E (Ed.). *Horace and Elizabeth Love and Death and Painless Dentistry – The Letters of Horace and Elizabeth Wells*. ISBN 9798622825798 Published independently and available from online book stores, 2020.

WRIGHT & HALL'S 'VETERINARY ANAESTHESIA'

The first edition of *Veterinary Anaesthesia* by Professor John George Wright appeared in 1941. In this he laid the foundations of modern veterinary anaesthesia and it soon became the most recommended textbook on the subject. There was a second edition in 1947 and a fourth in 1957. For the fifth edition published in 1961, Wright was joined by Leslie W. Hall as co-author. From the sixth edition (1966) it was titled *Wright's Veterinary Anaesthesia and Analgesia*.

Wright died in 1971 and the seventh edition that year was under the sole authorship of Lesley W. Hall. By this time, it was recognised not only as *the* textbook for veterinary students and as a reference manual for practising veterinary surgeons, but as a reference manual for experimental anaesthesia of domestic animals. Hall shortened the title to *Veterinary Anaesthesia* for the eighth edition (1983) for which he was joined by Kathy W. Clarke as co-author. In 2001, for the tenth edition, a third co-author, Cynthia M. Trim joined the team. The book reached its eleventh edition in 2013, having been the leading text- book on veterinary anaesthesia for decades.

John George Wright (1897-1971)

John George Wright was born in Newport, Wales and educated at Newport High School. At the outbreak of the First World War he volunteered for the Royal Field Artillery and served on the Western Front, rising to the rank of sergeant. Then he was sent to the Officer Cadet School in London, passing out as best cadet and a commission in June 1918. His posting until 1919 was to a British division in South Russia in support of the "White" anti-Bolshevik forces.

In 1919 Wright was admitted to the Royal Veterinary College (RVC), London where he was a brilliant student and graduated in 1923. He then went into private veterinary practice around London until 1928, when he returned to the RVC as Professor of Materia Medica. The following year he moved to the Chair of Surgery and over the next ten years he transformed small animal anaesthesia and introduced the use of chloral hydrate in horses and other large animals. At the Beaumont Animal Hospital there was a large through-put of small animals and he introduced intravenous barbiturates, revolution-izing their anaesthesia. In 1934 he was the first to be awarded the British Veterinary Association's highest honour: the Dalrymple-Champneys Cup and

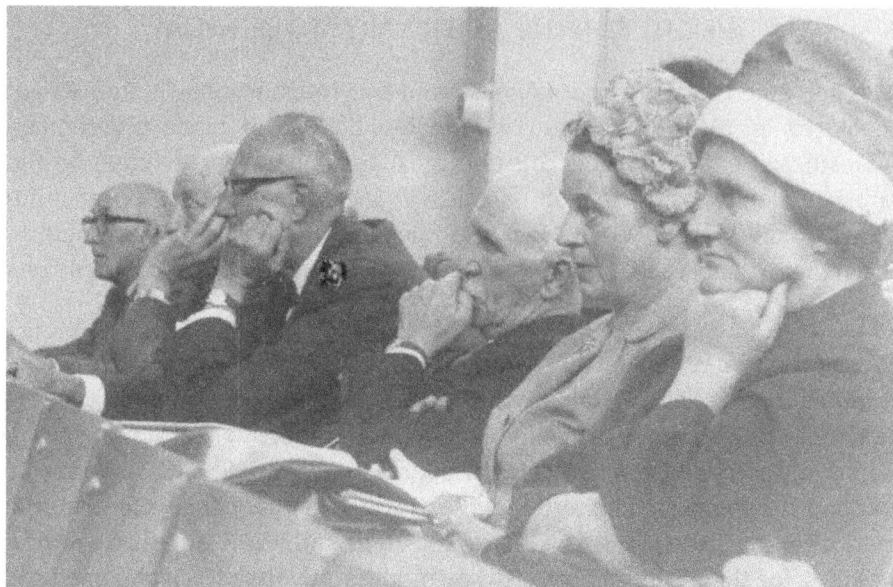

John George Wright (4ᵗʰ from left) at the Veterinary Pathology Lecture Room in 1963. Image (Ref. A031/57) by courtesy of the University of Liverpool.

Medal. After the outbreak of the Second World War, the RVC was evacuated to Streatley-on-Thames where Wright became enthused about a country establishment being integral to a veterinary school. He also felt that the study of veterinary medicine should be offered at universities, rather than confined to a few veterinary colleges. In 1941 the first edition of his classic textbook *Veterinary Anaesthesia* was published by Bailliere, Tindall & Cox, London.

Wright accepted an invitation to take the Chair of Veterinary Surgery at the Liverpool Veterinary School in 1941, perhaps persuaded by the commitment of the University of Liverpool to set up a veterinary field station at Leahurst in rural Cheshire. Under Wright's guidance, the Leahurst scheme flourished. He published the second edition of *Veterinary Anaesthesia* in 1947 and in 1950 he was co-author to Franz Benesch of *Veterinary Obstetrics*. The following year he was elected President of the Royal College of Veterinary Surgeons (RCVS). In 1952 his School was accorded the status of a separate Faculty of Veterinary Science by the University of Liverpool. Next, the Liverpool veterinary degree became the first to be registerable as it was recognized by the RCVS.

Wright retired in 1963 and stepped down from the Council of the RCVS on which he had served since 1939. Soon after retiring he was honoured by being elected a Fellow of the RVC. In retirement he continued input into *Wright's Veterinary Anaesthesia and Analgesia*. A heavy smoker, he died of lung cancer in 1971.

Leslie Wilfred Hall (1927-2010)

Leslie Hall was brought up in Sutton, Surrey, England and educated at the local grammar school. He began studies at the RVC in 1945 and qualified BSc and MRCVS in 1950. Then, instead of going into clinical practice, he stayed on to complete a PhD. With Barbara Weaver he set out to upgrade the standard of anaesthesia for small animals to that expected for humans. In 1954 they published a paper on balanced anaesthesia for the dog and cat, pointing out that further research was required to achieve a similar upgrade for the horse.

After the RVC, Hall went to Cambridge University to be a lecturer in the veterinary school. Initially he taught several aspects of veterinary medicine, but soon was able to concentrate on anaesthetics, both as a teacher and as a clinician. In 1961 he joined

Leslie W. Hall. Image courtesy of the History of Anaesthesia Society.

Professor John George Wright as co-author of *Veterinary Anaesthesia*. Notably, he liaised with medical anaesthetists locally and became a member of the AAGBI, the East Anglian Society of Anaesthetists and the Anaesthetic Research Society. He founded with six colleagues the Association of Veterinary Anaesthetists (AVA) in 1964.

Again, with Barbara Weaver it was Hall who pushed the establishment of the Diploma of Veterinary Anaesthesia of the RCVS. Later this was taken over by the Diploma of the European College of Veterinary Anaesthesia and Analgesia. In 1977 Hall was awarded the Faculty Medal of the Faculty of Anaesthetists, Royal College of Surgeons – the first veterinary surgeon to achieve this honour. Hall was renowned as an excellent teacher and researcher, progressing to be Reader in Comparative Anaesthesia at Cambridge University; he refused Professorships at other Universities. In 1982 he organised the first World Congress of Veterinary Anaesthesia, held in Cambridge.

Hall received numerous honours: the Francis Hogg Prize of the RCVS in 1955 for "the most serviceable work for the advancement of small animal practice"; the Livesey Medal of the RCVS in 1967 for "the alleviation of pain and fear in

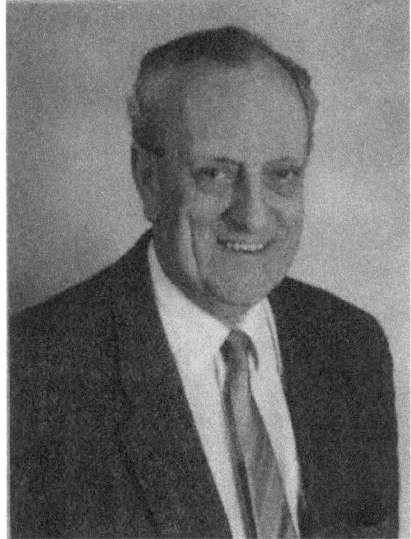

animals"; also in 1967 the Blaine Award of the British Small Animals Association. On retirement he became an Honorary Fellow of the AVA. The final accolade was his election as Honorary Fellow of the Royal College of Anaesthetists in 2001.

Further reading

Obituary John George Wright. *Veterinary Record* 1971; **89**: 514-15.

Clarke KW. Obituary Leslie W Hall, MA, BSc, PhD, DVA, Dr (Hons Causa) Utrecht, Dip ECVAA, DACVA (hon) FRCA, FRCVS. *Veterinary Anaesthesia and Analgesia* 2010; **37**: 387-9.

Hall LW, Weaver BMQ. Some notes on balanced anaesthesia for the dog and cat. *Veterinary Record* 1954; **66**: 289-93.

YAMAMURA MEMORIAL AWARD

Hideo Yamamura (1920-2017)

Hideyo Yamamura was born in January 1920. He graduated from the School of Medicine, Tokyo Imperial University in 1943. Then he began further training in surgery. At that time in Japan, anaesthetics were administered by the surgeons as anaesthesia was not recognised as a specialty. All surgery below the umbilicus was done under spinal anaesthesia; upper abdominal surgery was performed under either spinal anaesthesia or local infiltration with heavy sedation; for neck and brain surgery, local anaesthesia was used. If these techniques were found inadequate, general anaesthesia was administered: ether by open drop or by insufflation – as directed by the professor of surgery.

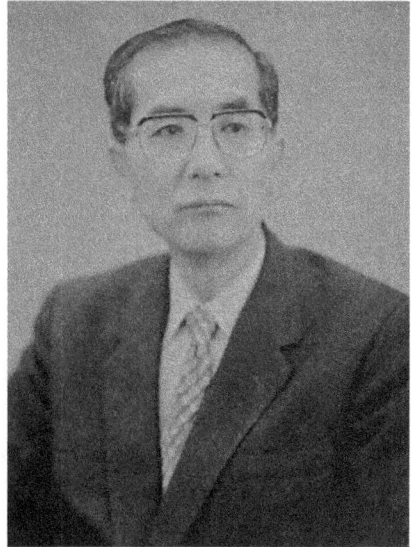

Hideo Yamamura. Image courtesy of Emeritus Prof. Kazuo Hanaoka.

After the Second World War during the occupation of Japan by the American Army, Brigadier General Crawford Sams, MD became concerned about the lack of postgraduate medical training there. He requested the Unitarian Service Committee (USC) of the American Unitarian Association to send a team of medical specialists to provide two medical meetings: one in Tokyo and the other in Osaka/Kyoto. Duly in 1950, physicians and specialists from the USA arrived in Japan. Meyer Saklad (q.v. page 7), Chief Anesthesiologist at Rhode Island Hospital, Providence RI represented anaesthesiology. Besides his lectures on all aspects of anaesthetic practice, he had joint sessions with a physiologist, a pharmacologist and a surgeon; this impressed the leading Japanese surgeons and stimulated the young doctors (including Hideyo Yamamura) to take an interest in anaesthesiology.

Kentaro Shimizu, the Professor of Surgery at the University of Tokyo, translated Saklad's lectures and asked his junior faculty member Yamamura, to switch from surgery. Despite having spent eight years training in surgery, Yamamura agreed. A second USC mission came in 1951: it visited 12 medical schools throughout Japan and included workshops and demonstrations. In this mission, Perry Volpitto, Chair of Anesthesiology in Augusta, Georgia represented anaesthesiology. Of course, Yamamura attended. In 1952 the first independent Department of Anaesthesiology in Japan was established at the University of Tokyo with Yamamura as Associate Professor. Then Yamamura was sent to the USA to train further in anaesthesia, which he did at Albany Medical College.

In 1954 the Japanese Society of Anesthesiologists (JSA) was founded and adopted *Masui* (later the *Japanese Journal of Anesthesiology*) which had begun two years earlier. The six founding members, including Yamamura, were all surgeons. A third USC mission went to Japan in 1956 – this time the presentations were mainly on research, with encouragement of the Japanese physicians to participate; again, Yamamura attended. In 1959 he became the sixth President of the JSA, the first full-time anaesthetist to be elected.

The JSA became a member of the World Federation of Societies of Anaesthesiologists (WFSA) in 1960 and was represented by Yamamura at the Second World Congress of Anaesthesiologists in Toronto. The Asian and Australasian Regional Section of the WFSA was established in 1962 and Yamamura was elected to the first executive board. In September 1966 he was congress President at the 2nd Asian-Australasian Congress of Anaesthesiology, held in Tokyo.

Naturally, Yamamura became an editor of the *Japanese Journal of Anesthesiology*. He was also much involved in establishing the Diplomate system of the JSA, which set up the regulations for training and examinations of the Board of the JSA. In September 1972 he was congress President of the 5th World Congress of Anaesthesiologists, hosted in Kyoto. This was held in the brand-new Kyoto International Conference Hall and the opening ceremony was graced by His Imperial Highness Crown Prince Akihito (later Emperor of japan) and the Crown Princess. The Congress was well attended and successful.

Yamamura was elected Chairman of the executive board of the 4th Asian-Australasian Congress of Anaesthesiology held in Singapore in September 1974. He retired in 1980, but he attended the First International Symposium on the History of Anaesthesia held in 1982 in Rotterdam, where he presented a paper on the history of modern anaesthesia in Japan.

In 1982 the JSA inaugurated its annual Yamamura Memorial Awards for best research work published in the previous year.

Table 1. Yamamura Memorial Award winners

Year	Recipient	Year	Recipient
1982	S. Kato *et al*; Y. Kamiyama, S. Maruyama *et al*	2001	N. Kotani
1983	K. Tsuno; Y. Koga	2002	M. Yamakage
1984	K. Yasumoto *et al*; H. Sakio	2003	M. Matsumoto
1985	H. Umegaki; F. Goto	2004	H. Kinoshita
1986	N.Myounaka *et al*; Y. Kadota	2005	S. Hagihara
1987	H. Usuda; T. Yusa	2006	H. Higuchi
1988	Y. Niimi; R. Kawade *et al*	2007	M. Kawamata
1989	S. Saeki *et al*; H. Saito *et al*	2008	E. Obata
1990	K. Doi *et al*; M. Okuda *et al*	2009	N. Matsuda
1991	H. Hirota *et al*; K. Okamoto *et al*	2010	M. Nishikawa
1992	M. Konno; K. Miyasaka *et al*	2011	C. Kawamata; K. Hirota
1993	T. Kanamaru *et al*; T. Akata *et al*	2012	K. Tanak
1994	N. Sibuya *et al*; A. Tanaka *et al*	2013	T. Kpuno
1995	S. Nishimi *et al*; S. Isono *et al*	2014	F. Amaya
1996	T. Sakai *et al*; A. Ogura	2015	NIL
1997	NIL	2016	A. Kojima
1998	H. Iida	2017	S. Kouno; M. Sumitani
1999	S. Tanaka	2018	Y. Takeda
2000	N. Kotani	2019	S. Ogawa; J. Kura

Acknowledgement

Prof. Hirosato Kikuchi kindly provided the list of Yamamura Award winners and procured the image of Hideo Yamamura.

Further reading

Yamamura H. History of Modern Anesthesia in Japan. In: Rupreht J, van Lieburg MJ, Lee JA, Erdmann W (Eds) *Anaesthesia Essays on Its History*. Berlin: Springer-Verlag, 1985; 217-19.

Ikeda S. The Unitarian Service Committee Medical Mission. Contribution by the United States to Post-World War II Japanese Anesthesiology. *Anesthesiology* 2007; **106**: 178-85.

Gullo A, Rupreht J. (Eds.) *World Federation of Societies of Anaesthesiologists 50 Years*. Milano: Springer-Verlag, 2004.

YANKAUER SUCTION NOZZLE

Sidney Yankauer (1872-1932)

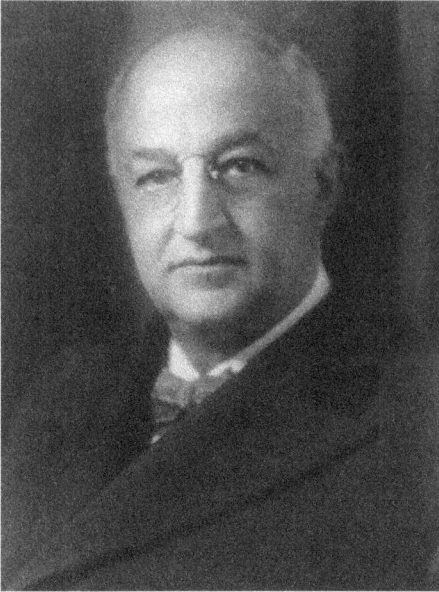

Suction apparatus is part of the ancillary equipment that practising anaesthetists check is ready and functioning before commencing the administration of anaesthesia. The most ubiquitous suction nozzle in the English-speaking world is the Yankauer sucker. Although made of metal in the 1970s, these suction instruments have since the 1980s usually been made of plastic and intended for single use.

Sidney Yankauer was born in New York City (NYC), the son of Jewish immigrants from Bavaria. He attended the free City College of New York, graduating in 1890 and then studied medicine at the College of Physicians and Surgeons, NYC. After qualifying in 1893, he proceeded to internship at Mount Sinai Hospital, where he then did surgical jobs. Next, he specialized in diseases of the ear, nose and throat (ENT) and was elected a Fellow of the New York Academy of Medicine in 1904.

Sidney Yankauer. Credit: The Arthur H. Aufses, Jr., MD Archives, Icahn School of Medicine at Mount Sinai/ Mount Sinai Health System, New York, N.Y.

Yankauer was interested in anaesthesia, to which he also turned his inventive skills. In 1904 he designed a wire mesh mask with a spiral spring for clamping the gauze or lint, onto which ether or chloroform would be dripped. It incorporated a gutter to prevent any surplus overspill onto the patient's face (like the Schimmelbusch mask) – see Figure 1. This mask became very popular in the USA and was also used in the UK.

Yankauer first published on use of the bronchoscope to remove a foreign body from the bronchus in 1905, the start of many surgical papers. In 1907 he designed the (later eponymous) sucker for keeping the operating field clear during tonsillectomy. Made of polished metal, this had a perforated rose end, which prevented soft tissue damage; the angles and handle of the instrument were ergonomically excellent – see Figure 2.

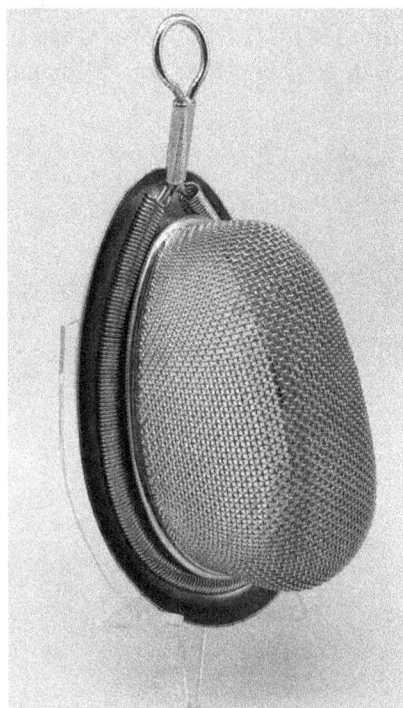

Figure 1. Yankauer wire-frame mask
c.1910. Image courtesy of The
Anaesthesia Heritage Centre, AAGBI.

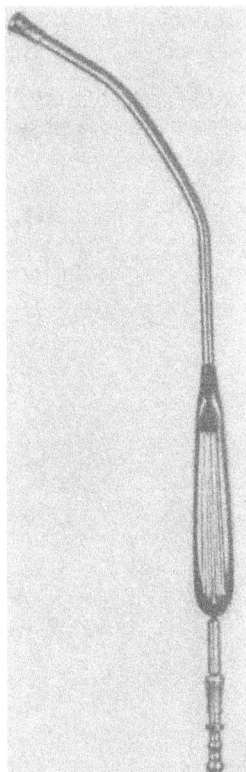

Figure 2. Yankauer metal
suction nozzle c.1910.

By 1917 Yankauer was appointed Attending Laryngologist at the Mount Sinai Hospital. From 1918 he served in the First World War by going with the Mount Sinai Unit as a medical officer (Captain) to Vauclair on the Western Front in France. The American Expeditionary Force set up Base Hospital No. 3 there in a Trappist monastery with personnel provided largely from Mount Sinai Hospital. In its period of service from May 1918 to January 1919, they cared for 9127 patients with 54 surgical deaths; the 118 medical deaths were mostly from the Spanish influenza pandemic. Yankauer was soon promoted to Major and was discharged with the rank of Colonel.

On return to NYC in 1919, Yankauer resumed his career as an ENT surgeon. He was on the editorial staff of *The Laryngoscope*. In 1920 *The American Year-Book of Anesthesia & Analgesia 1917-1918* was published with an advertisement of the portable Yankauer Combination Pressure and Suction

Outfit, manufactured by C.M. Sorensen Co. Inc. N.Y. – designed for tonsil and adenoid operations. One tube delivered ether vapour to an ether hook, mouth gag or face mask, while simultaneously a Yankauer sucker could be used to extract blood and secretions through a second tube into a vacuum bottle – see Figure 3.

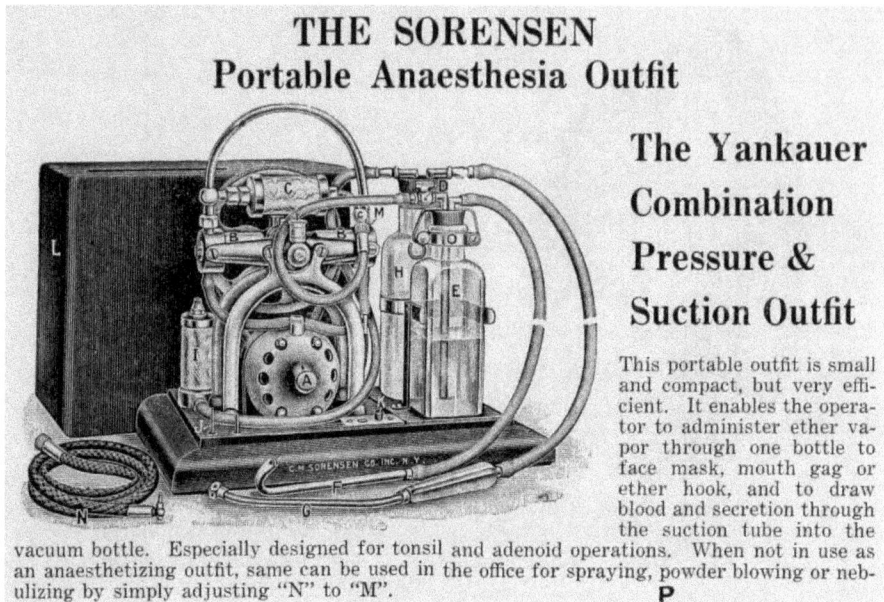

THE SORENSEN
Portable Anaesthesia Outfit

The Yankauer Combination Pressure & Suction Outfit

This portable outfit is small and compact, but very efficient. It enables the operator to administer ether vapor through one bottle to face mask, mouth gag or ether hook, and to draw blood and secretion through the suction tube into the vacuum bottle. Especially designed for tonsil and adenoid operations. When not in use as an anaesthetizing outfit, same can be used in the office for spraying, powder blowing or nebulizing by simply adjusting "N" to "M".

Figure 3. Advertisement in *The American Year-Book of Anesthesia & Analgesia* 1917-1918.

In addition to being Laryngologist to Mount Sinai Hospital, Yankauer was Consulting Laryngologist at the Beth Moses Hospital, Brooklyn and Peroral Endoscopist to Montefiore, Broad Street, Beth David and Beth Israel Hospitals, New York. He was a Fellow of the American Medical Association, a Fellow of the American College of Surgeons, a member of the County and State Medical Societies, a member of the American Laryngological, Rhinological and Otological Society, the American Society of Thoracic Surgery, and the American Academy of Ophthalmology and Otolaryngology. Two contributions he made in the mid-1920s were particularly valued: a radium needle for carcinoma of the oesophagus, and the treatment of lung abscess by bronchoscopy. He was elected President of the American Broncho-esophageal Association in 1927 and was also President of the American Bronchoscopic Society in 1928-1929.

Yankauer-type suction nozzles featured in catalogues of anaesthetic apparatus from the 1930s. By the 1980s the Yankauer-pattern metal suction nozzles were largely replaced by plastic suction tubes – see Figure 4. In 1990 the Association of Anaesthetists of Great Britain and Ireland published the first edition of its Checklist for Anaesthetic Machines, which included suction equipment. By 2002 it was estimated by one manufacturer (Tyco Healthcare) that over 17 million of its Yankauer suction instruments were used worldwide in one year.

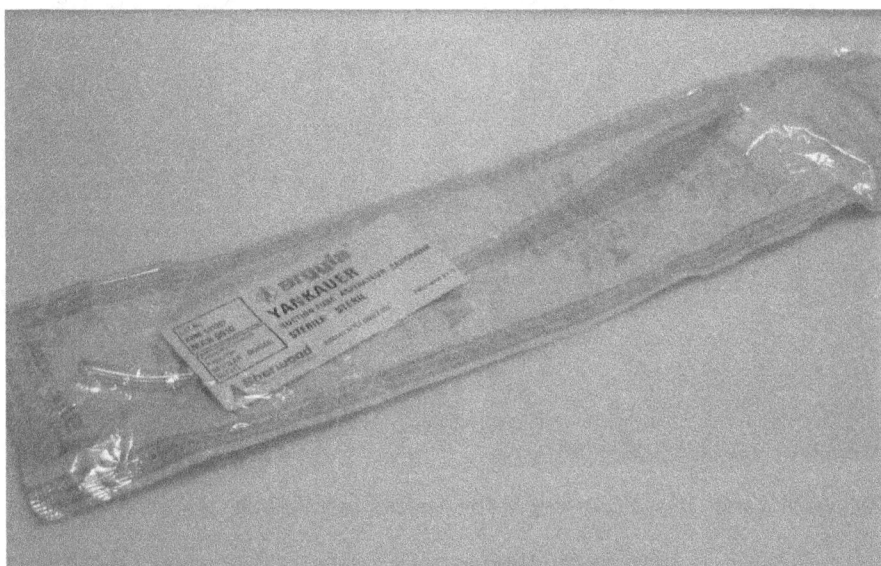

Figure 4. Sherwood Medical Industries' plastic Yankauer suction tube 'argyle'. Image courtesy of The Anaesthesia Heritage Centre, AAGBI.

Further reading

In Memoriam Dr. Sidney Yankauer. *The Laryngoscope* 1932; **42**: 819.

Smith T. Sidney Yankauer 1872-1932 – the man behind the mask. *The History of Anaesthesia Society Proceedings* 2012; **45**: 73-77.

Dickinson MC, Klein A. A faulty Yankauer suction catheter. *Anaesthesia* 2002; **57**: 310.

JOHN ZORAB PRIZE

John Stanley Mornington Zorab (1929-2006)

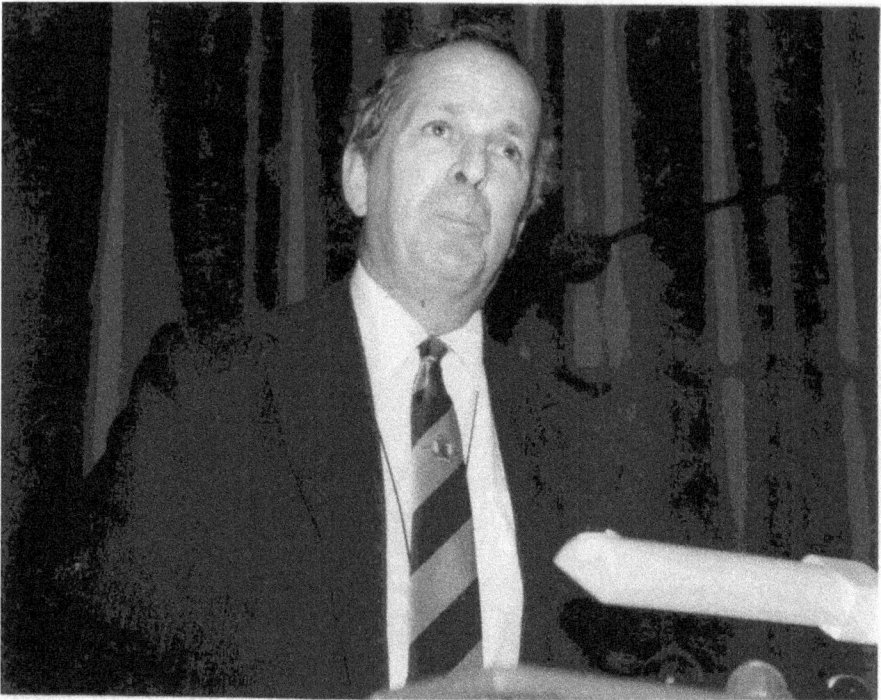

John S.M. Zorab. Image courtesy of The Anaesthesia Heritage Centre, AAGBI.

John Zorab was born in Southampton, England in 1929 and educated at Cheltenham College. After school, he did military service in the Royal Corps of Signals Regiment. From 1949 he trained in medicine at Guy's Hospital in London and qualified MRCS LRCP in 1956.

Zorab pursued training in anaesthesia at Guy's and Westminster Hospitals as well as in Southampton, obtaining the DA in 1958 and the FFARCS in 1962. He was appointed a Consultant Anaesthetist in 1966 at Frenchay Hospital in Bristol. There he befriended Peter Baskett and the two set up the Intensive Care Unit. Zorab took a great interest in training, setting up pre-examination courses and stimulating the building of the hospital's Postgraduate Medical Centre.

Zorab was elected to the Council of the Association of Anaesthetists of Great Britain and Ireland (AAGBI) in 1968 and served as Honorary Secretary for 1972-74. He was also elected Vice Chairman of the Board of the European Regional Section (ERS) of the World Federation of Societies of

Anaesthesiologists (WFSA) in 1974. He embraced this role with enthusiasm, publishing a special article in the journal *Anaesthesia* to cover the cessation of the WFSA newsletter. From 1976 to 1982 he was the representative of the AAGBI to the European Union of Medical Specialists.

In 1977 Zorab published with Peter Baskett a book *Immediate Care*. The following year he was appointed Chairman of the Examinations Committee of the European Academy of Anaesthesiology – a position he would hold for 21 years. This Committee established the multi-lingual European Diploma in Anaesthesiology and Intensive Care, which examination became the recognized specialist qualification in Europe. In 1979 Zorab was Chairman of the AAGBI's International Relations Committee, which promoted aid for developing countries. He was Vice President of the AAGBI in 1980.

Zorab was elected Secretary General of the WFSA in 1980. One of the first things he did was to revive the WFSA newsletter, getting it sponsored and produced in four languages. Then he was responsible for organizing the sixth European Congress of Anaesthesiology held in London in 1982. It was opened by HRH the Princess Margaret, Countess of Snowden and was a great success. Also in 1982, the World Health Organisation (WHO) wrote to Zorab requesting the WFSA to comment on anaesthetic drugs to be included in the WHO list of essential drugs. He realised the opportunity to better this by giving advice also on the equipment and training involved in the safe administration of these drugs in developing countries! So, a meeting was convened between the WHO and the WFSA represented by Zorab and colleagues, including Michael Dobson. This led to Dobson writing the manual *Anaesthesia at the District Hospital*, which was published by the WHO in 1987. Zorab took on a second term as Secretary General from 1984, in which period he published in association with the WFSA *Lectures in Anaesthesiology*. From 1986 he stimulated WFSA Refresher Courses, including those begun in Kenya and other African countries by Roger Eltringham (q.v. page 80).

In 1988 Zorab was elected President of the WFSA for a four-year term. Notably in 1991 he collaborated with Elena Damir, President of the All-Russian Society of Anaesthesiologists and Reanimatologists, and a member of the WFSA Executive, to organise the first Refresher Course in Europe, which was held in Moscow.

In the latter years of his career, Zorab became involved in management at Frenchay Hospital, and he was appointed the Clinical Director for Anaesthesia and Intensive Care, performing most effectively. He was President of the Society of Anaesthetists of the South-west Region for 1990-91. Although retiring officially from clinical work in 1994, his popularity with anaesthetists, surgeons and emergency staff was such that he stayed on as Medical Director for a further two years.

Honours received by Zorab included in 1992 the John Snow Silver Medal from the AAGBI and being Pinkerton Memorial Lecturer. He was made an Honorary Member of the AAGBI in 1996. After retirement he devoted much of his time to studying the history of medicine. He contributed a lot to the book *World Federation of Societies of Anaesthesiologists 50 Years*, published in 2004. At the age of 76, he passed the Diploma in the History of Medicine of the Society of Apothecaries.

Since 2005 the European Society of Anaesthesiology (now named European Society of Anaesthesiology and Intensive Care) has granted the John Zorab Prize to the candidate who obtains the best score at the European Diploma in Anaesthesiology and Intensive Care Part 1 examination (Table 1).

Table 1. John Zorab Prize winners

Year	Recipient	Year	Recipient
2005	Svetoslav Ivanov Iolov	2013	Asiam Sher Khan Akbar
2006	Robert Pongratz	2014	Thomas Chloros
2007	Jörg Maier	2015	Christopher Gergely
2008	Magdalena Wujtewicz	2016	Bernd Schälling & Florian Sator
2009	Laura Becker	2017	Petr Vrtny
2010	David Freiermuth	2018	Matthias Kainz
2011	Benjamin Müller	2019	Andrea Angi
2012	Christian Beilstein		

Further reading

Basket P, Simpson P, Carter J. Obituary John Stanley Mornington Zorab. *Anaesthesia* 2006; **61**: 1024-5.

Zorab JSM. The World Federation of Societies of Anaesthesiologists (W.F.S.A.) *Anaesthesia* 1976; **31**: 285-92.

Zorab JS, Baskett P. *Immediate Care*. London: WB Saunders, 1977.

Gullo A, Rupreht J (Eds). *World federation of Societies of Anaesthesiologists 50 Years*. Milan: Springer-Verlag, 2004.

DAVID ZUCK MEMORIAL PRIZE

David Zuck (1923-2016)

David Zuck was born in Birmingham, England into the Zhukovsky family of Jewish immigrants (pre-World War I) from Suwalki, Russia (now in Poland). Later the name was shortened to Zuck. He was educated at King Edward VI Grammar School, Birmingham and in 1940 entered the Medical School of the University of Birmingham. Graduating MB, ChB in 1945, he then worked as house physician in the local Selly Oak Hospital until March 1946, when he joined the Royal Army Medical Corps (RAMC).

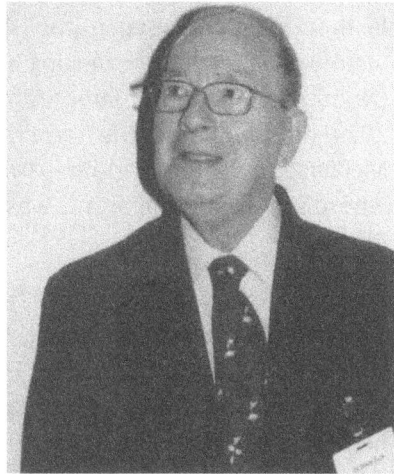

David Zuck. Photograph by Dr Alistair McKenzie.

Zuck was posted to Germany where he did anaesthetic duties, initially as a trainee, then promoted to Lieutenant in 1946 and Captain in 1947. He was demobilised in 1948, returning to be Resident Anaesthetist at Birmingham Accident Hospital. He passed the DA (RCP&S) at this time, just after the two-part examinations were introduced. Next came Registrar and Senior Registrar appointments in the London area and he qualified FFARCS without further examination in 1953. He was appointed as a Consultant Anaesthetist at Chase Farm Hospital and Enfield District Hospitals (North London) in 1954.

In 1955 Zuck designed a cuffed oesophageal tube to guard against aspiration of stomach contents during the induction of anaesthesia in emergencies. Although his design appeared novel, his publication in the *Lancet* carried the statement "However, no originality is claimed". It seems that even at this early stage of his career, Zuck was reading the early literature in depth: he realised that Blomfield's *Anaesthetics in Practice and Theory* (1922) mentioned that an inflatable rubber oesophageal/stomach bag had been described before the Society of Anaesthetists in 1905.

Zuck designed and published several more pieces of apparatus: Barts-Enfield drip indicator (1955), a transistorized time marker (1958), a ripple-mattress for the operating table (1959) and a non-return valve for use with intermittent positive pressure respiration during paediatric surgery (1964). He embraced teaching and in the late 1950s participated in the Colombo plan, training junior doctors from the Indian subcontinent. In 1969 he published a book *Principles of Anaesthesia for Nurses*.

In the 1970s Zuck began publishing some excellent papers relating to the history of anaesthesia – ranging from physics (Reynolds' number) to apparatus (Nooth) to biography (James Simpson, William Harvey and John Hunter). In 1974 he completed the requirements for the Diploma in the History of Medicine, Society of Apothecaries with a thesis on John M. Nooth, part of whose soda water apparatus was used to make the first ether inhaler in Great Britain.

Zuck was keenly interested in the early personal computers. He developed programming skills (self-taught) and produced multiple choice questions for trainees on a Sinclair ZX81 in 1982. He became a great collector of books on the history of science and medicine, particularly historical methodology, and he continued to publish on the history of anaesthesia through the 1980s and indeed for the rest of his life. In 1986 he was a founder member of the History of Anaesthesia Society. He continued working at the Enfield Hospitals and chaired several medical and anaesthetic advisory committees until his retirement in 1988.

By the 1990s Zuck was recognised as an expert historian and he was requested to review new books on the history of anaesthesia: his reviews were forthright to say the least, but always with wit and wisdom. He was elected President of the History of Anaesthesia Society for 1994-96. He helped to organize a series of historical exhibitions for the Association of Anaesthetists of Great Britain and Ireland (AAGBI), which awarded him the Pask Certificate of Honour in 1998 for his services and promotion of the history of the specialty. The History of Anaesthesia Society (HAS) elected him to Honorary Membership in 1999.

In 2002 Zuck was invited by the editor of the *Bulletin* of the Royal College of Anaesthetists (RCoA) to write an occasional history column, entitled 'As we were'. This turned out to be a regular feature: Zuck contributed an article for every issue from September 2002 until March 2017 – a total of 88 articles! He provided much research for the book *Cholera, chloroform, and the science of medicine; a life of John Snow* which was published by Peter Vinten-Johansen *et al* in 2003.

Further honours were awarded to Zuck in the new millennium. He was elected an Honorary Member of the AAGBI in 2004, and in 2008 he delivered the Blessed Chloroform Lecture, the organization of which was taken over from the John Snow Society by the HAS. His lecture was entitled "John Snow's

London". In 2012, when he had been doing the 'As we were' column for the RCoA's *Bulletin* for ten years, he was awarded the RCoA President's Commendation.

After his death, in 2018 the History of Anaesthesia Society established an annual David Zuck Memorial Prize for the best paper or chapter in a book (in the English language) published in the preceding year on the history of anaesthesia, resuscitation, intensive care or pain management.

Table 1. David Zuck Memorial Prize winners

Year	Recipient	Article
2018	George S. Bause	America's Doctor Anaesthetists (1862-1936) – Turning a Tide of Asphyxiating Waves.
2019	Michael G. Cooper *et al*	The Corfe-McMurdie anaesthetic inhaler of 1918 and the 2nd Australian Casualty Clearing Station.
2020	Adam Keys	Dr Ian Hamilton McDonald, MB BS, DA, FANZCA: The evolution of paediatric anaesthesia and intensive care at the Royal Children's Hospital, Melbourne.

Further reading

https://www.rcoa.ac.uk/dr-david-zuck (Accessed 27 April 2020).

Connor H. Obituary Dr David Zuck FRCA, DHMSA. *The History of Anaesthesia Society Proceedings* 2017; **50**: 157-60.

Rollin A-M. As we were … Dr David Zuck (4 June 1923 to 2 November 2016) An appreciation. *The Royal College of Anaesthetists Bulletin* 2017; **106**: 58-59.

Connor H. The Wit and Wisdom of David Zuck. *The History of Anaesthesia Society Proceedings* 2019; **52**: 98-109.

INDEX

www.ingramcontent.com/pod-product-compliance
Lightning Source LLC
Chambersburg PA
CBHW081459200326
41518CB00015B/2317